Nietzsche's Therapeutic Teaching

Bloomsbury Studies in Continental Philosophy

Bloomsbury Studies in Continental Philosophy presents cutting-edge scholarship in the field of modern European thought. The wholly original arguments, perspectives and research findings in titles in this series make it an important and stimulating resource for students and academics from across the discipline.

Other titles in the series:

Adorno, Heidegger, Philosophy and Modernity, Nicholas Joll
Between the Canon and the Messiah, Colby Dickinson
Castoriadis, Foucault, and Autonomy, Marcela Tovar-Restrepo
Deconstruction without Derrida, Martin McQuillan
Deleuze and the Diagram, Jakub Zdebik
Deleuze and the History of Mathematics, Simon B. Duffy
Derrida and the Future of the Liberal Arts, edited by Mary Caputi and Vincent J. Del Casino, Jr
Derrida, Badiou and the Formal Imperative, Christopher Norris
Derrida: Ethics Under Erasure, Nicole Anderson
Emmanuel Levinas, Abi Doukhan
From Ricoeur to Action, edited by Todd S. Mei and David Lewin
Gadamer and Ricoeur, edited by Francis J. Mootz III and George H. Taylor
Heidegger and Nietzsche, Louis P. Blond
Immanent Transcendence, Patrice Haynes
Jean-Luc Nancy and the Question of Community, Ignaas Devisch
Kant, Deleuze and Architectonics, Edward Willatt
Levinas, Storytelling and Anti-Storytelling, Will Buckingham
Lyotard and the 'figural' in Performance, Art and Writing, Kiff Bamford
Michel Henry, edited by Jeffrey Hanson and Michael R. Kelly
Performatives After Deconstruction, edited by Mauro Senatore
Place, Commonality and Judgment, Andrew Benjamin
Post-Rationalism, Tom Eyers
Rethinking Philosophy and Theology with Deleuze, Brent Adkins and Paul R. Hinlicky
Revisiting Normativity with Deleuze, edited by Rosi Braidotti and Patricia Pisters
The Movement of Nihilism, edited by Laurence Paul Hemming, Kostas Amiridis and Bogdan Costea
The Time of Revolution, Felix Ó Murchadha

Nietzsche's Therapeutic Teaching

For Individuals and Culture

Edited by
Horst Hutter and Eli Friedland

BLOOMSBURY
LONDON • NEW DELHI • NEW YORK • SYDNEY

Bloomsbury Academic
An imprint of Bloomsbury Publishing Plc

50 Bedford Square
London
WC1B 3DP
UK

1385 Broadway
New York
NY 10018
USA

www.bloomsbury.com

First published 2013

British Library Cataloguing-in-Publication Data
A catalogue record for this book is available from the British Library.

ISBN: HB: 978-1-4411-2533-0
ePDF: 978-1-4411-1540-9
ePub: 978-1-4411-0772-5

Library of Congress Cataloguing-in-Publication Data
A catalogue record for this book is available from the Library of Congress.

Typeset by Deanta Global Publishing Services, Chennai, India
Printed and bound in Great Britain

Contents

Note on the Contributors

Babette Babich is professor of philosophy at Fordham University (New York) and executive editor of *New Nietzsche Studies*.

Béatrice Han-Pile is professor of philosophy, University of Essex (England).

Bela Egyed received his M.A. and Ph D. in philosophy at McGill University. Over the years his interest has shifted from analytic philosophy to nineteenth century German and twentieth century French philosophy.

Eli Friedland is a doctoral student in political science at Concordia University (Montréal).

Graham Parkes taught Asian and comparative philosophy for thirty years at the University of Hawaii before taking up his present position as professor and head of the Department of Philosophy at University College Cork (Ireland).

Horst Hutter is professor of political science at Concordia University (Montréal).

José Daniel Parra is a doctoral student in political theory at the University of Toronto.

Keith Ansell-Pearson is professor of philosophy at the University of Warwick (England).

Lawrence J. Hatab is Louis I. Jaffe professor of philosophy and eminent scholar at Old Dominion University.

Martine Béland is professor of philosophy at Collège Édouard-Montpetit (Longueuil) and associate researcher at the Canadian Centre for German and European Studies (Montreal).

Michael Ure is lecturer at the School of Political and Social Inquiry, Monash University, Australia.

Nandita Biswas Mellamphy is associate professor in political theory in the University of Western Ontario's department of Political Science, as well as a core faculty member in the Centre for the Study of Theory and Criticism (UWO). She is the founder and coordinator of *The Nietzsche Workshop @ Western*, an annual international conference devoted to exploring Nietzsche's thought.

Nathalie Lachance teaches German and German literature at Bishop's University in Sherbrooke (Québec). She received her PhD from McGill University in 2010 (Department of German Studies).

Rainer J. Hanshe is the founder of Contra Mundum Press. He is the author of *The Acolytes, The Abdication*, and most recently the editor of Richard Foreman's *Plays with Films*. His writings have appeared in *Literatura, Jelenkor, The Pennsylvania Literary Journal, ChrisMarker.org*, and elsewhere. Hanshe's essay on the synesthetic dimension of Nietzsche's thought is forthcoming from Fordham University Press. He is working on two new novels, *Now, Wonder* and *Virtualize!*

Willow Verkerk is a doctoral candidate at the University of Leuven in Belgium working with Paul van Tongeren on Nietzsche's ethics of friendship.

Yunus Tuncel is a co-founder of the Nietzsche Circle based in New York City and serves on its Board of Directors and the Editorial Board of its electronic journal, The Agonist. He has been teaching philosophy at the New School University's General Studies Division since 1999.

Acknowledgments

We wish to express our deep gratitude to all the students, colleagues, and friends who have been instrumental in bringing this book to fruition. We could not have done this without you.

Eli Friedland wishes to thank the Social Sciences and Humanities Research Council of Canada for the generous funding for the completion of this project.

1

Introduction

Horst Hutter and Eli Friedland

The human being is, Nietzsche wrote in *The Genealogy of Morality*, "*the* sick animal" (Nietzsche's emphasis).[1] That is, inasmuch as we humans are self-conscious, time-conscious, causality-conscious creatures[2] who are no longer—and can no longer be—ruled by mere instinct, we are permanently ill (cf. *A* 14). The way back to an instinct-ruled life, a pre-self-conscious (i.e., "healthy") life in which the human animal can be imagined as a predatory "blond beast" like a lion—with as little "responsibility" or "blame" or "credit" or "courage" as a lion—is closed to us, though its powerful drives surge up through us from time to time with almost irresistible force. The fact that when this happens, we tend toward seeking answers as to *why* it happened, not to mention toward regret and anxiety *that* it happened, bespeaks the rift between the self-conscious human and her predecessors.

Given this, what can therapy mean or do for this permanently sick animal? To understand Nietzsche's answer(s) to this question, we must first recognize that he did not see himself as the first philosophical therapist, but rather as an inheritor of the work, and the human material, of several powerful philosophers, and in particular Plato—"the most beautiful growth of antiquity," and "the philosopher with the greatest strength of all time" (*BGE* Preface and 191). As the heir to Plato and to Platonisms—in particular Christianity—he has inherited human beings (including most especially himself) whose illness has been made *deeper*, almost to the point of self-annihilation, but whose new depth of illness also contains the capacity for never before possible self-transformations. Nietzsche's own therapeutic approaches therefore address two major "peaks" of the illness at once, one "the most dire" (*furchtbarsten*), the other "the most sublime" (*sublimsten*): the possibility of the illness as lethal, and the possibility of the illness as illness "in the same way that pregnancy is an illness" (*GM* II, 19).

This volume is composed around the Nietzschean insight, which has its roots in the Hippocratic tradition of ancient medicine, that beliefs, behaviors, ideals, and patterns of striving are not things for which individuals or even cultures are responsible. Rather, they are symptoms of what an individual or culture *is*, which symptoms require diagnostic interpretation and evaluation; they are manifestations that signify—but do not thereby completely *reveal*—the vast, subtle, and powerful forces that underlie them, and whose momentum requires their appearance. Two such forces could provisionally be identified as the unfolding of history and the shaping of human souls by unconscious drives.

In this regard, we can isolate three principal approaches, or facets, of Nietzsche's philosophy: diagnostic, prognostic, and therapeutic. For Nietzsche, diagnosis does not mean to discover what or who is to *blame* for a malady, but what is *included* within it, together with what might be called the functional operation that each aspect has performed and continues to perform. Such a method allows him to honestly (i.e., not just wishfully) assess potential prognoses of that malady, as well as develop therapeutic practices by which to achieve a new health. Only as such can what is self-destructive in it be recognized, and perhaps more importantly, what is fruitful in it explored. Thus, for example, the time and figure of Socrates are not to blame for nihilism, nor is Christianity, but they are certainly to be included within its progression—and so is Nietzsche himself. All contain elements that extend the reach of nihilism, to greater or lesser degrees, but all also contain elements that can be directed toward the self-overcoming of that same nihilism.

Each author contributing to this volume takes up this essential insight of Nietzsche's therapeutic philosophy from a different perspective. Many of these perspectives hinge on Nietzsche's varied relationships with ancient therapeutics, while others explore his keen interest in his contemporary environment and its specific quandaries.

As editors, we have attempted to gather in this volume a wide variety of perspectives on Nietzschean therapy, in the hopes of stimulating broader interest in this approach. Our selection criteria were based largely on the fruitfulness of a perspective, and not, in general, whether or not we completely agreed with it. Indeed, drawing together competing perspectives seemed, in this regard, to be quite necessary, though the reader must therefore keep in mind that the opinions of the authors and the editors are independent and in some cases, diverge to a serious degree. But bringing disagreements into the light of day is particularly appropriate for a volume on Nietzsche's therapeutic philosophy, a philosophy that attempted as no other to dig out and retrieve the essential tensions that have been buried both in grand "noble lies" and banal politeness. Certainly, no one knew better than Nietzsche that a deliberately provocative gesture could (which of course does not necessarily mean *would*) jolt a reader into self-reflection and self-work. We have done our best not to undermine this aspect of a Nietzschean approach to therapy, with our selections for the present compilation: *caveat lector*.

Notes

1 "*Das* kranke Thier" (*GM* III, 13; KSA 5, 367).

2 What is decisive here is the *consciousness* of self, time, and causality and *not* whether that experience actually means that such things exist, or exist in the way we experience them to exist (*hôs estin*, to use Protagoras' formulation).

2

The Nietzsche Cure: New Kinds of "Gymnastics of Willing"[1]

Horst Hutter

Few Nietzsche scholars have paid any attention to the theme of the philosopher as a therapist. Yet this theme dominates his entire opus, from his earliest writings through to the *Zarathustra* period and beyond, to the writings of his final active year. They have not seen, or simply ignored, due to certain preconceptions about what philosophy is, that Nietzsche wished to hasten the coming and future sanctification of a new type of synthetic human being. In addressing his specific audience of "free spirits," he aimed for them to transform themselves into physicians, priests, teachers, and leaders in one. Only such human beings would be able to become cultural healers and leaders on the model of the pre-Socratic thinkers. The pre-Socratic philosophers were educators, teachers, and physicians and were thus able to address the problems and disorders of their times. On such an understanding of Nietzsche, we may read in Camus' *L'homme révolté*: "Mais on ne peut rien tirer de Nietzsche . . . tant qu'on ne met pas au premier plan dans son oeuvre, bien avant le prophète, le clinicien."[2]

The lack of attention to such a major theme in Nietzsche implies that modern scholars and philosophers were and are perhaps themselves infected by the dis-eases of their times. Thus, they were unable to contribute any significant diagnosis and far less any curative suggestions for the modern, cultural and psychological malaises of nihilism. Many modern philosophers might thus not be philosophers for themselves, that is to say, to be both patients and physicians in one, but only manage to assume the image of philosophers in the eyes of fellow citizens in their roles as academics and as functionaries of political orders.

Nietzsche's entire teaching is shaped by his struggles against his own many illnesses that he traced to his upbringing as a Christian and to the embodiment of punitive Christian moralism in his character, in an age in which the Christian moral order is undergoing dissolution. This dissolution is induced by its own internal developments. His teaching hence does not offer any "doctrines" valid for all times and for all circumstances. The contradictory doctrines in his writings are historically situated at this particular point in the evolution of Christianity and do not aim to provide logically coherent "eternal verities." They are Janus-faced, looking backward to Christian origins, with an intention of deconstruction, and looking forward to the future, with an intention of eventual reconstruction and the creation of new types of human orders. They are oriented toward new kinds of ascetic practices, which hopefully might eventually be incorporated in new forms of religiosities that are "loyal to the earth." These new religions would not set the goals for human striving in some nebulous "beyond" to which "souls" should escape as quickly as possible. Nietzsche's teachings proceed from a negation, even if phrased affirmatively, and then proceed to an affirmation, even if phrased negatively.

This yes/no structure was identified by Nietzsche to reside in his own immense suffering, deeply rooted in his Christian "second nature," as well as his unsuccessful attempts to heal himself through writing. The attainment of what he envisioned as the "great health" was impossible for his own lifetime and only seen as tentatively possible for his future free-spirited disciples. His critical analyses of the nihilistic disorders of the modern Christian soul are both intensely personal and endowed with far-reaching emotional and mental implications. In his vision, the personal is thus both the philosophical and the political. Indeed, from this perspective, the understanding of philosophy as an abstract and impersonal theoretical discourse on the model of the natural sciences is both a symptom of the underlying malaise and a major factor contributing to its continuation.

A core idea of Nietzsche's diagnosis of current forms of Christianity as a malady involves a critical deconstruction of the soul/body division, implied by the anthropology of most Abrahamic religions. He proposes a new vision of the human totality that sees whatever may be understood as "mind," "soul," "spirit," seen as separate from a "body," and understood as a "monad," as an inherited cultural and political fiction. He prefers the German term "Leib" with its close etymological connection to "life," to the alternate German term "Koerper," which already suggests that humans are beings in which an at least potentially "'good' soul" temporarily inhabits a "bad" body, which already should be seen as a corpse (= Koerper). The Christian moral code is based on what St Paul called the "mortification of the flesh." The consequence of such an ascetic program has been to render sexuality sinful and something that needs to be hushed up. And just as the "body" may be thus despised, the material environment of life may also be neglected and treated with contempt—for after all, from this perspective, the world is going to disappear with the coming of the "savior." Against these harmful visions, Nietzsche has proposed a new focus that sees the "Leib" as an enspirited material entity that needs to renew its sundered connection with the earth and all of its living forms. In this sense, he proposes a vision of a "cosmos anthropos" that sees soul, mind, and spirit to be everywhere, completely connected to their material bases. Indeed, the very distinction between material base and inherent spirit is never more than a sometimes necessary conceptual fiction. Human selves and egos would be envisioned as temporary managerial entities with the task of assuming the "imperative of responsibility" for the Leib and its environment. They need to become responsible "masters of the earth" and cease to despoil and ruin nature.[3]

Every culture may be seen as a multifaceted and dynamically embodied program of thought and action: it is, to borrow a term from cybernetics, a "difference engine," something with a unified and finite structure with possibilities for infinities of developments. It is like a natural language that has finite sets of grammatical and syntactical rules that yet permit the construction of an infinite number of sentences. The culture that has proceeded from the Paulinian religious vision, supported by Platonic/Aristotelian reasonings, is also such a difference engine, but one that has served its evolutionary purpose and now is dissolving from within. This requires a new understanding of the human totality as "Leib," in which soul, mortal body, mind, and spirit, are seen as parts and aspects in antagonistic cooperation with one another. They need to be reordered and retrained.

To be sure, any new reordering also is based on a poetic/political fiction, but one more appropriate in its life-affirming tendencies, designed to resolve the crisis that is engulfing the planet. Nietzsche, in this manner, has proposed a new set of mythologies that are meant to beneficially guide human conduct. From the perspective of this new mythology, all elements of the old myths that can be adapted to serve in the new order are to be transformed and reused. Thus, the "Christian ascetic ideal," the last form of the Christian will-to-power as a will-to truth, is to be overcome in both its religious and scientific variants. Yet some of its practices, which in any case will still last for generations, may be integrated into new modes of askesis. A frequent error in interpreting Nietzsche's teaching has been not to see that his attack on the "ascetic ideal" is not his final word in regard to askesis. Thus, he has called for new modes of ascetic practices that will enable enspirited human totalities to survive and prevail in the coming "age of barbarism," in which the sciences will be in the service of barbarism,[4] which he has foreseen and predicted. This new version of an "ascetic ideal" calls for new kinds of ascetic practices that will lead to new kinds of "gymnastics of willing." Since we live in the era of globalization, the great wealth of ascetic practices to be found in the various religious traditions may be adapted to new requirements. Hence these practical aspects of Nietzsche's teaching have often been likened to a new kind of Buddhism, or, to use the title of a recent book, a "Euro-Taoism."[5] The new ascetic practices all would involve a mental focus by its practitioners on their embodied "souls," here and now, during movements, very much on the model of Eastern spiritual practices, such as Yoga or Tai Chi. They would not aim to attain a good position for its practitioners in any "beyond."

General human evolution has led to the development of a great variety of cultural programmings of animal bodies that have warred with one another across history. They may be seen as experiments made necessary and enabled by the "eccentric positionality"[6] of the human species: humans have left or "fallen," or perhaps been torn out of instinctual guidance and hence have needed emotional and spiritual guidance by culturally designed, embodied programs of conduct. These programs have been initiated by the shamanistic and spiritual poet-thinkers of the past, who have created the various religious and spiritual dispensations that have shaped human history hitherto. All such programs, once they are educated into bodies, provide goals and directions for human strivings and show how humans may increase and use their limited freedoms of choice. They are guides to the development of lines of willing and as such imply a terminus a quo (= from which), the animality of the human, and a terminus ad quem (= to which), often seen as "divine."

These cultural programs affirm distinctions between right and wrong, good and evil, or good and bad and thus define the in-between status of the human animal, defined

Platonically as the metaxy, but more relevantly in Nietzschean term, as the in-between the animal and the "over-human." They are the "golden loosings"[7] that have initiated the human evolutionary trajectory from animality to the "divine," or rather, the present stage of the "super-animal."[8] As an interesting aside it may be remarked here that Nietzsche's term "Uebermensch" is a direct translation of the Greek "hyperanthropos." One of the first uses of the latter term was the description of the nature of Jesus, as not an incarnate God, but as a hyperanthropos, by Montanus in the so-called Montanist heresy in the second century A.D.[9] These "golden loosings" have done so by imposing punitive moralistic chains on human animals. These involve a consciousness of sin and the memory of a fall from grace (of instinctual nature). The way backward is barred and the way forward is enabled by rules of conduct, the various moralities. With the disintegration of religiosities in this age of nihilism, new moral codes need to guide humans from the stage of super-animals to the stage of the over-human. Humans furthermore now are frequently in ignorance of what they should do, or when knowing what to do, are unable to do it. Other animals are innocent, as it were, and without "sin." But for humans "sin is behovely."[10] But the way up is only half-done, and the super-animals need further guidance from a new "golden loosing."

The rules that enable the transition of the in-between require incentives, threats, rewards, and punishments. They need to be "burned into the flesh" as it were, hence the great importance of cruelty in human history, so frequently both negated and affirmed by Nietzsche in his attempt to transfigure cruelty. Thereby the human will comes to be created and formed, with the suspension of all lines of willing from a summum bonum, a highest good that orients human conduct. The line of willing thereby created can only be sustained through spiritual and ascetic practices. Many of these askeses were developed in ancient philosophical schools of conduct, which in their times were schools for the reeducation of diseased groups of individuals in need of healing. The Christian religion has also provided such spiritual and ascetic practices, by way of selectively adopting them from philosophical schools, such as the Stoa and the Epicurean Garden. But these have now been, and continue to be, undermined by the metaphysical developments that have proceeded from within the enormous successes of Christian spirituality. The empirical sciences have their origins in this spiritual base, frequently by way of its dialectical negations.

Nihilism is for Nietzsche a part of the internal logic of the development of Christian history. With the loss of credibility of its metaphysical grounding via the development of the empirical sciences, the ascetic practices that had sustained religions also have lost their cogency and suffered a serious decrease in meaning. The aim of self-struggle and obedience to rules, seen to lie in salvation in the beyond, is no longer believable. Simultaneously, the fear of eternal damnation has become less and less real, leading to a tremendous loss of power for Christian authorities. A telling measure of these changes may be seen in the fact that, when the Nazi regime instituted a special tax for members of churches, many so-called Christians simply left the churches, so as to avoid this tax. When the regime then was defeated, many of those who had left returned to the churches so as to establish their de-nazification credentials. Such actions would have been unthinkable in the ages of faith, when the fear of damnation was strong and suffused the whole souls of believers.

These developments may be seen as terrible losses, but also as tremendous opportunities for the creation of new lines of willing, new spiritual practices, and new forms of askesis. These new "disciplinae voluntatis," as Nietzsche envisions them, will have the double task of undoing fully embodied doctrines which have now become harmful in their destructive impact on planetary nature. They need to be replaced by newly embodied rules and interpretations, even in the form of new modes of religiosity, "new gods," as it were. The philosophical schools that Nietzsche wished to create in his lifetime, but could only foresee for his posthumous future, would revolve around spiritual and ascetic practices that renounce any orientation to the "beyond," but center on the love of finite life. Like the ancient schools that Nietzsche admired, such as the Epicurean Garden and the Platonic Academy, these new schools would also be schools for the reeducation of humans. Some of these then would evolve into new forms of religiosity over several generations. Since Nietzsche conceived the human totality, the "Leib," as a labyrinth, escape from the sufferings that human totalities will have to endure, will require a new kind of Ariadne, with a new kind of thread, and her successful marriage with a new kind of kind of Theseus, who is sufficiently inspired by Dionysus and thus will no longer abandon Ariadne on Naxos. And Naxos in turn will have to evolve into a new kind of nurturing Gaia (= earth).

These processes will take a long time and will require sustained efforts by millions of reeducated humans, humans that have been conceived and nurtured in completely different kinds of erotic regimes. This new regime can naturally no longer be based on any vilification of the "flesh," but must valorize sexual pleasure as a genuine goal for human striving, without any intention of conception. Access to sexual pleasure must become free from the fear of disease and from inevitable and unwanted pregnancies. Only then will "conception" of children become the sacred task that it is meant to be; it may even become immaculate again. Then only wanted children will populate the earth and will be raised by parents, able and willing to sustain these efforts, unencumbered by rage and anxiety. Meanwhile, however, these latter thumotic soul formations will have to be transfigured through appropriate askesis that do not just engage the "body," but involve dancing and new forms of festivals, in which communities are sustained and members thereof rejuvenated, in such a manner that the inner divinity of each and every human is fully awakened. An excellent description of such a new founding of a tolerably good city, called Magnesia, may be found in Plato's *Laws*. It appears that Nietzsche read this text in one of the happiest moments of his life, when he sojourned in Sorrento, together with Paul Ree, in the house of his friend Malwida von Meysenbug, and paid frequent visits to the Wagner residence, borne by his still relatively undisturbed friendship with the Wagners.

Conception of children would have to become conscious and fully willed by both mothers and fathers, who in the act of love intend to conceive a child together, in an environment that is as benign and as stress-free as possible. This too is a suggestion to be found in Plato's *Laws*. Nietzsche functioned within a Christian context, and being strongly educated as a Christian, he was naturally aware of the concept of original sin and of the Christian doctrine that original sin is transmitted through the act of conception. His healing vision would seem to foresee an overcoming of the consequences of original sin that are present in the hatreds and anxieties transmitted from generation to generation. Only with an overcoming of original sin, is a new society, based in loyalty to the earth, even conceivable. Only such a society would have overcome the hatred of the "body" and of "nature," so deeply rooted in the second natures of all humans raised within the confines of Abrahamic religions. This process would naturally take a long time, and it would have to begin with a program of education that targets already the fetus in the mother's womb. At this stage, the "sounds of life" become crucially important, as the work of the French otolaryngologist Alfred Tomatis has shown. Dr Tomatis has been able to measure the responses of fetuses to benign and adverse sounds in the pregnant woman's environment. Ultrasound measurements have shown the responses of fetuses to be different to benign sounds than to adverse sounds. From this it would follow that, what is usually called second nature, is already programmed into humans at their fetal stage.[11] Naturally, Nietzsche did not know of the Tomatis effects, but these recent scientific results fit entirely within Nietzsche's program for building a better and higher human species and thereby also to save the earth.

The Tomatis method has been very successful in healing the condition of autism by way of introducing calming music at an early stage of life and even at the fetal stage. Certain kinds of music, in particular Mozart, have proven to be especially curative, a fact well-attested in Tomatis institutes. The odd thing about this is that Mozart's "The Magic Flute" is meant to convey a form of healing sound rooted in ancient Egyptian traditions. It may be a bit far-fetched, but one might speculate that Christian souls are in a way deeply autistic, and that what is needed is a new form of music, based in a new kind of Pythagorean understanding of human totalities. In any case, given the fact that Nietzsche held life to be a mistake without music, the above speculations would not seem to be so far-fetched.

Once the overall structure of the reeducative gymnastics and reeducative forms of music, and their role in preventing anxiety already in fetuses, for example, has been understood as involving both negations that imply affirmations, and affirmations that imply negations, specific techniques may then be envisioned. The great variety of spiritual and ascetic practices to be found in the philosophers of antiquity, as well as in Eastern spiritual disciplines, may serve as sources and guides for adaptation to modern humans. They need to be adapted to current forms of decadence, that is to say, weakness of wills, and would need to be adjusted to individual specificities. They would provide exercises designed specifically for the parts of human beings called "mind" and/or "spirit," as well as specific forms of askesis involving "body work." Such bodywork may be learned from Eastern schools to involve conscious attention during movements to that part of the human totality, so maltreated by the Paulinian "mortification of the flesh." Thereby a new type of human self would slowly be formed and re-formed by free spirits in themselves. These would transmit their embodied visions to their physical and spiritual descendants. But, currently, we still live (following categories described in *Zarathustra*) in the stages of the camel, and of the lion, with their emphasis on either blind obedience or misguided deconstruction. Few may have attained the stage of the child, at which a new beginning in a reconstruction becomes conceivable.

The present age of nihilistic disintegration is characterized by terrible confusion and by the strong resistances by the old orders of acculturation to any kind of change in regimes of the soul. Thus, at a recent population conference in Cairo, the representatives of the three monotheistic religions made common cause against any kind of innovation in erotic regimes. They strenuously insisted on maintaining moral codes that forbade any kind of erotic activity that did not intend conception. All artificial means of pregnancy prevention and interruption were vigorously rejected.[12] This resistance will continue for a long time yet, and this despite the fact that the human population of the planet is already too large, in terms of quantity, but even more in terms of quality. Similarly, resistance against reeducating girls in matters of erotics seems to be vigorously resisted in many parts of the world. It seems that humans are in love with oppression and oppressors.

The most significant part of the regime of human souls concerns erotic matters, as Eros is the strongest and completely unconquerable force in the soul. But this force has been shaped variously by taboos and restrictions that have become embodied in second natures, and which as such remain mostly unconscious. Humans are governed and willed from deep within themselves by age-old prohibitions and restrictions that are transmitted from one generation to the next. In such a situation, even if individuals feel the need to reeducate themselves, motivated by conflicts and deep suffering, all such reeducation has to proceed within the terms of embodied norms. The very terms of striving to overcome one's selves are defined by that which needs to be overcome. Thus, Christians struggle against Christian conditioning, while Muslims need to struggle against Muslim conditioning. The "enemy" is within and defines the very goals sought. The struggle is one between conditioned reactivities, one of these conditioned by education, and the other by suffering experienced due to a now increasingly useless education.

As stated above, human animals have been severed from instinctual guidance and hence need cultural modes that define lines of willing. Such lines of willing are defined for the few by philosophical practices and for the many by religions. The shamanic healers and philosophers, the paradigmatic individuals such as Jesus, the Buddha, Laotse, Muhammad, and Socrates, as well as many others before these, have established the patterns that then have been infused into religions for the masses. At all stages of these evolutionary developments, the human soul has revealed itself as a most complicated structure of command/obedience, as a conflictual and conflicted multiplicity, with a strong tendency to chaos. This tendency to chaos becomes very obvious in times of cultural disintegration, such as our era of nihilistic transition. The signs and concepts that have served to organize the dissolving order of the soul have become largely untenable and no longer serve their purposes. Chief among such concepts is the idea of a separate faculty of the soul, called "free will," which has been at the core of what Nietzsche has called the "metaphysics of the hangman."[13]

The foundation of this metaphysics seems to be the fear of death and of the horrors that might await the disobedient after death. An entirely phobocratic structure of command/obedience has been erected on these psychic factors, frequently nourished throughout Christian history by horrible acts of cruel punishments and ghastly public executions. Punishment in this life has often served as an anticipation of what might await "sinners" in the other life. In this manner, a structure of willing has been established in souls, in which the interior and inborn commands, such as sexual desires, have warred with the commands proceeding from imposed moral codes.

This has made the human soul rich in thoughts, feelings, and volitions. This very complicated structure of willing has then been ideologically fortified by the doctrine of "free will." As Nietzsche points out, the one word will has been used to hide an enormous complexity.[14] The basic chaotic nature of the soul has been manifesting itself with the waning in the fear of the metaphysical beyond. Cruel punishments and tortures still occur, but they are no longer publicly performed as spectacles on high religious holidays.

With the disappearance of the metaphysics of the hangman, its positive effects have also waned. Nihilism is characterized by decadence, and decadence may be defined as weakness of will. The chaos of the human animal soul is becoming visible in tremendous cultural confusions and in the search for substitute religions in the form of political ideologies such as Nazism, Marxism, and the various forms of Fascism. These ideologies order the chaos of the soul and straighten the lines of willing, by introducing new command centers and new forms of obedience. Naturally, these deep processes in the soul are accompanied by conflicts that are unimaginable in their extent and in their violence. There are "wars like there have never been wars before."[15] The current lack of any clear goals for human striving has also then led to serious emotional disorders that manifest themselves in events such as the drug culture and its lovely little "war on drugs."

Nietzsche's therapeutic teaching aims to diagnose the etiology of the above disorders and then to prescribe healing visions and actions. Chief among his curative suggestions is his call to his free-spirited followers to form political orders and small societies of sane and life-affirming ways of living. It seems to me that the model for such new healing communities might well be the garden communities, initiated by Epicurus in antiquity. Members would need to define their lines of willing entirely in this-worldly terms, and rule would be exercised in terms of joy and pleasure, and no longer in terms of fear and anxiety. Indeed, the latter might be the main motives for joining or forming such benign gardens. In such a garden community members would relate to one another in terms of agonistic friendships. They would dance, chant, and sing and thus aim to reestablish in their conscious lives, the unconscious rhythms of the Dionysian within. But, as the saying goes, the way is long and life is short.

Bibliographical note

My reasoning in the above is guided primarily by two sources:

(A) The Nietzsche dictionary, of which only the first volume is so far available. It is meant as a comprehensive subject index, and volume one contains every mention in all of Nietzsche's writings of the word Askesis in its various forms: Paul van Tongeren, Gerd Schank and Heinrich Siemens, eds. *Nietzsche –Woerterbuch*. Band 1. Berlin, New York, de Gruyter, 2004. Guided by this subject index, I have examined every mention and every discussion of the concepts of askesis and ascetic practices.

(B) Heinrich Schipperges. *Am Leitfaden des Leibes; zur Anthropologik und Therapeutik Friedrich Nietzsches*. Stuttgart: Ernst Klett Verlag, 1975.

Notes

1 The phrase "Gymnastik des Willens" is to be found in KSA, 12, 387.
2 Albert Camus. *L'Homme révolté*. Paris: Editions Gallimard, 1951, p. 88.
3 KSA 12 (9), 93 and 165.
4 KSA 9, 395.
5 Peter Sloterdijk. *Eurotaoismus*. Frankfurt: Suhrkamp Verlag, 1987.
6 The concept of the excentric positionality of the human animal is the key concept of Helmuth Plessener's major study in philosophical anthropology: *Die Stufen des Organischen und der Mensch. Einleitung in die philosophische Anthropologie* (Goschen, 1928). See also Ferdinand Fellmann. "Das Paar als Quelle des Selbst," *Deutsche Zeitschrift fuer Philosophie* 57 (2009): 745–56.
7 Der Wanderer und sein Schatten, # 350; KSA 2, 702.
8 "Ueberthier," in *Menschliches-Allzumenschliches* #40; KSA 2, 64.
9 Heinrich Mueller, a professor of Greek theology at the University of Rostock in the seventeenth century, in translating the theological writings of Montanus, was the first to render the Greek Hyperanthropos into the German Uebermensch, in his *Geistliche Erquickunsstunden* (1664).
10 The phrase is attributed to the highly mysterious, fourteenth-century English anchorite Juliana of Norwich.
11 Alfred Tomatis. *L'Oreille et la Vie*. Paris: Editions Laffont, 1987.
12 See the reports on the United Nations Cairo population conference, held in Cairo from 5 to 13 September 1994.
13 *Goetzendaemmerung*; "Die vier grossen Irrtuemer"; KSA 6, 90.
14 *Jenseits von Gut und Boese* # 19; KSA 5, 31–4.
15 *Ecce Homo* "Warum ich ein Schicksal bin"; KSA 6, 365–74.

3

Vocation as Therapy: Nietzsche and the Conflict between Profession and Calling in Academia

Martine Béland

It is our vocation that disposes of us,
even when we don't yet know it.

– Nietzsche, *HH* I, Foreword, § 7

As an academic at the University of Basel Nietzsche was no different than scholars of today: he was expected to keep himself informed of the latest results in his discipline, to publish review essays, to represent his institution during congresses, to train future specialists, and to publish original work in his field. But Nietzsche found no pleasure in these endeavors: he stopped publishing reviews in the early 1870s; he hated to bear the "face of a university-representative," as he wrote in July 1872 while going to the University of Munich's jubilee; rather than training pure philologists, he exhorted his students to take up philosophy; and rather than building his reputation as a serious scholar, he published a first book that "lacked all the usual signs of classical scholarship," that is, footnotes, quotations from Greek sources in the original, and references to scholarship.[1]

In fact, at the outset of his career in philology, Nietzsche rapidly became conscious of the ever-widening gap between the demands of his profession and his "natural" inclination toward philosophy.[2] In a late letter, Nietzsche told of an important crisis that happened in the middle of his decade-long career.[3] But he spoke of such a crisis as early as January 1871, when he said that his profession was contradicting his "task" and keeping him away from his "path," while a "conflict" "wore him down" even "physically."[4] Nietzsche's writings from the early 1870s show that while he was pondering the disciplinary constitution of knowledge and criticizing specialization in the humanities and social sciences, he was in a state of conflict between his profession and what he considered to be his vocation. This crisis entailed many repercussions. Indeed, Nietzsche interpreted his illnesses—both moral and physical—as the result of his having not followed his calling from an early point on.

As this paper sets out to show, this conflict asked for a radical therapy: an early retirement from academia. Nietzsche's decisive transfer to philosophy was a curative step in the construction of himself while fulfilling his vocation. His decision to leave academia and become a "wandering" philosopher—to use his friend Erwin Rohde's expression—was not motivated strictly by physical health issues: this decision was first and foremost a philosophical one, whereby Nietzsche sought to recover his moral health. His definition of philosophy as vocation can thus be considered as a therapy for the illnesses caused by the paradoxes of scholarly professions.

The following pages describe the structural conflict between profession and calling according to Nietzsche. I first situate Nietzsche within academia by showing what his profession as philologist entailed at the time he started his career. I then move on to describe Nietzsche's conception of classical philology through his Basel correspondence and essays on his profession: his May 1869 inaugural lecture, printed as *Homer and Classical Philology*; his 1871 summer semester introductory course to philological studies, *Encyclopedia of Classical Philology*; and his 1875 unfinished notes for an essay that would have been entitled *We Philologists*. I thereafter pinpoint three attempts made by Nietzsche to reconcile profession and vocation—to no avail. To explain these repeated failures, I clarify Nietzsche's concept of profession (*Beruf*) and his definition of a philosophical calling. This serves to show that his understanding of the demands of a profession, on the one hand, and of the requirements of philosophy, on the other, made it impossible for him to be a philosopher while holding an academic chair: philosophy for Nietzsche cannot be a profession. To finish this paper, I turn to two sources of Nietzsche's conception of a nonprofessional philosophical life.

Nietzsche in academia: Philology as a profession

Nietzsche's perspectives on his profession are somewhat neglected by scholars, who often simply remark upon his criticisms of academic philology. Carl Pletsch, for instance, writes that Nietzsche "announced himself to the intellectual world of Basel" with "ambivalence about himself and his profession" and adds: "Luckily, Basel was a quiet and unpretentious place for Nietzsche to work out his ambivalence." This is surely a simplification of the paradoxes of Nietzsche's early professional life. These professional issues, though, are extremely revealing, if one considers that Nietzsche was less interested in consolidating his career than in "the construction of himself as an intellectual."[5] Some scholars, though, have strived to contextualize Nietzsche's perspectives on his profession. In a convincing paper, James Whitman stresses that while publishing *The Birth of Tragedy*, Nietzsche identified with a magisterial tradition that flourished in German philology as of the 1830s. He shows that "Nietzsche's sense of artistic vocation would [not] have been at odds with his profession as classicist," especially as regards the importance of a scholar's personal experiences: "The philological tradition in which Nietzsche was trained required, and indeed celebrated, the display of a professor's powerful personality."[6] But Whitman does not speak of the conflict between Nietzsche's profession and his calling. Before turning to this issue, it is important to clarify Nietzsche's position within his academic field.

According to his letters, the young professor arrived in Basel in the spring of 1869 with enthusiasm, but also apprehensions regarding his decision to devote himself entirely to philology and to undertake a heavy workload. Upon his arrival, he taught for 14 hours weekly: 8 of university lectures plus 6 of secondary courses at the Basel Pädagogium.[7] Not surprisingly, he found his task most tiresome. He was nevertheless content with the appointment that transformed him from a "shooting star" into a "fixed star."[8] After but 5 months in Basel, he wrote to his friend Carl von Gersdorff: "I am quite satisfied with my academic activity, of which I have now happily finished the first semester. I notice that my students participate avidly and have a real sympathy for me, in that they often and gladly seek advice from me."[9] Nietzsche was simultaneously satisfied with his recent philological research (papers and reviews published since 1867), worried by the fatigue caused by his professional activities, and convinced of his pedagogical mission. Indeed, he was conscious of being the rising star of the Leipzig school of German classical philology. Some clarification as to what this meant will be useful here.

In the midst of a rationalization and bureaucratization of the universities and academies in Germany during the second half of the nineteenth century, classical philology was among the first disciplines to become specialized and professionalized.[10] "Specialization" can be defined as "the degree to which scientific work is concentrated narrowly in one or a few areas, rather than broadly diffused over many," whereas "professionalization" "refers to the possibility of making a career out of scientific work, both in the sense of earning a livelihood and achieving a collective identity with other practitioners in the field."[11] In this context, philology rapidly rose to the forefront of scientific disciplines, thanks to a series of innovations in the field: professional associations (the first was formed in Leipzig in 1837), scientific journals (of which there already existed four in 1846), and uniform professional training for future professors (through the Seminar developed by philologist August Boeckh in 1810).[12] As the historian of science Lorraine Daston puts it, "What had been the ancillary sciences of the eighteenth-century universities became the certification of the serious scholar in the nineteenth-century university seminar."[13]

One must not conclude from these processes that nineteenth-century academia as a whole was enthusiastically embracing this new stance. Indeed, many criticisms of specialization emerged, and they mostly came from the Berlin Academy of Sciences, whose members—in the spirit of German classicism and idealism—strived to maintain the "fundamental," "organic" unity of knowledge.[14] Historian Theodor Mommsen's 1895 lecture to the Academy gives a telling example of this attitude: "We do not accuse nor complain; the flower withers and the fruit must ripen. But the best amongst us sense that we have become specialists." In the 1880s, Hellenist J. G. Droysen diagnosed the same problem: "The humanities' privilege is shaken, philology's era has past; philologists are no more than monograph writers of classical Antiquity."[15]

In fact, German historical sciences were then going through an important crisis. Classicist Karl Reinhardt described what he considered the tragic dilemma of German classical philology in a 1941 conference. While the early nineteenth century had "tremendous hopes for the 'rebirth of Antiquity in the German spirit,'" the rapid subsequent development of historical sciences revealed the dilemma that was at the heart of philology: "The 'classical' . . . must be recognized at the same time as a historical value bound to a specific epoch, and as an eternal value."[16] In fact, once that "historical truth" became the guiding criteria for philological research, the "chief value of classical studies" could not continue to be based on aesthetic grounds (as was the case for Goethe or Schiller).[17] Philology, as Reinhardt put it, was facing "the dilemma between the classical ideal and the historical reality of its undertaking."[18] To quote philologist and Nietzsche scholar James Porter: "In this new uncertainty was encapsulated the whole of modernity's relationship to the classical past, and so too its own historical self-image."[19]

It was in this context of crisis amid rapid professionalization and specialization that Nietzsche became professor of classical philology. He is in fact representative of the issues facing German historical sciences in the last quarter of the nineteenth century. But he is original in that, whereas philology did not seek to ponder its theoretical issues, Nietzsche readily reflected upon them. In most of his early essays, he addressed the crisis of classical studies: its sociological causes (the transformation of the learned class as a consequence of increasingly technical disciplines in the context of industrialization), its pedagogical consequences (the transformation and perhaps disappearance of the classical education [*Bildung*]), and its political context (that of nation-building in the aftermath of the Franco-Prussian war).[20]

Nietzsche's classical philology

At the outset of a career, after long research studies, it is habitual, as philosopher Wilhelm Wundt noted in an 1876 article, to consider the task at hand and the means with which one hopes to accomplish it.[21] That is what Nietzsche's inaugural lecture intended to do. His entry in professional philology, as Porter noted, is a reflection on "the entire attitude of modernity to the study of the 'so-called "classical" antiquity.'"[22] Nietzsche was conscious of the importance and difficulty of founding and defending the absolute value of the classical. As an admirer of Goethe and Schiller, he argued for a classical vision of Antiquity: philology's pedagogical mission is "to uncover a buried, ideal world and to show the present the mirror of the classical as an eternal model."[23] This task required that philology open up to other areas of knowledge. In this respect, Nietzsche's perspective recalls that of Schelling's 1803 *Lectures on the Method of Academic Studies*. Schelling stressed that the philologist must work with artists and philosophers: "Its task is the historical construction of the works of art and science, whose history the philologist must seize and represent within a living conception."[24] In Greek Antiquity, "all public actions were but different paths to a general, objective, and vital work of art."[25] That was precisely Nietzsche's thesis in 1869: to guarantee the status of the classical, philology must define itself as a "scientific-artistic movement."[26] Nietzsche would go on to develop his thoughts on the relationship between historical knowledge and culture in his famous second *Untimely Meditation* (1874): rather than to achieve a "complete" knowledge of the past, history must strive to be recognized as an artistic or symbolic force.[27]

In today's terminology, Nietzsche's perspective on his profession would be viewed as "interdisciplinary," though, in this regard, it was not particularly original in its time. In Germany, classical philology has always been conscious of integrating different disciplines such as history, linguistics, literary studies, archeology, and the arts.[28] As Reinhardt has said in words that could well have been Nietzsche's or Schelling's, "the classical—one cannot research it as a scientific object without it starting to crumble or to evaporate. For it to make sense, it must be depicted, felt, embraced, it must become spirit and body—but that was and remains a task for other spirits than philologists."[29] Nietzsche's distinctiveness in this respect is that he gave all the importance to philosophy's contribution to classical studies. As he told his first-year students, one must emphasize the intimacy between philology and philosophy so that the claim "to the classicality of Antiquity against the modern world does not sound like a laughable pretention."[30] A broader philosophical perspective would enable philology to overcome its internal crisis, and for this to be achieved, the classicist's personal attitude was of utmost importance. Nietzsche thus defended ideas that were also held by academicians such as Mommsen and by pioneers of classical philology. Indeed, Boeckh, founder of the philological Seminar, insisted that the "philologist give unity to his material by reliving it in his own mind."[31]

Following his classical and "interdisciplinary" conception of philology, Nietzsche's courses directed classical studies toward philosophy. He enthusiastically traced philosophical issues in the Greek texts that his students were to read, as he wrote to his former professor Friedrich Ritschl on 10 May 1869: "By making them read Plato's *Phaedo*, I can inoculate my pupils with philosophy."[32] He explained that it would be profitable "if every future expert first studied *philosophy* for one year, so that he would not resemble the factory worker who screws his bolts day in day out."[33] Once more, Nietzsche thereby voiced worries that were common in German academia. Physiologist Emil Du Bois-Reymond described similar concerns in his 1882 lecture to the Berlin Academy: "Relinquishing their claims to fame, a thousand diligent, scientific workers daily put forth innumerable details, unconcerned with internal and external completeness, only eager to attract instant publicity and gain the best price for their commodities."[34]

Nietzsche's harsh appraisal of professional research, which he shared with many German scholars, is rooted in his thoughts regarding the disciplinary constitution of knowledge. At the start of his career, he noticed an inner contradiction in all knowledge-oriented professions. This contradiction can be summarized by two opposite assertions: "Life is worth living," and "Life is worth knowing."[35] The 1869 lecture accordingly opposed two impulses: one that leads the professional classicist's scientific work, and one that leads the instinctive pleasure which enticed him to precisely research the Greeks rather than another field of knowledge. Nietzsche showed that as the scholar does his scientific work, he overlooks the initial pleasure he first took in Greek works, ideas, or objects:

> When we consider Antiquity scientifically, when we try to take hold of its becoming with the eye of the historian, or when, like the naturalist, we try to categorize and compare the linguistic forms of ancient masterpieces to relate them to morphological laws, then we always lose the wonderful form, the particular

> atmosphere of Antiquity, we forget the nostalgic impulse that brought us toward the Greeks with the power of our instinct, this sublime guide of ours.[36]

Nietzsche thus pointed to an incompatibility between the instinctive impulse—the passion—that had initially determined the choice of his career, and the scientific impulse that guided his professional research work. While both impulses feed on the same ideal, one expression of this ideal tends to extinguish the other.

The inner contradiction of philology as a profession is thus double. On the one hand, the philologist's professional activity rests upon a classicist ideal that is slowly obliterated by the "historicist" perspective resulting from scientific historical data. This disciplinary contradiction entails the general problem of the historical conscience in nineteenth-century Germany, as mid-twentieth-century philologists such as Reinhardt have remarked. On the other hand, the scientific impulse toward knowledge that motivates the scholar tends to deaden the passionate drive that brought her to a particular field of knowledge. This personal contradiction causes a malaise within the scholar, whatever her discipline. Nietzsche suggests that this second contradiction characterizes the disciplinary constitution of knowledge as such. It is thus impossible for a scholar to escape it and the problems, the difficulties, and—eventually—the crises that it causes. He who has chosen a scholarly career will necessarily be confronted to the contradiction between passion and knowledge impulse. Nietzsche's Basel writings indeed show that he did not escape this existential difficulty: he rapidly felt the contradiction between his profession and his "instinctive passion" and "inclination" toward the Greeks.[37]

Towards a therapy: Three attempts at reconciling profession and vocation

Although his inaugural lecture showed that a scholar could not escape the contradiction between passion and science, it seems that Nietzsche did not immediately grasp the practical—and radical—implications of this thesis. Indeed, in the first half of the 1870s, he made three attempts at reconciling his profession with his vocation. We will now turn to these failed attempts at healing what he interpreted as an existential illness.

(1) In January 1871, Nietzsche applied to the chair of Philosophy at the University of Basel. His long and inauspicious letter to the principal of the University, philologist Wilhelm Vischer-Bilfinger, illustrates the conflict between his profession and what he deemed to be his proper task (his "*eigentliche Aufgabe*"), his "natural" calling:

> I live here in a most peculiar conflict that has exhausted and physically worn me down. Naturally I am strongly inclined to philosophically unify my reflections and to dwell undisturbed and with sustained reflection on one problem. I feel myself always thrown hither and thither, and driven off my course, by my daily variegated professional work and by the way it is disposed. This juxtaposition of Pädagogium and university I cannot in the long run tolerate, because I feel that my real task, to which I *must* necessarily *sacrifice any profession*, my *philosophical* task, is being made to suffer by it, and is even being reduced to an activity on the side.[38]

Nietzsche cherished many hopes regarding this new position, but his project—which included proposing his close friend Erwin Rohde as successor to his chair of philology—did not work out: the University of Basel hired yet another Aristotelian, Rudolf Eucken. Nietzsche's attempt at becoming a professional philosopher entails two observations. First: his initiative was an attempt to unify profession and task—in other words, to fulfill his vocation within a profession. This project thus ignores the final implications of the contradiction between scientific drive toward knowledge and passionate attraction toward the Greek world. Second: Nietzsche singled out his Schopenhauerian philosophy as the cause of his application's rejection. He wrote to Rohde on 29 March 1871: "Think how much one has me [*mich in der Hand hat*], when one refers to my never withheld Schopenhauerianism!"[39] Nietzsche said nothing of his unusual attempt to change faculties and to be recognized as a scholar of a discipline that he had not specialized in. He simply concluded that in order to maintain the possibility for him to eventually become a professional philosopher, *he must prove and legitimize his identity as one*. He announced to Rohde that his next step in this direction was his upcoming book on tragedy. Let us now turn to this second attempt.

(2) While his first attempt sought to engage in a profession that would respect his vocation, Nietzsche's second attempt rather sought to unify profession and vocation within his philological career. He told Rohde in March 1871 that *The Birth of Tragedy* was his strategy. Nietzsche's first book was an effort to renovate the field of philology[40]: in the spirit of his inaugural lecture, he guided scientific philological endeavors toward philosophy and art as curative forces, in order to develop a newly self-conscious practice of philology. The book's reception, though, reveals that its author incorrectly foresaw its effects. *The Birth of Tragedy* was indeed echoed mostly by silence.[41] During its first year, it gave way to only two responses in the press: Rohde's celebratory review in the 26 May 1872 *Norddeutsche allgemeine Zeitung*, and young doctor of philology Ulrich von Wilamowitz-Möllendorff's two-part critical pamphlet (spring 1872, winter 1873). In both pamphlets, Wilamowitz made "out as if Nietzsche was arguing from philological fact, or that he was at the very least arguing on the basis of philological knowledge," which he was not: in *The Birth of Tragedy*, Nietzsche did not defend theses on the grounds of scholarship, "but on some other level, which we might variously call rhetorical, aesthetic, or cultural grounds, with a heavy dose of imaginative invention besides."[42] Yet some classicists did recognize the usefulness of Nietzsche's intuitions. For instance, amid the criticisms that he addressed to Nietzsche, philologist Ernst Leutsch of the University of Göttingen nevertheless wrote that here was a "scholar who does not lack spirit, as several insights in the book show."[43] But most scholars in the field deemed that with *The Birth of Tragedy*, Nietzsche "was indeed risking academic notoriety."[44] In a broader perspective, one can see that Wilamowitz was criticizing Nietzsche's philosophical stance inasmuch as he was arguing against the possibility of doing classical philology in any other way than a purely scholarly one. Wilamowitz considered philology as a science whose solid, critical method yielded definite results that enabled scholars to make precise, substantial progress in the historical knowledge of the past.[45] His second pamphlet against Nietzsche ended with these words:

> If he [Mr. Nietzsche] now were to reply to me that he simply did not want to know anything of "so-called world history," nor of "history and criticism," that

> he merely wished to create a Dionysian-Apollonian work of art, a "metaphysical consolation" . . . then I revoke my critique and lower its import. . . . then I will gladly permit his gospel, for my weapons are unable to touch it. . . . but one thing I would then demand: that Mr. Nietzsche keep his word and withdraw the thyrsus and move from India to Greece, and climb down from his pulpit on which he is meant to teach scientifically.[46]

Wilamowitz's conclusion was clear: as his first book—an unscientific essay written by a bad scholar—showed, Nietzsche was not worthy of his position.

Interestingly, while "the immediate response of the profession" to Nietzsche's book was silence,[47] Nietzsche's answer was the same. The 1872–73 quarrel about *The Birth of Tragedy* was between Rohde, Wagner, and Wilamowitz: Nietzsche did not answer directly to Wilamowitz. In fact, Nietzsche decided to keep away from all future disputes. After reading Wilamowitz's first pamphlet, he wrote to Gersdorff on 3 June 1872: "I will never get involved in a polemic."[48] However, his first book did have an important consequence as to Nietzsche's disciplinary status: as of this publication, he was considered mostly as a philosopher (and more often than not, as a Wagnerian philosopher). A short column in the *Philosophische Monatshefte* even named Nietzsche among the Philosophy Professors of Basel![49] Ironically, he was listed precisely between two holders of the Basel chair of Philosophy, one of which was the recently appointed Eucken. Nietzsche wrote on 30 April 1872, that he was most happy to be "included within the 'professors of philosophy.'"[50] This shows that he still ignored the final consequences of the contradiction between profession and vocation. It is certain that this attempt at realizing his task within his profession failed because the philological profession was not open to his methodological, philosophical, and cultural perspectives. But it also failed, on the one hand, because of the structural contradictions between passion (vocation) and science (scholarly profession), and on the other hand, because of the inner tensions of a philosophical vocation. We will turn to this last point shortly, but let us first describe Nietzsche's third attempt.

(3) While he was thus confronted with two public failures early on in his career, it is telling that Nietzsche's third attempt at reconciling profession and vocation remained private. During the winter of 1875, he took notes for an essay on philology that he entitled *We Philologists*. He never published nor even finished this project that would have been another of the *Untimely Meditations*. In these notes, Nietzsche reflected upon his profession in a more personal manner than in his inaugural lecture. He noticed that like marriages, successful careers are extremely rare because "one *chooses* a profession when one is not yet able to choose: one does not know the different professions, one does not know oneself." He thereby identified a cause of the failure of a career: one can choose the wrong profession when one does not yet know oneself. While he was speaking on his own behalf, Nietzsche was also considering that most scholars do not have the right job for them: they sit in their chair because they wrongly interpreted their passion. They mistook their drive toward a particular type of knowledge for their true vocation. In other words: most academics' careers reveal that they ignore, or are ignorant of, their vocation. Nietzsche was sour as to the outcome of such a personal mistake: the scholar "uses his active years in this profession, he

uses all of his capacity to reflect upon it, then he becomes more experienced; but should he reach the height of his professional insight then it is usually too late to begin anything new."[51] He considered that this situation contributed to his own moral and physical illness.

The structural conflict between profession and vocation in philosophy: Nietzsche and the definition of "profession"

I have situated Nietzsche within the context of his profession in the last quarter of the nineteenth century and described his failed attempts at reconciling scientific impulse and intuitive passion. I will now turn to the structural conflict between profession and philosophical vocation. To better understand Nietzsche's position on this matter, one can consider the Lutheran tradition—of which he was well aware—that infuses the concepts that he used. For this task, I believe it is not an anachronism to examine Max Weber's exemplary definition of profession. While speaking of the Lutheran usage that recognizes the vocational meaning of a professional activity, Weber explains that the German word *Beruf* names a particular area of work but also a position that one holds for life.[52]

This concept has both an external and internal signification: a *Beruf* is a profession and at the same time a vocation or calling. As Weber stressed in his famous 1917 conference *Science as a Vocation*, the scholar's *Beruf* as a profession (in its external sense) follows the demands of disciplinary specialization and method.[53] As for its internal sense, the scholar's *Beruf*, according to Weber, is necessarily linked to a passion for knowledge per se. Passion and work, "both together,"[54] are the prerequisite for the scholar's inspiration—which Weber assimilates to an "intoxication" (*Rausch*)—and thus for his ideas. Without an inspiring passion and conscientious work guided by method, one cannot make a profession out of knowledge as science. Now as work and passion, a profession has exterior and interior effects. Through her profession, a scholar participates to the progress of knowledge in her particular field, but she also makes considerable progress as to the knowledge of herself. That is why Weber's 1917 conference ends on his saying that science as a vocation entices the individual to work so that the "the 'demands of the day' are fully met, both professionally and humanly."[55] *Beruf* is a "profession-calling": in this Lutheran-Weberian sense, the scholar's task or vocation is his profession.

Rather than following on this "existential" understanding of profession as a calling (a *Berufung*), Nietzsche dissociates *Beruf* and *Aufgabe*. He considers "profession" in its external sense as a concept that has to do only with work. To quote Weber again, one can say that, for Nietzsche, profession is "the activity defined by the division of labor which both constitutes for an individual his source of income and thereby the lasting source of his livelihood and his survival."[56] Weber adds that this meaning of *Beruf* characterizes Latin languages that lack a word for the German concept that encompasses both ideas of "profession" and "calling." But Nietzsche precisely distances himself from the Lutheran concept: the "organic" unity of profession is impossible for he who recognizes his vocation as a philosophical calling. On the basis of his reading of Schopenhauer and of his Greek definition of philosophy—more on this shortly—Nietzsche proposed that philosophy cannot be an academic endeavor. In other words, inner philosophical passion and the calling that it ignites cannot be exteriorized in a career socially and economically speaking. Nietzsche's task thus led him toward a "philosophical life" independent from a profession. Before we turn to his philosophical path, let us make three remarks on this structural conflict between profession and vocation in philosophy according to Nietzsche.

First, it is clear that to change careers would not be a solution to this conflict. Indeed, the problem does not reside in the passion—be it understood as a "drive" (*Trieb*), an "enigma" or an "intoxication"[57]—that prompts an individual to apprehend a particular field of knowledge. Rather, *the problem lies in the disciplinary constitution of this passion*. Nietzsche suggests that if it engages with the demands of a scholarly discipline, one's drive toward knowledge will unavoidably become inclined to seek its own accomplishment above all else, as is the case with philology: "classical philology pursues only the final end of its own being, which is the fusing together of the initially hostile and violent impulses that have only forcibly been brought together. Let us talk as we will about the unattainability of this goal, and even designate the goal itself as an illogical pursuit—the pursuit of it is very real."[58] This goes to say that disciplinary endeavors do not primarily function so as to quench the scholar's passion, but rather so as to define, circumscribe, limit, and preserve the academic discipline itself. This observation precisely refers to the activities of the bustling scientific laborer whom Nietzsche, like Berlin academicians, criticized as dangerously resembling more and more a factory worker.[59] The scientific laborer shuns his passion for the "enigma" as he turns to more practical objectives. Some of these objectives contribute to maintain the discipline (such as finding data that confirm the disciplinary constitution of knowledge), while others contribute to maintain the researcher's own status (such as building one's reputation and negotiating a salary). In fact, these practical objectives accomplish the specialization and professionalization of the discipline. One can understand Nietzsche's words in his 1875 notes accordingly: "When we observe how few philologists there actually are, except those that have taken up philology as a means of livelihood, we can easily decide for ourselves what is the matter with this impulse for antiquity, it *hardly* exists at all; for there are no disinterested philologists."[60]

Second, it appears that while a profession entails many public actions (lectures, conferences, publication of research, professional representations, social mingling, etc.), a vocation as Nietzsche understands it—that is, a philosophical vocation—rather commands some degree of private expression. Indeed, because "particularly sad facts lie in the essence of things," philosophy discovers disturbing truths that are not for all ears to hear.[61] In the early 1870s, Nietzsche cherished the idea of a gathering of philosophical spirits—he used the expression "cultural-educational sect" (*Bildungs-Sekte*)—akin to the philosophical communities of Antiquity, something like "a new *Greek* academy," as he wrote to Rohde.[62] Even in these dreams of private communion, Nietzsche's intellectual desires echo those of Mommsen and other academicians who felt part of a group of initiates at the Berlin Academy of Sciences. Through this multidisciplinary quasi "religious confraternity," the unity of knowledge could survive in spite of the increasing specialization of academic disciplines.[63] Nietzsche's peculiarity, though, is that he did not think of the universities or scholarly academies as places where the philosophical spirit could flourish.

Third, from what has been said above regarding his three failed attempts and his definition of profession, it follows that Nietzsche considered the conflict between profession and vocation as irreconcilable. This observation became concrete reality when he retired from academic life in 1879. He was not in favor of saying, as Rohde did, that an academic career "is in all circumstances the safest and most reliable one for confronting all dangers."[64] Because he considered that philosophy could not be a profession, Nietzsche opted for a nonprofessionalized vocation. He abandoned his profession to lead a philosophical life and became the "wandering doctor" that Rohde dreaded. Commentators do not hesitate to say that Nietzsche at this point was "liberated" by his physical illness. He indeed acknowledged this fact in 1888 when he wrote about the 1876–78 period: "Sickness *slowly liberated me*."[65] His bad health no doubt intervened in his decision to quit academia, but one must not conclude that this was the only or even major reason for his retirement. As I hope to have shown, Nietzsche's 1870s crisis was fundamentally philosophical: it pertained to a deeply reflected upon conflict between profession and vocation.

Nietzsche's definition of philosophical life: Sources

As we have seen, Nietzsche's understanding of this conflict and his parallel project to resign his chair progressed throughout the 1870s. His letters reveal that early on he considered the possibility of quitting academia. In 1872, he talked of long trips away from Basel, and he wrote to Rohde on 11 April: "For the purposes of this endeavor I now define my position so that you may be my successor in *every* respect."[66] But Rohde did not support his friend's anti-professional stance. He constantly reminded Nietzsche that "at no price" should he abandon the position that secured the financial, intellectual, and social means "to build his life in a grand style without fear."[67] Though he did believe that in an ideal world, philosophical spirits could shut themselves off from everyday life, Rohde held academia to be "without doubt the noblest among all professional duties."[68] He invariably tried to convince Nietzsche to keep his chair: as he wrote on 14 November 1872, in their common war against the new German culture "to give up *material* chances would be the greatest folly."[69] Rohde dearly hoped that Nietzsche would abandon his "wandering doctor plans" rather than his career, and he himself in no case wished to become a literary vagabond.[70]

Clearly, Nietzsche and Rohde defended two opposite visions not of the task at hand, but rather of the site from which this task could be fulfilled. Rohde wanted to pursue their cultural movement in the academic world, supported by professional titles, grants, and networks, whereas Nietzsche talked of "running away" from academia to "travel," of "abandoning" his career for new "philosophical sects," and of finding "radical truths" that would define a "philosophical life." Let us now turn to the definition of a philosophical life that Nietzsche developed while reflecting upon the disciplinary constitution of knowledge. There are two major sources for his considering it impossible to be a "professional" philosopher: the first is Schopenhauer; the second is the Greek conception of philosophy in the fifth century B.C. I will look briefly at both.

Nietzsche read Schopenhauer every year between 1865 and 1878.[71] His 15 December 1870 letter to Rohde shows how important Schopenhauer's 1851 essay *On University-Philosophy* was for him: "in the long run, I also realize what Schopenhauer's doctrine of university wisdom is all about. A completely radical institution for *truth* is not *possible* here."[72] Schopenhauer believed that "if profit is being derived from it, intention at once gains an ascendancy over insight and from self-styled philosophers we get mere parasites of philosophy."[73] According to him, the demands of a profession paralyze the mind in such a way that ideas simply cannot bloom: "hardly anything is so obstructive to the actual attainment of a thorough or very deep insight and thus of true wisdom, as the constant obligation to appear wise, the showing off of so-called knowledge in the presence of pupils eager to learn and the readiness to answer every conceivable question."[74] Schopenhauer indeed stressed that philosophy as a profession cannot be truly independent because it must answer to the authority that supports it: "a government will not pay people to contradict directly, or even only indirectly, what it has had promulgated from all the pulpits by thousands of its appointed priests or religious teachers, for insofar as such a proceeding were effective, it would inevitably render ineffective the former organization."[75] Schelling had already raised this issue in his lectures on academic studies: "The normal view of universities is that they should produce able servants and tools for all purposes of the state." And Wolf, the founder of classical philology, held the same conclusion about universities in 1787: "the State has little use for the mere humanist."[76] But Schopenhauer further suggested that philosophy simply cannot exist if a superior instance imposes a dogma upon it, whether it be the Christian religion, Hegelianism, the omnipotence of the Prussian state, or the disciplinary definition of knowledge. Schopenhauer stressed that "the atmosphere of freedom is indispensable to truth,"[77] and accordingly, he urged that philosophy should stop being a profession.

Nietzsche followed Schopenhauer's ideas on this issue. He noticed that scholarly work unfortunately does not serve the goal of defining one's own existence: "Just take a look at the activities with which a scientific person spends and thus kills his life: what does the Greek rule of particles have to do with the meaning of life?"[78] Because a philosopher "is meant to seek the truth for himself and not so as to write books,"[79] Nietzsche repeatedly returned to one of the first philosophical principles: "Know thyself."[80] This brings us to the Greek sources of his conception of philosophy. It goes without saying that Nietzsche as a philologist knew the Greeks very well. He gave lectures on Plato's dialogues, Aristotle's metaphysics and rhetoric, Diogenes Laërtius, Democritus, and the Presocratics. In his lectures, he reiterated Socrates' definition of the origins of philosophy: he stated that philosophical insights originate from "astonishment at everything that lies before one."[81] In fact, it is this fundamental wonder, this "enigma" of the unknown that ignites passion and determines the choice of a career. In philosophy, this impulse should take a practical form: Nietzsche believed that a philosopher must give an example by his or her life more than by his or her writings. "I am a philosopher inasmuch as I am able to serve as an example. . . . But this example must be given by outward life and not merely through books, in the way, that is, in which the philosophers of Greece taught, through one's expressions, attitudes, clothing, food, and way of life rather than through speaking or writing."[82] He further believed that "in a refuted system, the only thing of interest is the personal element," that is, the efforts toward philosophizing.[83] Philosophy is better represented by the verb than by the noun.

This reflexive activity encompasses all of the individual's existence, so much so that it defines a particular type of life—a philosophical life. As Nietzsche stressed, "The only critique of a philosophy which is possible and which proves something, namely trying to see whether one can live in according with it, has never been taught at universities."[84] That is to say that the most important philosophical attitude cannot take place within academia. As early as March 1871, Nietzsche wrote to Rohde: "I am gradually habituating myself to being a philosopher, and already I believe in myself."[85] As a philosopher, he wished to realize what he called a type, a "hitherto undiscovered highest *possibility of philosophical life*."[86] This life must be guided by a precept that defines philosophy since Socrates: "The Delphic God shouts out to you, at the very start of your wandering to that goal, his saying 'Know thyself.' It is a difficult saying."[87] The Delphic precept invites an individual to return to the first site of philosophical investigation, because the knowledge of oneself opens onto a knowledge of the world. Nietzsche tied his reflection to Heraclitus' motto: "I sought and consulted myself."[88] Because he followed the Delphic precept, Heraclitus showed that one must first turn toward oneself in order to learn what it means to be a human being. And as we have seen, Nietzsche believed that it was precisely this knowledge, this first stage of philosophical investigation that philologists lack—as most scholars in all fields: they chose their career out of lack of self-knowledge. Philologists failed to notice, as Dale Wilkerson rightly points out, that "all examinations of the past are explorations of oneself."[89]

Conclusion

Nietzsche did not stay a rising or even a fixed star of classical philology for long. With his early retirement from academia, he recovered his wandering star status and lived the philosophical life of a "literary vagabond" that his former kindred spirit dreaded. Perhaps "The loss was philology's," as some scholars today consider that Nietzsche must be remembered "as one of the more promising and least realized classicists of all time."[90]

Nietzsche was physically ill in the 1870s, but as we have seen his decision to resign from his career was essentially philosophical. It stemmed from his having identified the cause of his mental and physical illnesses as an irreconcilable existential conflict between his profession and his natural calling to philosophy—a conflict that he felt since starting his career. Turning away from academia and favoring a nonprofessional philosophical activity was a therapeutic process: the only possibility of healing was to quit the profession for the vocation. Nietzsche's understanding of both conflict and therapy rested upon his "material" definition of profession and his Schopenhauerian and Delphic conception of a philosophical calling and life.

Nietzsche's decision to leave academia was no doubt radical. In fact, it appears unique when one considers that the reflections behind it—regarding the limits of the disciplinary constitution of knowledge, the problems facing specialization in the humanities and social sciences, the structural paradoxes of knowledge-oriented professions, and the limits to philosophy as a profession—were actually shared by many nineteenth-century scholars, from Schelling to Schopenhauer to Mommsen.[91] But these did not turn away from their university chairs or their prestigious positions at the Berlin Academy. A contextual appraisal of Nietzsche's ideas thus enables one to grasp the true originality of this thinker. Contrary to what one too often reads in noncontextual Nietzsche commentaries, his originality lies not in his young age when he started his professorship, nor in his defense of artistic vocation in classical philology, nor in his longing for a global philosophical perspective to historical studies.[92] Rather, Nietzsche's true originality lies in the radical decision in favor of a philosophical life, following his experience in and assessment of the crisis in philological studies.

Once this is made clear, we can pursue for ourselves a reflection upon the issues raised by Nietzsche. Can science be reconciled with passion within a knowledge-oriented profession, in a more Weberian than Nietzschean sense? Can one practice philosophy in its existential definition as "*manière de vivre*"[93] from within academia? And perhaps more pressingly, does the disciplinary definition of knowledge in academia impose ultimately fatal limits to a scholar's "inspiring passion"?[94] Indeed, these are fundamental and pressing interrogations in an academic age dominated by the obligation for scholarly research to fit into predefined disciplinary categories, following which governmental organisms issue funding opportunities inasmuch as a research project can yield quantifiable and operational data, and this in all fields of inquiry—even philosophy.

Notes

1 On Nietzsche's published reviews and philological essays, see William H. Schaberg, *The Nietzsche Canon: A Publication History and Bibliography* (Chicago/London: University of Chicago Press, 1995); and James I. Porter, "'Rare impressions.' Nietzsche's Philologica: A Review of the Colli-Montinari Critical Edition," *International Journal of the Classical Tradition* 6(3), (2000): 409–31. On his going to the University of Munich's jubilee, see KSB 4, p. 37. On the philosophical orientation of his philology, see EKP (which I will discuss later in the paper). And on *The Birth of Tragedy*'s lack of scholarship apparatus, see James I. Porter, "'Don't Quote Me on That!' Wilamowitz Contra Nietzsche in 1872 and 1873," *Journal of Nietzsche Studies* 42 (2011): 73.

2 Nietzsche to Vischer-Bilfinger, January 1871, KSB 3, p. 175.

3 Nietzsche to Brandes, 19 February 1888, KSB 8, p. 260; see also EH, "Menschliches."

4 Nietzsche to Vischer-Bilfinger, January 1871, KSB 3, p. 175.

5 Carl Pletsch, *Young Nietzsche: Becoming a Genius* (New York: The Free Press, 1991), p. 106.

6 James Whitman, "Nietzsche in the Magisterial Tradition of German Classical Philology," *Journal of the History of Ideas* 47 (1986): 461.
7 On Nietzsche's workload, see Curt Paul Janz, *Friedrich Nietzsche: Biographie*, vol. 1, part 2: *Die zehn Basler Jahre (19 April 1869 bis 2. Mai 1879)* (Munich: Carl Hanser, 1978), ch. 4.
8 Nietzsche to Ritschl, 2 August 1869, KSB 3, p. 34.
9 Nietzsche to Gersdorff, 28 September 1869, KSB 3, p. 61.
10 See William Clark, *Academic Charisma and the Origins of the Research University* (Chicago/London: University of Chicago Press, 2006), pp. 9–10; and R. Steven Turner, "Historicism, *Kritik*, and the Prussian Professoriate, 1790 to 1840," in M. Bollack and H. Wismann, eds, *Philologie et herméneutique au 19e siècle* (Goettingen: Vandenhoeck & Ruprecht, 1983), pp. 468 and 475–76.
11 Lorraine Daston, "The Academies and the Unity of Knowledge: The Disciplining of the Disciplines," *Differences* 10(2) (1998): 69; see Turner, "Historicism, *Kritik*," p. 460.
12 See Daston, "The Academies," p. 74; Turner, "Historicism, *Kritik*," p. 461; and Clark, *Academic Charisma*, p. 171.
13 Daston, "The Academies," p. 77; see Turner, "Historicism, *Kritik*," p. 465.
14 See F. W. J. von Schelling, *Vorlesungen über die Methode (Lehrart) des akademischen Studiums* (Hamburg: Meiner, 1990), pp. 41–164; and Daston, "The Academies."
15 Droysen is quoted in Karl Reinhardt, "Die klassische Philologie und das Klassische," in Carl Becker, ed., *Vermächtnis der Antike: Gesammelte Essays zur Philosophie und Geschichtsschreibung* (Goettingen: Vandenhoeck & Ruprecht, 1989), p. 342. For previous quote, see Theodor Mommsen, "Ansprache am Leibnizschen Gedachtnistage," in *Reden und Aufsätze* (Berlin: Weidmannsche Buchhandlung, 1905), p. 198.
16 Reinhardt, "Die klassische Philologie," p. 339 and 336. On the crisis in the German historical sciences, see Hugh Lloyd-Jones, Introduction to Ulrich von Wilamowitz-Möllendorff, *History of Classical Scholarship* (trans. A. Harris, Baltimore: The Johns Hopkins University Press, 1982), pp. xxviii–xxix; and Christian J. Emden, "The Invention of Antiquity: Nietzsche on Classicism, Classicality, and the Classical Tradition," in P. Bishop, ed., *Nietzsche and Antiquity: His Reaction and Response to the Classical Tradition* (Rochester: Camden House, 2004), p. 372.
17 Lloyd-Jones, Introduction, p. x.
18 Reinhardt, "Die klassische Philologie," p. 342.
19 James I. Porter, "Nietzsche, Homer, and the Classical Tradition," in P. Bishop, ed., *Nietzsche and Antiquity* (Rochester: Camden House, 2004), p. 13.
20 See Emden, "The Invention of Antiquity," p. 378. On the transformation of the learned class, see Turner, "Historicism, *Kritik*." On philology's incapacity to confront its theoretical issues, see Reinhardt, "Die klassische Philologie," p. 342.
21 Wilhelm Wundt, "Mission de la philosophie dans le temps present," *Revue philosophique de la France et de l'étranger* 1(1876): 113.
22 Porter, "Nietzsche, Homer," p. 12.
23 HKP, KGW 2, 1, pp. 249–50.
24 Schelling, *Vorlesungen*, III, p. 40.
25 Schelling, *Vorlesungen*, XIV, p. 146.
26 HKP, KGW 2, 1, p. 253.
27 See NN § 3.
28 See Lloyd-Jones, Introduction, p. xi and xiv; and Turner, "Historicism, *Kritik*," p. 469.

29 Reinhardt, "Die klassische Philologie," p. 351.
30 EKP § 7, KGW 2, 3, p. 370.
31 Whitman, "Nietzsche in the Magisterial Tradition," p. 459.
32 Nietzsche to Ritschl, 10 May 1869, KSB 3, p. 7.
33 EKP § 7, KGW 2, 3, pp. 369–70.
34 Emil Du Bois-Reymond, "Über die wissenschaftlichen Zustande der Gegenwart," in *Reden*, vol. 2 (Leipzig: Veit, 1886), p. 450.
35 See HKP, KGW 2, 1, pp. 251–2.
36 HKP, KGW 2, 1, p. 252.
37 Ibid.
38 Nietzsche to Vischer-Bilfinger, January 1871, KSB 3, p. 175. Emphasis in all quotations in this paper is in the original.
39 Nietzsche to Rohde, 29 March 1871, KSB 3, p. 189.
40 See Whitman, "Nietzsche in the Magisterial Tradition," p. 463.
41 Ibid., p. 466.
42 Porter, "'Don't Quote Me on That!'" p. 75. Rohde's review and both of Wilamowitz's pamphlets are reprinted in Karlfried Gründer, ed., *Der Streit um Nietzsches Geburt der Tragödie* (Hildesheim/Zurich/New York: Olms, 1989).
43 l [Ernst von Leutsch], [Review of *Die Geburt der Tragödie*], *Philologischer Anzeiger* 5(3) (1873): 138; see Rohde to Nietzsche, 12 January 1873, KGB 2, 4.
44 Porter, "'Don't Quote Me on That!'" p. 74.
45 Ulrich von Wilamowitz-Möllendorff, *History of Classical Scholarship* (trans. A. Harris, Baltimore: The Johns Hopkins University Press, 1982), p. 1.
46 Ulrich von Wilamowitz-Möllendorff, "Zukunftsphilologie!," in K. Gründer, ed., *Der Streit um Nietzsches Geburt der Tragödie* (Hildesheim/Zurich/New York: Olms, 1989), p. 55.
47 Whitman, "Nietzsche in the Magisterial Tradition," p. 455.
48 Nietzsche to Gersdorff, 3 June 1872, KSB 4, pp. 5–6.
49 See Anonymous, "Die Vertreter der Philosophie an der Universität Basel," *Philosophische Monatshefte* 8 (1872): 93–5. For Nietzsche considered as a Wagnerian philosopher, see for instance Leutsch, "Review," pp. 137–8.
50 Nietzsche to Rohde, 30 April 1872, KSB 3, p. 314.
51 The two last quotes are from Nachlaß 3[19], March 1875, KSA 8, p. 20.
52 Max Weber, *Die protestantische Ethik und der Geist des Kapitalismus,* in Marianne Weber, ed., *Gesammelte Aufsätze zur Religionssoziologie* (Tuebingen: Mohr Siebeck/UTB, 1988), p. 63. On Nietzsche and Lutheranism, see Duncan Large, "'Der Bauernaufstand des Geistes.' Nietzsche, Luther and the Reformation," in N. Martin, ed., *Nietzsche and the German Tradition* (Bern: Peter Lang, 2003), pp. 111–37.
53 See Max Weber, "Wissenschaft als Beruf," in Winckelmann, ed., *Gesammelte Aufsätze zur Wissenschaftslehre*, vol. 1 (Tuebingen: Mohr Siebeck/UTB, 1988), p. 588 (as regards specialization) and 590 (as regards method).
54 Weber, "Wissenschaft als Beruf," pp. 590–1.
55 Ibid., p. 613.
56 Weber, *Die protestantische Ethik*, p. 64, note.
57 See, respectively, for "drive," Nietzsche, Nachlaß 3[62], March 1875, KSA 8, p. 31; for "enigma," Reinhardt, "Die klassische Philologie," p. 335; and for "intoxication," Weber, "Wissenschaft als Beruf," p. 590.
58 HKP, KGW 2, 1, p. 253.

59 See for instance EKP § 7, KGW 2, 3, pp. 369–70; and Du Bois-Reymond, "Über die wissenschaftlichen Zustande," p. 450.
60 Nachlaß 3[62], March 1875, KSA 8, p. 31.
61 EKP § 7, KGW 2, 3, p. 371.
62 Nietzsche to Rohde, 15 December 1870, KSB 3, p. 165. For "*Bildungs-Sekte*," see Nachlaß 32[62], early 1874-spring 1874, KSA 7, p. 776.
63 Daston, "The Academies," p. 82.
64 Rohde to Nietzsche, 6 May 1872, KGB 2, 4.
65 EH, "Menschliches" § 4, KSA 6, p. 326. For an example of a Nietzsche scholar attributing a liberating effect to Nietzsche's physical state, see Paolo D'Iorio, "La naissance de la philosophie enfantée par l'esprit scientifique," in P. D'Iorio, ed., Nietzsche, *Les philosophes préplatoniciens*, trans. N. Ferrand (Combas: L'Éclat, 1994), p. 41.
66 Nietzsche to Rohde, 11 April 1872, KSB 3, pp. 304–5.
67 Rohde to Nietzsche, April 1872, KGW 2, 2.
68 Rohde to Nietzsche, 6 May 1872, KGB 2, 4.
69 Rohde to Nietzsche, 14 November 1872, KGB 2, 4.
70 See Rohde to Nietzsche on 6 May 1872 and 14 November 1872.
71 See Thomas Brobjer, *Nietzsche's Philosophical Context: An Intellectual Biography* (Urbana/Chicago: University of Illinois Press, 2008), pp. 254–5.
72 Nietzsche to Rohde, 15 December 1870, KSB 3, p. 165.
73 Arthur Schopenhauer, "Über die Universitäts-Philosophie," in Schopenhauer, *Parerga und Paralipomena: Kleine philosophische Schriften*, vol. 1 (Zurich: Haffmans, 1988), p. 156.
74 Schopenhauer, "Über die Universitäts-Philosophie," p. 152.
75 Ibid., p. 141.
76 Wolf is quoted in Clark, *Academic Charisma*, p. 171. See Schelling, *Vorlesungen*, III, p. 23.
77 Schopenhauer, "Über die Universitäts-Philosophie," p. 152.
78 Nachlaß 3[63], March 1875, KSA 8, p. 32.
79 Nachlaß 32[73], early 1874-spring 1874, KSA 7, p. 780.
80 See NN § 10, KSA 1, p. 333.
81 VP I, KGW 2, 4, p. 215. Also see Plato, *Theae.* 155c-d, and Aristotle, *Meta.* A, 2, 982b.
82 SE § 3, KSA 1, p. 350.
83 PTZ I, KSA 1, p. 803.
84 SE § 8, KSA 1, p. 417.
85 Nietzsche to Rohde, 29 March 1871, KSB 3, p. 190.
86 MA § 261, KSA 2, p. 217; see also PTZ.
87 NN § 10, KSA 1, pp. 332–3.
88 FV I, KSA 1, p. 758.
89 Dale Wilkerson, *Nietzsche and the Greeks* (London/New York: Continuum Press, 2006), p. 3.
90 See Porter, "'Don't Quote Me on That!,'" p. 90; and Porter, "'Rare impressions,'" p. 410.
91 A parallel could perhaps be drawn here between Nietzsche and Swiss historian Johann Jakob Bachofen, who retired from his University of Basel chair in 1845 after holding it but 4 years. Bachofen pursued his research on archaic societies and published most of his works as an independent scholar. According to Hubert Cancik, Bachofen is to be counted among the four figures most important for Nietzsche in Basel (along with Wagner, Overbeck, and Burckhardt). See Hubert Cancik, *Nietzsches Antike: Vorlesungen* (Stuttgart: J. B. Metzler, 1995).

92 Regarding the rather common practice in Swiss and German universities of hiring very young scholars during Nietzsche's time, see Janz, *Friedrich Nietzsche*. For other examples of artistic vocations in philology, see Whitman, "Nietzsche in the Magisterial Tradition." And for another defense of a philosophical perspective in historical studies, see Schelling, *Vorlesungen*.

93 See Pierre Hadot, *Exercices spirituels et philosophie antique* (Paris: Albin Michel, 2002).

94 Weber, "Wissenschaft als Beruf," pp. 590–1.

Abbreviations to Nietzsche's texts

EH	Ecce homo
EKP	Encyclopædie der klassische Philologie
FV	Fünf Vorreden über fünf ungeschriebene Bücher
HKP	Homer und die klassische Philologie
KGB	Briefwechsel. Kritische Gesamtausgabe
KGW	Werke. Kritische Gesamtausgabe
KSA	Kritische Studienausgabe
KSB	Sämtliche Briefe. Kritische Studienausgabe
MA	Menschliches, Allzumenschliches
NN	Vom Nutzen und Nachteil der Historie für das Leben
PTZ	Die Philosophie im tragischen Zeitalter der Griechen
SE	Schopenhauer als Erzieher
VP	Die vorplatonischen Philosophen

4

Nietzsche's Ethics of Reading: Education in a Postmodern World

Nathalie Lachance

The Nietzsche reader cannot help but notice a tension in the philosopher's work between his concern for education and his postulate of the constructedness of all truths. What becomes of education if we accept this postulate? What is one to teach? How should one teach it? Nietzsche grappled with these questions – as did Zarathustra, whose tale can be interpreted as the therapeutic journey of an educator who has much to (un) learn. The chapter "The Convalescent" suggests that Zarathustra's journey is a kind of therapy.[1] How could one define the illness from which Zarathustra must recover? Without going into a detailed interpretation of the text, it is safe to say that it is as *educator* that he suffers: his convalescence is coined by a transformation of his task as *educator*, as it appears that he must relinquish or at least reassess his teaching of the Overman. As teacher of the Overman, he was mocked by men on the marketplace: what authority could Zarathustra and his teaching possibly possess in the eyes of those men who live in a world in which God is dead – in a world in which every discourse is but another construct? Zarathustra's illness originates from this crisis, as does Nietzsche's project.

This crisis of authority led, in philosophy of education, to the debate between liberal education and constructivism. Those who promote liberal education and the *transmission* of an existing body of knowledge are accused of indoctrinating pupils with the narratives of the established order. Those who champion constructivism – the *construction* of knowledge by pupils – are accused of indoctrinating these pupils with a dangerous relativism. This very tension permeates Nietzsche's work. The death of God may result in the emancipation of humankind, but if this means the emancipation from all that gives weight and meaning to the human experience, from all that has enabled it to survive thus far, humankind will perish. Survival is inextricably linked, as one reads in the chapter "On the Thousand Goals and One" of *Thus Spoke Zarathustra*, to the steadfast belief in certain values: "Man alone assigned values to things, to preserve himself."[2] A humankind confronted by the thought that its values are only constructs might very well find itself in a pedagogical impasse: why value anything, why transmit anything, why learn anything? The crisis of authority arises from the devaluation of the concept of value itself and is a potentially fatal illness. How does Nietzsche, as an *author* who shuns *authority*, address this? What does he suggest to the reader—and how?

Inspired by Keith Ansell Pearson's suggestion that an ethics of reading lies at the center of Nietzsche's pedagogy,[3] I will explore the points of intersection, in Nietzsche's work, between education and reading, to show that Nietzsche devises an ethics of reading coined by agonistics and which functions as therapy for a culture suffering from the pedagogical impasse produced by the death of God. In his study *The Ethics of Reading*, J. Hillis Miller defines the ethical moment in the act of reading as follows: "On the one hand it is a response to something, responsible to it, responsive of it. . . . On the other hand, the ethical moment in reading leads to an act."[4] This definition has been interpreted as a response to attacks on deconstruction, which its detractors deem nihilistic and relativist.[5] Postmodern theory, with its deconstructive approach revealing the unstable foundations of language, has indeed insisted upon the *unreadability* of texts – on textual indeterminacy, on the impossibility to determine anything at all that is *definitive* in texts, including Nietzsche's.[6] Confronted to this *unreadability*, the reader has a great textual *response-ability*, to use a coinage by Alan D. Schrift.[7] In Nietzsche's work, as I will show, the reader is constantly reminded of this textual response-ability.

For Nietzsche, the act of reading is an agon, a contest with and against philosophical, cultural, and literary traditions, a process which does not consist in a systematic deconstruction for deconstruction's sake but which seeks to educate and emancipate readers by means of a rigorous confrontation with worthy opponents. Nietzsche's whole philosophical project itself can be interpreted as his own education and emancipation—and those of the reader—through and against the great opponents that are Socrates, Jesus, Schopenhauer, Kant, and Wagner, to name a few. As Hutter puts it: "We cannot begin to understand Nietzsche if we do not see his writings as expressions of a personal quest for autonomy and wisdom that call on readers to engage in a similar struggle."[8] Nietzsche's utterances regarding reading suggest that his reader himself must enter in a contest and educate and emancipate himself through and against the texts of his worthy opponents, including Nietzsche's. Nietzsche's pedagogical project, his ethics of reading, consists in an incessant agonistic movement between transmission, deconstruction, and creation. Nietzsche would not side with those who transmit knowledge like a faded hand-me-down, robbing their pupils of the joys of discovery and experimentation, but he would not side with the proponents of constructivism either, whose pupils are meant to create their reality *ex nihilo*, robbing them of the chance—and of the responsibility—to engage with history. This agonistic movement between transmission, deconstruction, and creation is the contest, which Nietzsche proposes to his reader. In order to explore this contest, I will present Nietzsche's early texts *On Truth and Lie in an Extra-Moral Sense*, *On the Future of Our Educational Institutions*, and *Homer's Contest*. These will serve as theoretical framework, enabling me to interpret other passages from Nietzsche's work in which he engages with Socrates and Kant, criticizing their pedagogical methods and developing, in opposition to these, his own style and ethics of reading. I will end with a reading of *Ecce Homo*, in which Nietzsche's thoughts on education and health converge, revealing the relationship between reading, agonistics, and health.

Nietzsche's preoccupation with agonistics has received much attention, in the last decade or so, in the works of Acampora, Appel, Hatab, and Siemens, in Lungstrum's and Sauer's collection of essays *Agonistics: Arenas of Creative Contest,* and in Schrift's *Why Nietzsche Still?* These studies have looked at the agonal problematic in Nietzsche's work in existential, aesthetic, and political terms, yielding enlightening results. As for the signification of agonistics for education in Nietzsche's thought, Murphy, in his study *Nietzsche as Educator*, identified the contest as "the pivotal element of educational practice."[9] Murphy also wrote that Nietzsche's books "beautifully exemplify the spirit of the contest between master and student, between author and reader."[10] This is what I propose to explore in this paper, namely: the implications of the agonal problematic for Nietzsche's writing itself and for the act of reading Nietzsche, a problematic which Nietzsche scholarship has neglected thus far but which is vital to our understanding not only of Nietzsche's thoughts on education but of his contribution to what Keith Ansell Pearson calls modernity's "project of developing and securing humankind's intellectual maturity."[11]

Intellectual maturity requires, according to Nietzsche, that we question and challenge language itself: in his early text *On Truth and Lie in an Extra-Moral Sense*, Nietzsche depicts language as a supple construction, seemingly made of a "spiders' webs," in which we are all entangled.[12] The whole structure of concept is described as a "web of concepts."[13] The acts of reading and writing necessarily rely on a plethora of terms which are not "things-in-themselves" (which are not only inconceivable but not even worth conceiving, writes Nietzsche) but rather metaphors for those "things-in-themselves," conventions on which speakers have agreed in order to communicate with one another.[14] What is truth, then, asks Nietzsche? "Truths are illusions about which we have forgotten that they are illusions, metaphors which are now worn out and without sensuous power, coins which have lost their picture and which count only as metal, no longer as coins."[15] As Lacoue-Labarthe expresses it in an essay in which he investigates Nietzsche's early lectures and fragments (dating from 1872 to 1875) on language and rhetoric: "Language is thus originally figurative, tropical, that is originally metaphorical."[16] This metaphorical language is, however, the very tool used in the elaboration of discourses, in the writing of texts. Nietzsche's critique of language thus reveals the unstable foundations of all discourses, of all texts, including his own—suggesting to the reader that he or she must engage, seriously and cautiously, with texts.

Nietzsche's study of language and rhetoric transformed his relationship to writing, as Lacoue-Labarthe points out: it is after this period that one notices a certain fragmentation in his style.[17] He is aware that his own work is entangled in a spider web, and that, as such, it might lull the reader into blindly accepting and believing what it suggests. Nietzsche therefore wants a vigilant reader who keeps the text at a distance, and his style after his study of language and rhetoric can be interpreted as an attempt to avoid indoctrinating such a reader. Nietzsche wishes to write as Thucydides, about whom he writes: "One must read him inside out, line by line, and read his unuttered thoughts as much as his words: there are few thinkers who are so rich in unuttered thoughts."[18] What I translate here as "unuttered thoughts" (*Hintergedanken*) could also be translated as "ulterior motives": Thucydides, according to Nietzsche, hides his true message between the lines. Nietzsche believes such a strategy to be highly educational, as one of his aphorisms, titled "The Incomplete as the Effective," indicates: here, Nietzsche insists on the educational benefits of letting a reader complete a thought, a task which would not be possible had the author exhaustively exposed his own views.[19] He thus favors a fragmentary style in order to encourage his reader to be an active reader—to pause and ponder not only what is written but also upon that which is left unsaid.

Nietzsche will embrace the aphorism as narrative strategy, the aim of which is to engage the reader in a contest for meaning, a contest which can be not only highly educational and emancipatory, but therapeutic as well. Danto reminded us of the relationship between the aphorism as genre and medicine, explaining that the earliest collection of aphorisms is attributed to Hippocrates. They were maxims regarding health and well-being which were meant to be learned by heart by interns. As Marsden writes in her study of aphorisms in Nietzsche: "It seems significant that the aphoristic style should be developed in Nietzsche's thought at a time when he is exploring the extent to which ideas can transform and redirect the energies of the body."[20] If language is a spider web in which one is entangled, then a fragmentary style that leaves much unsaid might afford the reader a greater freedom of thought and movement. In *Thus Spoke Zarathustra*, aphorisms are described as mountain peaks: one's task is to embark on a journey leading from one peak to the next,[21] or, as Nietzsche writes elsewhere, to (re) construct a "chain of thoughts," [22]supplementing what Nietzsche writes in order to bring his narrative to completion—perhaps better, to fruition. This is undoubtedly what Nietzsche enjoyed as reader of Thucydides: the possibility to explore, develop, and challenge his own thoughts, using Thucydides as raw material and impetus. Nietzsche even claims that reading Thucydides was *therapeutic* in his case, *curing* him of all Platonism.[23] Nietzsche will thus prefer writing in a fragmentary fashion, in order to elicit such a reception from his own readers: instead of systematically laying down concepts and theories, theses and arguments, he will favor that which leaves itself open, thus avoiding the exertion of (too much) authority on his reader. Nietzsche leaves these open spaces for the reader to occupy them.

Nietzsche's early praise of Schopenhauer has much to do with such a reading experience, as one gathers from *Schopenhauer as Educator*. One learns very little about Schopenhauer and his philosophy in this text, in which Nietzsche reveals much about *himself*. In *Schopenhauer as Educator*, Nietzsche criticizes institutions of higher learning and the scholars who are responsible for educating the students attending these institutions. To these scholars and their methods, Nietzsche opposes Schopenhauer—or rather: his reading of Schopenhauer. Nietzsche's portrayal of his Schopenhauer experience exemplifies his thoughts on reading and writing, acts which should aim at liberating the reader by revealing him to himself. This is a feat which universities, he claims, cannot achieve, as they transmit knowledge in the shape of tables and charts, whereas Schopenhauer is one of those educators who reveal the core of one's self, that which cannot be educated nor shaped, that which is latent but accessible only with difficulty. Nietzsche concludes: "Your educators can be nothing else but your liberators."[24] This quote is important as it reveals what the concept of education means for the young Nietzsche: education is not the transmission of knowledge per se. It is the revelation and liberation of one's true self, as it were. Educators ought to make this emancipation possible. Education thus appears here as the process by which one becomes what one is.

Later in his life, Nietzsche will famously reject Schopenhauer and his philosophy; this rejection, however, does not lead him to recant the views on education that he expressed in this early text. One must remark that the young Nietzsche's relationship to Schopenhauer, as he describes it in *Schopenhauer as Educator*, does not seem to be coined by agonistics. He seems to blend with his educator, as the following passage reveals: "I understood him as if he had written for me."[25] Does Nietzsche just blindly accept and embrace whatever Schopenhauer wrote? A passage from *Ecce Homo* might provide an answer to this question. Here, Nietzsche discusses the limits of the knowledge which one can glean out of books, concluding: "In the final analysis, no one can get more out of things, including books, than one already knows."[26] Nietzsche's reading of Schopenhauer thus helped him formulate his own thoughts on education. If there is an agon in *Schopenhauer as Educator*, it is thus not that between Nietzsche and Schopenhauer but rather that between Nietzsche and the academic world. Nietzsche was shaped by institutions of higher learning and was now struggling to break free from them. He found in Schopenhauer, who had had his share of problems with the academic world, a kindred spirit whom he could recuperate for his attack on this academic world, which, Nietzsche contended, did not truly serve the education of humankind.

In *Schopenhauer as Educator*, Nietzsche addresses problems which he had already explored in his lectures *On the Future of Our Educational Institutions*, written 2 years earlier and which consist in an even more vehement attack on the academic world. It is necessary to discuss these lectures briefly, as they enable Nietzsche to present his own views not only on education but also on reading. Here, Nietzsche casts a damning light upon German institutions such as high schools and universities. He identifies two drives that are seemingly contradictory but which, however, merge or coalesce in the academic world, namely: "the drive toward a greater extension of education" and "the drive toward a lessening and weakening of it."[27] On the one hand, education is no longer the stronghold of a minority: the spreading of democratic ideals in nineteenth-century Germany is transforming its educational establishments. On the other hand, the democratization of education leads not only to a lowering of academic standards, according to Nietzsche, but also to a deplorable revaluation of the very function of education and higher learning: "Every education is hated, which isolates, which sets goals beyond money and gain, which requires time."[28] These institutions, Nietzsche adds, prepare their students for the world, that is, for the world *as it is*: they transmit a consensual knowledge, loading onto the backs of their pupils and students—as if they were camels, Zarathustra might say—the safe weight of tradition. It is quite clear why the education system is controlled by the state, Nietzsche claims, and why the state offers such an education in its institutions: in order to instill in students values that not only do not threaten the state, but that actually reinforce its hold on them.[29] Nietzsche thus envisions a time when it might become necessary, for the sake of education, to radically reform institutions of education, or even abolish them altogether,[30] in order to offer a completely different kind of education, namely, one that would turn these human beings into what he defines here as truly practical human beings, "who have good and new ideas and who know that true genius and true practice must necessarily converge in one individual."[31]

Against the backdrop of Nietzsche's critique of German institutions of education, it is enlightening to analyze his preface to these lectures, a preface titled "Preface to be read before the lectures, even though it does not really relate to them." Contrary to Nietzsche's suggestion, this preface has much to do with his subsequent critique of the academic world: Nietzsche depicts his ideal reader in opposition to the pupil and student of German institutions of education. In this preface, Nietzsche describes the three features which characterize his ideal reader, or, as he writes, *the reader from whom he expects something*: "He must be calm and read without haste, he must not always bring everything back to himself and his 'education,' finally he must not expect results and tables as conclusion."[32] Nietzsche then unpacks this list of features, and one can readily see that his ideal reader is *untimely*. He is untimely first and foremost because, being a calm and slow reader, he goes against the grain of his times by making a different use of his time: "This book is intended for calm readers, for people who have not yet been seized by the dizzying haste of our fast-paced epoch."[33] A slow pace enables the untimely reader to reflect upon that which he reads: "Such a man has not yet unlearned to reflect while he reads, he can still read the secret between the lines, he is so wasteful that he still reflects about what he has read, long maybe after putting down a book."[34] Secondly, this reader is untimely because he has not been corrupted by modern educational and cultural tenets: as previously mentioned, the reader must keep texts at a critical distance but he must also keep his world at a distance when reading. This reader does not believe that his *Bildung* is the measure of all things, as Nietzsche writes: "We rather hope that he is educated enough to think little of his education, to even despise it."[35] Thirdly, the Nietzsche reader is untimely, because he does not expect knowledge to be fed to him, he does not want to learn by heart but is rather eager to reflect critically and creatively upon what he reads. The timely product of German institutions of education bends under the weight of tradition; Nietzsche's untimely reader, in contrast, will stand up to it, (re) evaluating it, challenging it, supplementing it, renewing it.

On the Future of our Educational Institutions is thus a key text in Nietzsche's early attempts to formulate an ethics of reading coined by agonistics. From the introduction to the very end, Nietzsche suggests that his text is not about transmitting knowledge as educational institutions do, and that the act of reading his text will thus be a learning experience which radically differs from what one experiences in these institutions. As Deleuze stated in his essay *Pensée nomade*, Nietzsche's style enables him to decodify the world without recodifying it:[36] Nietzsche's reader is not given codes, he is given the space to decode Nietzsche's text on his own. Already in his introduction, Nietzsche announces that he will not provide the reader with a text that contains all the answers, as his whole pedagogical endeavor opposes the very sort of knowledge that fits nicely into tables and charts. Nietzsche writes that his readers will only understand him "when they immediately guess what can only be suggested, complete what had to be withheld, when they only need to be reminded, not taught."[37] Nietzsche thus admits that his text is fragmentary, that he left gaps purposefully, challenging the reader to meet him half way, to do half the work. Nietzsche is thus seeking to educate the reader, challenging him to wage a war against—and to emancipate himself from—textual claims and assertions, including his own.

The relationship between agonistics and education is also the subject of Nietzsche's early text *Homer's Contest*, in which Nietzsche celebrates a healthy agon as pedagogical strategy, a strategy that he then recuperates for his ethics of reading. Nietzsche investigates here a text by Hesiod in which the poet explains that there are two kinds of envy, each represented by a different goddess, and each called Eris. The one Eris, whom Hesiod describes as evil, instills an envy into men that leads them to enmity, to wars of annihilation, whereas the other Eris, the good one, instills an envy which encourages men "not to a war of annihilation, but rather to a *contest*."[38] Nietzsche explains that the Hellenic world was coined by competitiveness: "Every talent must unfold in a struggle, as suggested by Hellenic popular pedagogy."[39] Poets envied each other and thus wanted to outdo each other; so did philosophers, politicians, singers, carpenters, and beggars. They would greatly develop their skills in their desire to surpass one another—a competition which benefited the whole community. Nietzsche then reminds the reader of the former meaning of the term *ostracism*. The Ephesians once banned a member of their community, justifying this ostracism, according to Nietzsche, as follows: "No one should be the best amongst us; should one be the best, then he should be elsewhere, with other people."[40] Nietzsche explains that the Ephesians thus ensured that the contest would go on: should a contestant be overwhelmingly superior to all others, the contest would lose of its relevance. Lungstrum and Sauer remark regarding the contest: "It is in the nature of the agon neither to render its participants mute nor to attain the conquering finality of *telos*."[41] The fight must go on, it must never end, as it is only in the agonistic movement itself that learning, surpassing, and overcoming oneself is possible. The Hellenic state needed such ongoing contests, which, as stimulant, promoted development and excellence among its citizens, in order to thrive and flourish. Ostracism was thus a way to eliminate all-too powerful individuals who could, because of their superior qualities and talents, ultimately become a threat to the state, as their superiority would bring the contest to a standstill. Nietzsche thus explains: "That is the core of the Hellenic understanding of the contest: it loathes the autocratic rule and fears its dangers, it demands, as *protective measure* against a genius – a second genius."[42] The Hellenic contest, as Nietzsche interprets it here, is thus a pedagogical strategy ensuring the health of the whole community.

This early text which celebrates a healthy agon as pedagogical strategy must be taken into consideration when one interprets, for instance, the martial metaphors which abound in Nietzsche's work: Nietzsche does not promote wars of annihilation, but rather agonal education. He proclaims his admiration for this pedagogical strategy of the ancients, who put their pupils' envy to good use, whereas modern educators "fear, above all, the unleashing of what they call ambition."[43] These modern educators, who dread the unbridling of envy in their pupils, stem from the Judeo-Christian tradition, in which envy is a deadly sin. Hellenic educators, in contrast, redeem envy, as it were, by stimulating it for what Nietzsche might call noble purposes, that is: for educational purposes. Pupils who are envious of their gifted peers feel challenged by these and work all the harder, hoping to surpass them, thus developing their own skills and talents. For the reader of *Homer's Contest*, a chapter such as "On War and Warriors" in *Thus Spoke Zarathustra* provides examples of passages in Nietzsche's work which have an undeniable martial tone, but which really promote agonal education:

> By our best enemies, we do not want to be spared. . . . My brothers in war! I love you deeply; I am and was your equal. And I am also your best fiend. . . . I know your heart's hatred and envy. You are not great enough not to know hatred and envy. Be great enough, then, not to be ashamed of them! . . . I see many soldiers: I wish to see many warriors! 'Uniform' we call what they wear: may it not be uniform, what they hide under it! . . . You must be proud of your enemy: because your enemy's successes are your own.[44]

In *Homer's Contest*, when Nietzsche praises agonal education, he observes that, were one to remove the contest from the Hellenic world, what would remain would be the abyss "of a gruesome fierceness of hatred and lust for annihilation," as envy would then be channeled into wars of annihilation. In the sentences quoted above from *Thus Spoke Zarathustra*, Nietzsche promotes enmity between equals as a healthy challenge, suggesting that we (Christians) reconcile with envy and use it not only to better ourselves but also to emancipate ourselves, breaking free from uniforms and uniformity by means of the contest. As in *Homer's Contest*, the enemy here is to be admired as he reveals our own measure and as the sum of successes arising from the contest ensures the vitality of the whole community.

As writer and philosopher, Nietzsche will never cease to criticize texts or methods that, according to him, seek to foreclose the possibility of a contest, such as those of Socrates and Plato, for instance. Nietzsche criticizes Socrates as educator, because the latter seeks to impose his own views onto others instead of *liberating* them—which is, in Nietzsche's view, the task of a true educator, as quoted earlier. Socrates explains, both in *Phaedrus* and in *The Republic* that the educator's task is to give a new direction to the soul, by turning the pupil's gaze toward the light, to *enlighten* the pupil, literally. In the parable of the cave, as the enlightenment process of the prisoner who ascends toward the light is described, one cannot help but notice the plethora of terms which betray the educator's controlling attitude. About the prisoners of the cave, Socrates explains: "When one of them was freed and suddenly compelled to stand up, turn his head, walk, and look up toward the light, he'd be pained and dazzled and unable to see the things whose shadows he'd seen before."[45] Socrates goes on to describe the prisoner's enlightenment process using terms and phrases such as "if we . . . compelled him to answer," "if someone compelled him to look at the light itself," "if someone dragged him away from there by force, up the rough, steep path, and didn't let him go until he had dragged him into the sunlight," among others.[46] The educator is removing the pupil from "a sort of barbaric bog"[47] in order to enlighten him; he does so, however, by "compelling" the pupil to follow him by "dragging" him along—terms that remind one of cavemen, if anything, not of educators. In *Phaedrus*, Socrates describes the oratory art, which he practices as educator as a way to "direct the soul."[48] Nietzsche will thus condemn Socratic pedagogical methods, dismissing dialectics as the expression of a will to power, which does not truly seek to educate and emancipate: "One chooses dialectics only when one has no other means."[49] Only he who cannot assert himself by means of force, money, or any other power makes use of this method, which enables him to rule over others. Nietzsche does recognize the fact that Socratic dialectics is a kind of contest between two interlocutors[50] but this strictly logical method which Socrates masters as no one else and which negates all other kinds of knowledge ultimately fails to educate: "The dialectician *disempowers* the intellect of his opponent."[51] As Acampora puts it: "Nietzsche thinks Socrates' contestants do not have even a remote chance to win."[52] And indeed: a dialogue with Socrates typically ends with a resigned nod and admission, by his interlocutor, that Socrates was absolutely right. The Socratic method is thus, in Nietzsche's view, the opposite of a healthy agon, which calls for enmity between equals, if true education is to take place, if the contest is to go on.

Similarly, Nietzsche will criticize Kantian philosophy, in particular the categorical imperative, which disempowers the individual, in his view. It is the practicality of this absolute practical law, which Nietzsche questions. In *Human, All Too Human*, for instance, Nietzsche criticizes the idealism of Kant's position. The following is a long quote but is worth quoting at length, as it reveals what it is, exactly, that Nietzsche considers to be harmful in Kantian philosophy:

The older moral, namely that of Kant, wants from the individual actions which one would want from all human beings: that was a beautiful, naive idea: as if everybody readily knew which actions would benefit the whole of humankind, and thus which actions would be desirable at all; it is a theory like that of free trade, which assumes that universal harmony would necessarily unfold on its own, according to innate laws of improvement. Maybe a future perspective on the needs of humanity will show that it is not desirable at all that all human beings act in the same way, but rather that in the interest of ecumenical goals, special tasks, maybe even evil tasks, under certain circumstances, will be required of whole stretches of humankind.[53]

Nietzsche insists here upon the fact that it is impossible to know whether one's actions are propitious for the whole species or not, claiming that categories such as good and bad, or good and evil, are neither eternally stable nor universally valid. Beyond this, however, it is the practicality of Kant's categorical imperative which Nietzsche questions here, suggesting that one would certainly feel disempowered by such an imperative, which endows every decision with so much meaning, with so much weight, that decisions become impossible to make. Nietzsche vehemently rejects the claim to truth and universality on which the categorical imperative is based, writing in *The Antichrist*:

> A virtue must be *our* invention, *our* most personal self-defence and need: otherwise it is only a danger. That which does not serve our life *harms* it: a virtue solely out of respect for the concept of 'virtue,' as Kant wanted it, is harmful. 'Virtue,' 'duty,' 'the good-in-itself,' the good that is impersonal and universally valid – fantasies which reveal decline, the last weakening of life, and the Chinese spirit of Königsberg.[54]

Nietzsche cannot believe that life could ever be made fruitful by obeying a law which leaves little to no room for self-assertion, originality, invention, desire, passion, etc. After this passage, a seemingly bewildered Nietzsche exclaims: "That one has not felt that Kant's categorical imperative is a *mortal danger*!"[55] Elsewhere, he will go as far as claiming that Kant's categorical imperative "smells of cruelty:"[56] in Nietzsche's view, it reeks of the cruel scent of Christian asceticism and self-mortification as it demands, just as Judeo-Christian commandments do, that one blindly obeys a moral law which reason cannot grasp, repressing or denying parts of oneself in doing so. Nietzsche will thus consider Kant to be an underhanded Christian:[57] his categorical imperative being an offspring of Judeo-Christian commandments, it undermines Kant's narrative of enlightenment and emancipation in both form and content. It is fairly evident that Nietzsche's harsh criticism of Kant—and of Socrates—does not do justice to the works of these two philosophical giants and is not devoid of contradictions: Nietzsche's critique is rather meant to serve a specific function, namely, to educate the reader with and against (these) texts and (their) assertions, claims to universal truths and imperatives.

Nowhere in his work, however, does Nietzsche formulate the commandment or imperative *thou shalt not read* but he does make the reader aware of the uses and abuses of reading, often giving philologists as examples. Philological methods—reading slowly, carefully, and closely—can only appeal to a philosopher who is so preoccupied with language. Philologists are, however, guilty of an all-too intense reading activity as well as of taking themselves and their discipline all-too seriously: they are among the "most educated and conceited of all scholars."[58] There is no doubt that Nietzsche holds philology and a philological approach to reading in high regard. He describes philology as "the art of reading well—to be able to read facts *without* falsifying them through interpretation, *without* losing, in the desire to understand, caution, patience, subtlety."[59] He claims that "science has only acquired continuity and steadiness when the art of reading well, i.e. *philology*, arose."[60] Philologists, just as scientists and scholars, run the risk, however, of falling prey to these virtues of circumspection and patience, of seeing their task as an end, not a means. This is typical, Nietzsche claims, of (German) scholars, who think more "about science than about humanity"[61] and indeed, Nietzsche often portrays them as beings who have lost touch with humanity or humaneness. As educator, for instance, the philologist "teaches grinding"[62]—in German, Nietzsche uses the term *ochsen*, a term which reminds one of cattle (*Ochs*, or *Ox* in English) rather than of humans. A famous fellow philologist is said to be endued "with the venerable assurance of a worm dried up between books."[63] Philologists have a tendency to become obsessed with their work, Nietzsche writes, sometimes *handling* 200 books per day: "I have seen this with my own eyes: gifted, rich and liberal natures ruined by reading as early as in their thirties."[64] Nietzsche's portrayal of philologists suggests that there are limits to the knowledge one can glean from books: the most knowledgeable scholar may turn out to be a very unwise human being. Nietzsche's warning when it comes to books might read: *handle with care*, a warning that captures both the promise and the threat enclosed in every book.

When Nietzsche writes, in the quote above, that he has seen *with his own eyes* the terrible effects which reading had on certain young scholars, he hints at his own reading experience: in *Ecce Homo*, he will explain that he experienced pain *with his own eyes*, quite literally, as his own eyes were almost completely ruined by reading. *Ecce Homo*, more than any other text, I would argue, reveals the relationship in Nietzsche's thought between reading, agonistics, and health. In this text, he reveals how unhealthy his relationship to reading used to be, going as far as claiming: "My eyes alone put an end to my bookworm habits, in German: philology: I was freed from the 'book,' for years I did not read a thing – the *greatest* favour which I ever did myself!"[65] He seems to construct a relationship of cause and effect here (even though he warns the reader against such constructions[66]): the nearly complete loss of his eyesight is depicted as an eye-opening experience. This experience, according to him, led him to revaluate the value of philology and reading and to disavow his decision to study philology, calling it a mistake, an instinctual aberration, wondering why he became a philologist at all, "why not a doctor at least or something else which would have opened eyes?"[67] Reading, by directing the reader's gaze to the page, blocks everything else from his view, making him lose sight of what is going on around him. In this context, the following statement from *The Case of Wagner* might take on a new significance: "What is typical of all *literary* decadence? That life no longer dwells in the whole."[68] Literary decadence could thus also be that of the reader blinded by books, the reader who only lives through his eyes, the reader who has become one big eye. Such a reader would be, for Zarathustra, "an inverse cripple . . ., who has too little of everything and too much of one thing."[69] By enabling him to look at reading from a different perspective, or so he claims, Nietzsche's poor eyesight radically transformed his approach to books. Whereas he claims, in *Ecce Homo*, that his condition allowed him to break free from the yoke of the book, he then writes that reading has now become his main recreational activity—a statement that comes as quite a surprise in view of his harsh critique of reading. It is then most certainly his *attitude* toward reading, which has changed. Reading is something that he no longer takes seriously, he writes.[70] Whereas the act of reading was interpreted as a sign of decadence, it is now the curative properties of reading, which now come to the fore: "Reading is my recreation from *my* seriousness."[71] It is thus clearly a certain usage of books, and not reading books *per se*, that Nietzsche condemns. He writes as much when he claims that books are absent from his surroundings when he writes, and that a reading room makes him feel ill.[72] It is of utmost importance to discriminate when it comes to books: first, one must discriminate with regard to what one reads. As Nietzsche prides himself on being untimely, his attitude toward new books will not come as a surprise: he writes that, instinctively, he has always felt a certain "enmity against new books."[73] One must also discriminate in another regard: there is a time to read and a time to leave books behind. Nietzsche thus writes: "To read a *book* early in the morning, at daybreak, when one is fresh, in the dawn of one's strength – I call that depraved!"[74] A healthy reader who wishes to foster his vitality must know how, what, and when (not) to read.

To conclude, I would like to propose an interpretation of the title *Ecce Homo*: could it not be read as a statement by means of which Nietzsche yet again warns the reader against himself? It is a biblical reference, but tellingly, these are words spoken neither by the believers in Christ nor by the Jews who asked for him to be crucified. They are the words of Pontius Pilate, of whom Nietzsche writes in *The Antichrist* that he "has enriched the New Testament with the only word *which has value*,—which is its critique, its *annihilation*: 'what is truth!' . . ."[75] It is thus fitting that Nietzsche, who relentlessly attacks believers, would title his autobiographical text *Ecce Homo*, thus quoting the one character of the New Testament depicted as a skeptic. By quoting Pilate, who exclaimed *what is truth!*, a phrase which subversively undermines the Bible from within, Nietzsche undermines the claims to truth which his own text could suggest. As for the expression "ecce homo," Pilate pronounces it as he presents Christ to the crowd asking for his life. He famously washes his hands of Jesus, leaving the crowd the responsibility to sentence him. By calling a text in which he portrays himself *Ecce Homo*, words uttered by Pilate, Nietzsche thus, first, calls the truth of his text into question, and, second, indicates that his fate as a writer is in the hands of his readers. Confronted to what some may designate as the *unreadability* of the Nietzschean text, the reader has the *textual response-ability* not only *to supplement* it but also *to supplant* it.

Was Nietzsche trying, as Hutter argues, "to initiate a new authoritative tradition in which books had to carry readers beyond all books?"[76] It is tempting to claim so, but I would argue that Nietzsche wanted to carry his readers beyond *his* books. To carry readers beyond *all* books would put an end to the agon, keeping readers from striving for what Nietzsche calls *the great health*, which is a health which "one does not merely have, but rather which one wins and must constantly win, because one always gives it up and must always give it up . . ."[77] Nietzsche's reader must engage with what is out there, he is not to remain (too long) in his cave, on the mountain, dwelling on lonely heights, constructing narratives *ex nihilo*, without confronting his thoughts with the thoughts of others. He must descend, as Zarathustra does, and this descent will be, as Lampert explains it, "a descent to the things of the earth that gives them weight and importance again."[78] With this descent, the movement between transmission, deconstruction, and creation is given a new impetus. Nietzsche arms the reader with the very weapons needed to carry out this task, taking the reader beyond *Nietzsche*'s books—not for the agon to end but for the agon to resume on other, newer grounds, as Nietzsche suggests in his lectures on education:

Be at least readers of this book in order to annihilate and forget it later through your deed! Think of it as being meant to be your herald: when you, in your own armor, appear on the fighting ground, who will want to turn around and look at the herald which called you?[79]

Notes and references

1 Pettey indicates that the first recognizable narratorial passage in Nietzsche's notes written in preparation for what would become *Thus Spoke Zarathustra* is a narrative that sets the stage for this very chapter. See John Carson Pettey, *Nietzsche's Philosophical and Narrative Styles* (N.Y.: Lang, 1992), p. 65.

2 Z: I "On the Thousand Goals and One" (KSA 4, p. 75). I have worked exclusively with the German text. Translations are my own.

3 Keith Ansell Pearson, *An Introduction to Nietzsche as Political Thinker* (Cambridge: Cambridge University Press, 1994), p. 205.

4 J. Hillis Miller, *The Ethics of Reading: Kant, de Man, Eliot, Trollope, James and Benjamin* (NY: Columbia University Press, 1987), p. 4.

5 Éva Antal, "The Ethics of Reading – a Postmodern Theory?," *Pedagogy Studies (Pedagogika)* 71 (2004): 16.

6 See Paul de Man, *Allegories of Reading. Figural Language in Rousseau, Nietzsche, Rilke, and Proust* (New Haven, London: Yale University Press, 1979) and Jacques Derrida, *Éperons. Les Styles de Nietzsche* (Paris : Flammarion, 1978).
7 Alan D. Schrift, *Nietzsche and the Question of Interpretation. Between Hermeneutics and Deconstruction* (NY, London: Routledge, 1990), p. 193.
8 Horst Hutter, *Shaping the Future. Nietzsche's New Regime of the Soul and Its Ascetic Practices* (Lanham: Lexington Books, 2006), p. xiii.
9 Timothy F. Murphy, *Nietzsche as Educator* (Lanham, NY, London : University Press of America, 1984), p. 4.
10 Ibid., p. 48.
11 Keith Ansell Pearson, *How to Read Nietzsche* (London: Granta Books, 2005), p. 115.
12 TL 1 (KSA 1, p. 882).
13 TL 2 (KSA 1, p. 887).
14 TL 1 (KSA 1, p. 879).
15 TL 1 (KSA 1, p. 880f).
16 Philippe Lacoue-Labarthe, "Le détour (Nietzsche et la rhétorique)," *Poétique* 5 (1971): 64. This is my translation of the French text.
17 Ibid., 57.
18 TI "Ancients" 2 (KSA 6, p. 156).
19 HH 178 (KSA 2, p. 161f).
20 Jill Marsden, "Nietzsche and the Art of the Aphorism," in K. Ansell Pearson (ed.), *A Companion to Nietzsche* (Oxford: Blackwell Publishing, 2006), p. 24.
21 Z: I "On Reading and Writing" (KSA 4, p. 48).
22 KSA 8:20 [3].
23 TI "Ancients" 2 (KSA 6, p. 156).
24 SE 1 (KSA 1, p. 341).
25 SE 2 (KSA 1, p. 346).
26 EH "Books" 1 (KSA 6, p. 299f).
27 FEI "Introduction" (KSA 1, p. 647).
28 FEI I (KSA 1, p. 668).
29 FEI III (KSA 1, p. 710).
30 FEI "Preface" (KSA 1, p. 649).
31 FEI II (KSA 1, p. 673).
32 FEI "Preface" (KSA 1, p. 648).
33 FEI "Preface" (KSA 1, p. 649).
34 Ibid.
35 FEI "Preface" (KSA 1, p. 650).
36 Gilles Deleuze, "Pensée nomade," *Nietzsche aujourd'hui? Tome 1* (Paris: UGE 10/18, 1973), p. 165.
37 FEI "Introduction" (KSA 1, p. 644).
38 HC (KSA 1, p. 787).
39 HC (KSA 1, p. 789).
40 HC (KSA 1, p. 788).
41 Janet Lungstrum and Elizabeth Sauer, "Creative Agonistics: An Introduction," in J. Lungstrum and E. Sauer eds, *Agonistics: Arenas of Creative Contest* (Albany, NY: State University of New York Press, 1997), p. 25.
42 HC (KSA 1, p. 789).
43 Ibid.
44 Z: I "On War and Warriors" (KSA 4, p. 58f).

45 Plato, "The Republic," in J. M. Cooper (ed.), *Complete Works*, trans. G. M. A. Grube, and C. D. C. Reeve (Indianapolis/Cambridge : Hackett, 1997), p. 1133.
46 Ibid., 1133.
47 Ibid., 1149.
48 Plato, "Phaedrus," in J. M. Cooper (ed.), *Complete Works*, trans. A. Nehamas, and P. Woodruff (Indianapolis/Cambridge : Hackett, 1997), p. 548.
49 TI: "Socrates" 6 (KSA 6, p. 70).
50 TI: "Skirmishes" 23 (KSA 6, p. 126).
51 TI: "Socrates" 7 (KSA 6, p. 70).
52 Christa Davis Acampora, "Nietzsche's Agonal Wisdom," *International Studies in Philosophy* 35, 3 (2003): 173.
53 HH 25 (KSA 2, p. 46).
54 A 11 (KSA 6, p. 177).
55 Ibid.
56 GM II 6 (KSA 5, p. 300).
57 TI: "Reason" 6 (KSA 6, p. 79).
58 BGE 204 (KSA 5, p. 130).
59 A 52 (KSA 6, p. 233).
60 HH 270 (KSA 2, p. 223).
61 SE 2 (KSA 1, p. 344).
62 TI "Skirmishes" 29 (KSA 6, p. 129).
63 TI "Ancients" 4 (KSA 6, p. 158).
64 EH "Clever" 8 (KSA 6, p. 293).
65 EH "HH" 4 (KSA 6, p. 326).
66 TI "Errors" 1 (KSA 6, p. 88).
67 EH "Clever" 2 (KSA 6, p. 283).
68 CW 7 (KSA 6, p. 27).
69 Z II: "On Redemption" (KSA 4, p. 178).
70 EH "Clever" 3 (KSA 6, p. 284).
71 Ibid.
72 Ibid.
73 EH "Clever" 3 (KSA 6, p. 285). It is also quite fitting that the only journal which he claims to read on a regular basis is called *Journal des Débats*, the very title of which captures the spirit of agonal writing and reading. See EH "Books" 1 (KSA 6, p. 301).
74 EH "Clever" 8 (KSA 6, p. 293).
75 A 46 (KSA 6, p. 225).
76 Hutter, 6.
77 EH "Z" 2 (KSA 6, p. 338).
78 Laurence Lampert, *Nietzsche's Teaching. An Interpretation of 'Thus Spoke Zarathustra'* (New Haven, London: Yale University Press, 1986), p. 10.
79 FEI "Preface" (KSA 1, p. 650).

Works cited

Primary literature

Nietzsche, Friedrich. *KSA*. Eds. G. Colli and M. Montinari. München: DTV, 1999.
Plato. *Complete Works*. Ed. J. M. Cooper. Indianapolis/Cambridge: Hackett, 1997.

Secondary literature

Acampora, Christa Davis. "Nietzsche's Agonal Wisdom." *International Studies in Philosophy* 35(3), (2003): 163–82.

Ansell Pearson, Keith. *An Introduction to Nietzsche as Political Thinker*. Cambridge: Cambridge University Press, 1994.

—. *How to Read Nietzsche*. London: Granta Books, 2005.

Antal, Éva. "The Ethics of Reading – a Postmodern Theory?" *Pedagogy Studies (Pedagogika)* 71 (2004): 12–17.

Carson Pettey, John. *Nietzsche's Philosophical and Narrative Styles*. NY: Lang, 1992.

Deleuze, Gilles. "Pensée nomade." *Nietzsche aujourd'hui? Tome 1*. Paris: UGE 10/18, 1973. 159–74.

de Man, Paul. *Allegories of Reading. Figural Language in Rousseau, Nietzsche, Rilke, and Proust*. New Haven, London: Yale University Press, 1979.

Derrida, Jacques. *Éperons. Les Styles de Nietzsche*. Paris: Flammarion, 1978.

Hillis Miller, J. *The Ethics of Reading: Kant, de Man, Eliot, Trollope, James and Benjamin*. NY: Columbia University Press, 1987.

Hutter, Horst. *Shaping the Future. Nietzsche's New Regime of the Soul and Its Ascetic Practices*. Lanham: Lexington Books, 2006.

Lacoue-Labarthe, Philippe. "Le détour (Nietzsche et la rhétorique)." *Poétique* 5(1971): 53–76.

Lampert, Laurence. *Nietzsche's Teaching. An Interpretation of "Thus Spoke Zarathustra."* New Haven, London: Yale University Press, 1986.

Lungstrum, Janet and Elizabeth Sauer. "Creative Agonistics: An Introduction." *Agonistics: Arenas of Creative Contest*. Eds. J. Lungstrum and E. Sauer. Albany, NY: State University of New York Press, 1997, 1–32.

Marsden, Jill. "Nietzsche and the Art of the Aphorism." *A Companion to Nietzsche*. Ed. K. Ansell Pearson. Oxford: Blackwell Publishing, 2006, 22–37.

Murphy, Timothy F. *Nietzsche as Educator*. Lanham, NY, London: University Press of America, 1984.

Schrift, Alan D. *Nietzsche and the Question of Interpretation. Between Hermeneutics and Deconstruction*. NY, London: Routledge, 1990.

5

"Who Educates the Educators?" Nietzsche's Philosophical Therapy in the Age of Nihilism

José Daniel Parra

Introduction

Nietzsche's philosophy seeks to shape the future.[1] It is a way of confronting the nihilistic historical impulse in contemporary Western culture, resulting from the desacralization of Judeo-Christian metaphysics at the hands of its progeny, modern science. It is "post-Abrahamic" for it encompasses a critique of monotheism in its different manifestations, presenting the notion of "eternal recurrence" as a form of overcoming the "spirit of revenge." It is also a rejection of Hegel's notion of the end of history as a final dialectical synthesis where Spirit has come to complete self-consciousness and man has reconciled himself with the rational, modern-state, in the best of possible worlds. On the contrary, Nietzsche claims the Hegelian end of history leads to cultural decadence which he depicts with the image of the "last man." Nietzsche envisions a physicianship of culture that would procure the approximation of philosophical insight and political *praxis* by reshaping Platonic *paideia*.

Nietzsche attempts to induce modern *libre penseurs* to be skeptical of their skepticism.[2] Nietzsche's teaching is an enticement to self-examination, personal development, and spiritual self-overcoming. It is addressed to "free spirits"—"good Europeans" with the "will to free will"[3] to shape and cultivate themselves, to form a new nobility that leads a life of experimentation, compassion, and care for the world that makes our existence possible. Nietzsche is not a philosopher of history because history is not over—rather, Nietzsche attempts to propose a historical prelude to a philosophy of the future. It is the task of free spirits to understand their historical condition and begin to give shape and substance to a world that, as yet, has no name.[4]

Beyond Platonism

Nietzsche's *Beyond Good and Evil* is a deconstructive, "No-saying, No-doing" work[5] that deals with the nearest, the "timely." It is a polemic, a fishhook meant to entice and challenge modern readers, skeptics suffering from "the most spiritual expression of a certain complex physiological condition that in ordinary language is called nervous exhaustion and sickliness."[6] This is a result of the overwhelming success of Platonism (i.e., the doctrinal, nonironic interpretation of Plato's writings) in our spiritual history, becoming a popular prejudice through Christian doctrine.[7] Platonism is a sophistic belief in a dualistic conception of reality. Nietzsche's observation is that this cultural dichotomy has been in-bred into human beings in Western culture, providing them with a spiritual line of self-development (a what for, a purpose) at the expense of the "real." Furthermore, not only Christianity but also Judaism and Islam, the two other Abrahamic monotheistic faiths can be conceived as theological manifestations of Platonism for the people.[8] Their two-world distinction, Nietzsche claims, has been crafted and sociologically in-bred for the sake of consolation and political control of "masses" of human beings, making sense of their experience of injustice as results of Providential will that promises to provide atonement and retribution in the Messianic future or in the eschatological beyond.[9]

For Nietzsche the Judeo-Christian will to truth—or the ascetic cultivation of the virtue of honesty on the basis of this version of monotheistic cosmology— is the precursor of Western modern science. The practice of modern science has, in turn, undermined the very foundations of its own ontological source. This means, to use the dramatic expression of the Madman (*der tolle Mensch*) in *The Gay Science* that "God is dead. God remains dead. And we have killed him."[10] Now, if Platonism were refuted, we seem to be left with a degraded merely "mundane" reality that would not provide a source of meaning for men and women conceiving their distinct "human dignity" as derived from what is beyond the physical. To an enormous extent, Western culture has been shaped by the notion of individual responsibility as a consequence of our (metaphysical) free will. Particularly on the Augustinian version of free will, conceived as an emanation of the will of God in the human agent, which provides the metaphysical foundation for moral action among persons on the basis of a third, transcendent, and ultimate source.[11] Moral action (and the avoidance of the cycle of vengeance) under these conditions follows from intrinsic habituated moral virtue reinforced by the fear of punishment or retribution and desire for "eternal life" after we "pass away." But if metaphysics were untenable, then "becoming" would be sovereign, all concepts would be fluid—there would be no cardinal difference between man and animal. The immediate reaction following this line of logic leads, Nietzsche observes, to frustration and despair: nihilism.

For Nietzsche, this is an outcome of a misconceived (dualistic) vision of the nature of things, an untruth that was, however, the constitutive sphere of our human horizon for millennia, but which as a result of the triumph of modern empirical science seems to no longer be believable. Western culture stands at crossroads between the overcoming of an overripe tradition and the sowing of a new horizon.[12] In the words of Keith Ansell-Pearson: "But how is Christianity to be overcome? Nietzsche's argument is that Christianity and morality, like all great things, *overcome themselves*."[13] Nietzsche's affirmation attempts to repatriate the sacred back into the world, to embrace life as both eternally given and yet always masked to our awareness,[14] concealing and revealing within itself the future that will become the past (and vice versa?) by means of us in the present moment.

Nietzsche's teaching in *Beyond Good and Evil* is addressed to specific men and women who may have the insight and the endurance, to attempt to understand and experience the "nature of things" as will to power by means of self-examination. This, he tells us, is very dangerous: "in the end it must be as it is and always has been: great things remain for the great, abysses for the profound, nuances and shudders for the refined, all that is rare for the rare.—".[15] Nietzsche's task is to elicit new, genuine spiritual directions, a "new heart" that may justify human action in times of cultural anxiety and confusion.[16]

Askesis: Toward a morality for free spirits

A Nietzschean understanding of *askesis* (self-shaping as spiritual exercises[17]) implies a constant process of self-examination. It is an exercise of discipline following a particular line of willing to enact a chosen outcome. It is a spiritual "tyranny" over oneself substantiated by the joyous willingness to cultivate one's strength, seeking to experience the freedom of mastery. Moral codes, by the same token but on a large scale, are limitations set upon peoples in order to make possible for individuals to relate meaningfully with one another, to have the conditions for a shared communal life, to shape and limit the one-dimensional *laisser-aller* that would lead to anomie and social disarray.

Nietzsche elucidates the significance of moral codes making a parallel with syntactic norms. As he puts it one "just [has to] think of the coercion every language has employed up till now in achieving its strength and freedom—the coercion of metre, the tyranny of rhyme and rhythm."[18] Language is an artifice. So are orthography, calligraphy, semantics, syntax. However, these are constrains that also provide parameters without which no meaningful self-expression or communication would be possible—including the critique of the medium. The same allusion is pertinent, according to Nietzsche, to all human action. Anarchic *laisser-aller* in reality is unfreedom, for it curtails the "subtlety, daring, dance, and perfect sureness, whether it be in ideas, or in governance, or in oratory and rhetoric, in the arts as well as in manners," that follows from the willingness to achieve excellence in a given activity or endeavor.

Nietzsche, however, criticizes Kant's morality of the categorical imperative for positing morality as normatively given. Nietzsche understands the fundamental role of morality for the sake of human preservation and self-overcoming, but he is cautious not to take it for granted. It is something that has to be carefully inculcated through character-formation particularly in early education. For Nietzsche, every morality is a piece of "tyranny" against "nature," but also against "reason"; however, such tyranny is both natural and reasonable in the case of the human species given its spiritual and creative condition, and the high degree of *disciplinae voluntatis* it requires to unfold.[19] As the new unidirectional line of obedience, Nietzsche puts forward a noncategorical imperative, "thou shalt obey, obey somebody, and for a long time: *or else* you will perish and lose your last remnant of self-respect."[20] Nietzsche is addressing the "free spirits" as guardians of culture to be aware of the responsibility the species, "the whole animal human" has to be the guarantor of the continuation of life, together with the planet that, as far as we know, makes its appearance and manifestation possible.

Christian morality, according to Nietzsche, has bred the European spirit to be "strong, ruthlessly curious, and beautifully nimble"[21] and in that sense, he is thankful for the possibility of self-enhancement this sacred line of willing has provided humankind. However, at our historical juncture, Nietzsche proposes to embrace a different train of obedience, one that involves a consciously created morality based on "epistemic" knowledge of nature and compassion. Knowledge of nature is essential for the exploration of what constitutes the realm of "natural kinds," and therefore what can be created through "social kinds" grounded in but not determined by natural possibility. Compassion, according to Nietzsche, seems to be distinct from pity which he likens to passive-aggressive revenge.[22] Nietzsche finds pity undesirable, softly cruel, ignoble.[23] For Nietzsche, there is a fundamental distinction between the pity of the utilitarians that seeks to do away with suffering as the panacea to solve the problem of human alienation, and the compassion of the noble mind, which has respect for the contours of human emotion, and acknowledges the spiritual potential of "intentional suffering" as a delicate venue for soul-craft and self-overcoming.

One thing is clear: Nietzsche is not romanticizing destitution, or the spectacle of the "perennially depraved and downtrodden who lie around us everywhere." He puts forward an understanding of compassion that sees pleasure and pain as some of many emotional consequences, side effects, of more fundamental, more profound states of mind.[24] He embraces the "deep suffering that makes us noble [that] . . . separates,"[25] as an experience of human self-creation from a soul undergoing the "coexistence of clearmindedness and intoxication," following an informed awareness of the spectacle of what is. Nietzsche's "accursed *ipssisimosity*" involves an acknowledgment of the profundity of the suffering that fosters insight[26] (one of his four cardinal virtues), that makes possible the order of rank among human and nonhuman types, but which he fears may be lost due to man's conquering of nature, aiming at the abolition of suffering and beneficent kinds of inequality, which seems to have no assignable limits in contemporary Western culture. And yet suffering and inequality well understood—the *pathos of distance*—are the fundamental prerequisites for the self-overcoming of man.[27] Nietzsche's morality of the noble reenacts an order of rank along the lines of Aeschylian "learning through suffering." A shared human feeling or *pathos* can be explained or communicated on the basis of common experience. Now, when it comes to experiences that are not widely shared, or that are especially demanding or perhaps unique, communication becomes less commonsensical, potentially leading to meditative silence only broken by compassionate pedagogical communication: "whoever is a teacher through and through takes all things seriously only in relation to his students—even himself.[28]

Pathos is what men (and all other sentient beings) have emotionally in common—therefore, *pathos of distance* suggests a *quantitative*, not a qualitative distinction. Though its manifestations and intensities may vary, it points to a passive experience, not an action: *pathos* is something by which we are struck fatefully, like madness, anger, fear, rejection, or love.[29] The notion of *sympathy*, for instance, entails an understanding that a feeling of another is also part of what I have or may undergo, thus an identification of *self* with *other* becomes possible at an instinctive level, so to speak. Meaningful communication, as well as sound political deliberation depends on shared experiences.

Recall Machiavelli's claim that there are two fundamental human types—characterized by distinct *humors* that urge a few to rule, and that make the majority desire not to be ruled.[30] Is communication possible between these two distinct "natural" factions? Machiavelli's observation seems to reflect Nietzsche's dichotomy between master and slave moralities, though, as Nietzsche puts it, both human kinds are animated by the same will to power with varying strengths, repressions, and intensities.

Now, in modern democratic times:

> There [still] are master morality and slave morality—I add immediately that in all the higher and more mixed cultures there also appear attempts at mediation between these two moralities, and yet more often the interpenetration and mutual misunderstanding of both, and at times they occur directly alongside each other—even in the same human beings, within a *single* soul.[31]

Nietzschean compassion sees the importance of the suffering "that has created all human greatness to date,"[32] as a spiritual work on oneself, a delicate act of "self-remembering" from unconscious tension, reaction, and emotional association to ever subtler forms of attention. He is definitely not exhorting flagellation. Nietzsche disapproves of modern moralists who want to abolish suffering: he looks down on their pity as hypocritical *suffering with*, that instead of healing the malaise unconsciously reproduces misfortune in the observer.

Nietzsche wants to stimulate the creative unfolding of natural energy—testing how much insight into your inner forces you are able to endure while still retaining sway over your person. The Apollonian *principium individuationis* is challenged, tested, and recaptured, in a "dialectical dance" with Dionysian provocation.[33] This primordial understanding of fueling life opposes the tepid modern consensus on "compassion" so called, it is against the dissipation of pain into moderate pleasures, and as such, appears to be immoral.[34]

Sympathy is a virtue of the noble. The noble person is ready to give more than is owed. Nietzsche attempts to envision pain in a spiritual manner: the modern quest for the abolition of suffering entails not only a mistaken but a dangerous conception of "compassion" that could have the consequence of turning us all into predictable automata[35]. For the noble person *fitting tension* offers access to a spiritual reservoir [36] that embodies "heights of the soul from which vantage point even tragedy ceases to have a tragic effect."[37] Nietzsche further elaborates this experience on the basis of the notion of eternal recurrence.

Eternal recurrence: "*But thus I willed it!*"

Eternal recurrence is a spiritual reflection of love of self (*amor fati*) expanded as love of the whole. It is the manner through which the individual sees himself as embodying the Spirit's unfolding (coming from the past, extending itself into the future through him in the present moment) and as such directs the individual to redeem humanity's past through his way of living in the now. It embraces "the ideal of the most audacious, lively, and world affirming human being, one who has learned not only to accept and bear that which has been and is, but also wants to have it over again, *just as it was and is*."[38]

This insight however, entails according to Nietzsche "the greatest weight" for us spiritually fatigued modern humans. Nietzsche urges us to ponder on the following:

> This life as you now live it and have lived it, you will have to live once more and innumerable times more; and there will be nothing new in it, but every pain and every joy and every thought and sigh and everything unutterably small or great in your life will have to return to you, all in the same succession and sequence . . . If this thought gained possession of you, it would change you as you are or perhaps crush you. The question in each and every thing, 'Do you desire this once more and innumerable times more?' would lie upon your actions as the greatest weight. Or how well disposed would you have to become to yourself and to life to *crave nothing more fervently* than this ultimate eternal confirmation and seal?[39]

Nietzsche envisions eternal recurrence as a therapeutic, meditative notion (a poetic image if you will, expressing a philosophical idea) that could help postdualistic humans avoid the cycle of vengeance without appealing to compensation in an afterlife. Eternal recurrence is a nondualistic notion meant to replace heaven and hell. It also implies a "pagan" conception of "nature" that is cyclical, thus beginningless and endless, encompassing origin and purpose in the whole.[40] Eternal recurrence is a *pharmakon*, and thus depending on its dosage can be either poison or remedy in the healing of our historicist "consuming feverishness."[41] The notion of eternal recurrence could help temper the apocalyptic visions prophesied by the Abrahamic faiths, which now as a result of modern science have the means to bring about Armageddon: "I do not say this because I want it to happen—the opposite would be rather more after my heart . . . [but] the time for petty politics is over: the very next century will bring the fight for the dominion of the earth—the *compulsion* to large-scale politics."[42]

To respond to this pressing reality, Nietzsche urges "good Europeans" to "acquire one will" by means of a new natural aristocracy. This will require a careful preparation, a combination of manly, *zetetic*, "German" hard skepticism, with French *noblesse*, psychological nuance and inventiveness, a synthesis of north and south that once gave rise to Napoleon.[43] In this light, Nietzsche expects the coming to the fore of world-historical individuals[44]—men with the soul of "Caesar with the heart of Christ"[45]—leaders that particularly in times of crisis will have to rise through the ranks in democratic political culture.

At this juncture, Nietzsche returns to the perennial Platonic theme of education in philosophical and political guardianship. Platonic-Nietzschean education requires careful character-formation as preparation for mature science or philosophy "the most spiritual will to power" to eventually ground both statecraft and individual self-overcoming. Nietzsche's re-shaping of Platonic *paideia* responds to a major political challenge of our time—the problem of planetary rule.[46] Nietzsche's political philosophy links "Athens" and "Jerusalem-Rome": therefore philosophy, religion, and empire take a distinct role in his thinking.[47] Nietzsche claims that without the "Roman Caesars and Roman society Christianity would have never come to power."[48] Is a united Europe a political prelude to a religion of the future? The relation between democracy, empire, and the problem of tyranny has long been a theme of exploration in Platonic political philosophy.[49] Nietzsche seems to follow Plato in his understanding that both philosophy and tyranny are the consequence of "unnecessary desires" such as the erotic love of universal wisdom and the erotic love of universal political rule, both of which can potentially thrive under democratic freedoms.[50] For Nietzsche, the fundamental *political* predicament takes place in the difficult relation between philosophy and religion for ultimate authority in the guidance of world culture. The history of Hellenic Athens and imperial Rome points out that democratic rights are the result of political "realism": the people attain civic rights in exchange for their exertions in imperial expansion or contention. The multicultural affirmation of different traditions under democratic "imperial" tolerance and procedural law paradoxically creates the conditions for the rise of "primitive" religious and philosophical groupings (sects), whose eventual missionary aim will be to enlarge and impose a new universal line of willing on future generations. Nietzsche notes that the tolerance made possible by a powerful successful culture can become indolent relativism.[51] The decline of a coherent set of cultural institutions opens up the possibility for various public interpretations of natural, human and even divine right.[52]

In this "spiritual crisis" the philosophers of the future, "commanders" and "legislators" need to be prepared to perform their task of creation of values and the careful elaboration of horizons for the nurturing and protection of the "plant man." They embody, Nietzsche tells us, the highest responsibility for "their 'knowing' is creating."[53] The philosopher *has been* also *of necessity* a man of the future, step-son of his time, always in contradiction to his today, thus he is akin but different from the wise man in the Hegelian conception.[54] But the philosophers of the future are not to be confused with present day free spirits—afflicted misfits, burdened men confronted with rules they no longer believe in; the free spirits are free from the philosophy of the past (Judeo-Christian Platonism) but are not yet philosophers of the future: thus they are in a period of transition[55] and experimentation about Post-Christian "forms of time." The free minds may be "freer" than the philosophers of the future. The free spirits portrayed by Nietzsche seem to be sensible, solitary, vulnerable, confused, dangerous, but also noble, and always brave, daring: young *Raskolnikovs* undergoing the present drama of the Spirit in their own psyche.

What is noble?

The future morality of the noble acknowledges the exuberant innocence of becoming, of life—which is a woman. As such, Nietzsche suggests to envision and approach it—her—not as "physical or cosmic necessity but as a lover's necessity, erotic necessity"[56]. Likewise with "truth": for "supposing truth is a woman—what then?" Could truth and life be jealous of one another? And in that case: would religious monotheism[57] as well as philosophical dogmatism preclude "bigamy"? However this may be, Nietzsche envisions an eroticism of a new world affirmation—embracing and overcoming the negation of Platonism—so as to "come to terms with and learn to get along with everything that was and is [which] . . . means no longer to take revenge on the world or to seek deliverance from the world."[58] Nietzschean political philosophy incorporates spiritedness as the force behind the self-overcoming of life together with the pedagogical magnetism of *ta erotika* in the declaration of a transfigured cultural *agon* of life-affirming practices. Now, given his enthusiastic rhetoric, it seems fitting to pose the question: is Nietzsche a romantic? I would like to propose he is not. Nietzsche makes a distinction between shapeless fantasy and the manifestation of what is. For Nietzsche, the fundamental fact is will to power[59]—the *hypokeimenon* or groundless ground of every living "thing," which, although open to the process of self-overcoming within holistic recurrence, cannot be imagined away.

Nietzschean free spirits face now the need to live by new virtues: the *sublation* of Platonism implies that it's domesticating four cardinal virtues (plus the Christian virtues of faith, hope, and charity), now have to be conceived in terms of the present unfolding of the Spirit. In this nonfinal period of transition courage becomes the primary virtue, followed by insight, sympathy (giving more than is due), and solitude.[60] Nietzschean therapy for contemporary culture sheds light on the present need to repatriate the sacred back into life, and thus, to conceive of ways of living shaped by the incorporation of both cyclical, erotic, eternal recurrence and linear, spirited, willful self-overcoming. The aim is individual autonomy as *amor fati*, that is, the conscious realization of one's genuine vocation—not "missing yourself" and thus being mindful of "becoming who you are."[61]

Refounding the Platonic academy: Prelude to a philosophy of the future

Nietzsche's re-constructive critique of Platonism begins with a historical return to the sources of our tradition. Nietzsche distinguishes Plato from "Platonism" implying that nihilism is not a unique contemporary event, but exemplifies a disintegration of cultural standards, a spiritual crisis of which Plato, for his own time, had also been a diagnostician. Hence the model of the "Platonic academy" is a permanent idea for reeducation toward philosophical living. Nietzsche, much like Plato's Socrates,[62] does not aim to perform the role of prophet in the market place (*pace* Zarathustra), but rather seeks to be an educator of educators, a "genius of the heart" who's highest task is to encourage the gifted young into "becoming who they are." Nietzsche's writings propose the education of a new spiritual nobility that may, in private at first,[63] cultivate and reeducate itself for the task of creating and experimenting with future "lines of willing." Thus, like Plato, Nietzsche's teaching attempts to infuse philosophical light into "political" practice. It is a kind of "liberal education" in the ample sense of the term.

The idea of reviving some version of the Platonic academy is not new in Western history. It was a touchstone of Renaissance culture led by figures such as Gemistius Plethon (1355–1464), Marsilio Ficino (1433–99), among others. Ficino's villa in

Florence, under the auspices of Lorenzo de′ Medici, served as a place of learning that gathered and influenced some of the greatest figures of Renaissance culture "including Leone Battista Alberti, Angelo Poliziano, Christoforo Landino, Pico della Mirandola, Botticelli, Michelangelo, Raphael, Titian, and Albrecht Dürer."[64] In the same light, Nietzsche, perhaps inspired by the lived presence and scholarship of Jacob Burckhardt,[65] envisions with a high degree of both seriousness and self-irony, a new "postmodern" Renaissance of culture in the realm of future possibility: "supposing that someone believed that it would require no more than a hundred men educated and actively working in a new spirit to do away with the bogus form of culture . . . how greatly it would strengthen him to realize that the culture of the Renaissance was raised on the shoulders of just such a band of a hundred men." Nietzsche, however, immediately takes this lofty analogy with a grain of salt: "and yet—to learn something straightaway from this example—how inexact, fluid and provisional that comparison would be!"[66] Creative vision goes beyond antiquarian romanticism.

Nietzsche makes a claim for "active contemplation" manifested in "examined" practices. He poses the question: what obstacles would have to be removed so that above all the philosopher's example should produce its full effect, so that the philosopher should again educate philosophers?[67] Genuine culture procures action and struggle in the production of "genius" or true "authenticity." This may take place in two stages: (1). Master-pupil relationship for the transmission of "dispositional knowledge," and (2). Pedagogical *praxis:* "thought of a distant future and a possible revolution in education" through new kinds of institutions.[68] Education involves two types of tendencies: focus/specialization and harmonious development.[69] Can both be reconciled? Nietzsche's own condition, unfortunately, could not balance his powerful, epoch-making insights, with a ripe philosophical way of life. Here the Socratic way of living, as depicted by Plato and Xenophon, could provide a model of such "complementary man." Nietzsche's love-hate relationship with Socrates has a quite ambivalent character. It manifests deep skepticism of the "sophistic" side of Socrates that undermined tragic wisdom for ironic dialectical *aporia*, demanding that noble "instinctive" action be analyzed in the *human all too human* terms of craftsmanship and utility. On the other hand, Nietzsche is fascinated by the erotic counter-side of Socrates[70]: the pedagogical, seductive, "musical" dimension that, magnetically, drew toward him some of the most beautiful youths in classical Athens. But was the Socratic "elenctic mask" independent of his psychological finesse and erotic nature? However this may be, Nietzsche acknowledges the necessity of a master-apprentice *propaedeutic* for the "turning around"[71] toward philosophical insight and disposition:

> I see above me something higher and more human than I am; let everyone help me to attain it, as I will help everyone who knows and suffers as I do: so that at last the man may appear who feels himself perfect and boundless in knowledge and love, perception and power, and who in his completeness is at one with nature, the judge and evaluator of things. It is hard to create in anyone this condition of intrepid self-knowledge because it is impossible to teach love; for it is love alone that can bestow on the soul, not only a clear, discriminating and

> self-contemptuous view of self, but also the desire to look beyond itself and to seek with all its might for a higher self as yet still concealed from it. Thus only he who has attached his heart to some great man receives thereby the *first consecration to culture.*[72]

Nietzsche's radically individualistic thought would be very skeptical of the potential reinstauration of dogmatism from his philosophy.[73] A Platonic-Nietzchean academy would be a learning place for spiritual healing and communal tasks crafted for the sake of "self-remembering," soul-care, and soul-craft—but always providing spaces for intimate, nonintrusive solitude.[74] Solitary decantation can be balanced by a relearning of the value of friendship,[75] grounded, at first, on the common search for the self-overcoming of psychic nihilism. For "free spirits," Nietzsche's teaching takes the model of friendship from the dynamics in the Epicurean garden[76]; but his task for the "philosophers of the future" goes beyond Epicurean consolation and retreat: they will assume principles for "extra-moral" transformation in the far future.[77] Such philosophers of the future are to combine intellectual probity, cheerfulness, and the victory-loving desire to conquer the highest tasks. Nietzsche is a "pied piper of philosophy"—philosophy now understood as unconditional love to shape and tend to life's odyssey.

Notes and references

1 The expression comes from Horst Hutter *Shaping the Future: Nietzsche´s New Regime of the Soul and Its Ascetic Practices* (New York: Lexington, 2006). I would like to dedicate this chapter to Professor Hutter, with gratitude.

2 KSA 5, 60–63; *BGE* 44.

3 Nietzsche's conception of the will is akin to Schopenhauer's will as vital impulse—though, for Nietzsche, the will *is the representation* in the world. Contrary to the Augustinian conception of the will (*voluntas*) which is assimilated to the will of God, and thus to faith in a realm beyond material causality, Nietzsche conceives the will as will to power (*BGE* 13), as nondualistic force (*dynamis*), swarm of diverse drives composing all living things, spiritedness striving toward differentiated kinds of self-enhancement and self-overcoming.

4 KSA 5, 237; *BGE*, 295.

5 KSA 6, 350; *EH* "Beyond", sec. 1.

6 KSA 5, 138; *BGE*, 208.

7 KSA 5, 12; *BGE*, Preface.

8 KSA 5, 111–4; *BGE*, 190–1.

9 KSA 5, 208–12; *BGE*, 260.

10 KSA 3, 481; *GS*, 125. Michel Haar, *Nietzsche and Metaphysics,* trans. and ed. Michael Gendre (Albany: State University of New York, 1996), p. 133, analyzes this image from Christian confessional religion to nineteenth-century positivism. Haar notes that "the centuries-old religious practice of the examination of conscience gave birth to a spirit of scientific scruple, which itself engendered a methodological atheism, forbidding appeals to 'hidden causes' to explain phenomena, requiring adherence to facts." For an exploration of this theme in terms of the death of the

"Godhead," see Martin Heidegger, "The Word of Nietzsche: God is Dead", in *The Question Concerning Technology*, translated and with an introduction by William Lowitt (New York: Harper, 1977), pp. 53–112, together with Nietzsche Vol. I. Trans. David Farrell Krell (New York: Harper, 1984), especially pp. 156–7.

11 KSA 5, 70–1; *BGE*, 50.

12 KSA 5, 237–9; *BGE*, 295.

13 Keith Ansell-Pearson *An Introduction to Nietzsche as Political Thinker* (Cambridge: Cambridge University of Press, 1999), pp. 142.

14 KSA 5, 57; *BGE* 40.Consider the notion of "panentheism" as the identity of identity *and* nonidentity, a qualified nondualism, in Tom Darby *The Feast: Meditations on Politics and Time* (Toronto: Toronto University of Press, 1990), p. 75, footnote 54.

15 KSA 5, 60; *BGE*, 43.

16 KSA 5, 207–8; *BGE*, 259. For an analysis of the different accounts of nihilism as a spiritual crisis in the nineteenth and twentieth centuries, see Franco Volpi, *Il Nichilismo* (Roma: Laterza, 2004).

17 My rendition of philosophical *askesis* is informed by Pierre Hadot *Exercises Spirituels et Philosophie Antique*. Préface d'Arnold I. Davidson (Paris: Albin Michel, 2002), as well as Horst Hutter *Shaping the Future*, pp. 2–25; 65; 176; 182–6; 192–93, with "Philosophie et religions comme gymnastiques de la volonté dans la pensée Nietzschéenne," *Conjonctures, (2008)*, No.45/46, Été-Automne, 2008, pp. 89–120. For an important complementary position in favor of the ontological dimension of philosophy, see Waller Newell, *Tyranny: A New Interpretation* (Cambridge: Cambridge University Press, 2013), pp. 8–9.

18 KSA 5, 108: *BGE*, 188.

19 KSA 2, 371; WP, 132.

20 KSA 5, 110; *BGE*, 188.

21 KSA 5, 109; *BGE*, 188.

22 KSA 4, 45–7; *Z* I "On the Pale Criminal."

23 KSA 5, 47–8; *BGE*, 29.

24 Consider Plato *Gorgias* 497a-b.

25 KSA 5, 225; *BGE*, 270.

26 "Like the sick man, the religious man is projected onto the vital plane that shows him the fundamental data of human existence, that is, solitude, danger, hostility of the surrounding world. But the primitive magician, the medicine man, or the shaman is not only a sick man; he is, above all, a sick man who has been cured, who has succeeded in curing himself" thus learning by *pathic* experience and informed practice how to guide and heal others in the community. Mircea Eliade, *Shamanism: Archaic Techniques of Ecstasy* (Princeton: Princeton University of Press, 1964). pp. 27; 314.

27 KSA 5, 208–12; 175–8; *BGE* 260, 239.

28 KSA 5, 85; *BGE* 63.

29 C.f. Plato *Gorgias* 481b10-d3.

30 Machiavelli *Prince* Ch. IX.

31 KSA 5, 208; *BGE*, 260. In connection to this point cf. volume two of Alexis de Tocqueville's *Democracy in America*. For a contrast between Tocqueville and Nietzsche on the democratic soul, see Joshua Mitchell, *The Fragility of Freedom: Tocqueville on Religion, Democracy and the American Future* (Chicago: University Chicago Press, 1999), pp. 87–101.

32 KSA 5, 161; *BGE*, 225.

33 KSA 1, 25–38; *BT*, sections 1–3.

34 KSA 5, 162; *BGE* 226.
35 *WP*, 866.
36 Cf. the "bow image" in *BGE*, Preface; KSA 5, 12–13.
37 KSA 5, 48; *BGE*, 30.
38 KSA 5, 75; *BGE*, 56.
39 KSA 3, 570; *GS*, 341.
40 Jean Seznec, *The Survival of the Pagan Gods: The Mythological tradition and Its Place in Renaissance Humanism and Art*, trans. Barbara Sessions (Princeton: Princeton University Press, 1972).
41 From this perspective, monotheistic culture can be conceived as a world-shaping monumental effort to counter the fatalism of pagan astrological "idolatry" through the psycho-political gymnastics of willing of community-forming religion. This linear-historical remedy for fatalism seems to have become excessive in contemporary Western culture, however, and needs now a counter corrective in the form of "Dionysian" holistic constitution that may give roundedness to natural destiny, to soothe the emancipatory drive of "Apollonian" linear, individual, and historical agency. (*BT*, Sections 9–12). See Roy Bhaskar, *From East to West: Odyssey of a Soul* (London: Routledge, 2000). Ronald Beiner *Civil Religion: A Dialogue in the History of Political Philosophy* (Cambridge: Cambridge University Press, 2011), pp. 371–94.
42 KSA 5, 140; *BGE*, 208.
43 KSA 5, 140, 199; *BGE*, 209, 254.
44 Hegel, *Philosophy of History*, trans Sibree (New York: Dover, 1956), pp. 29–32.
45 WP, 983.
46 On this point consider the Strauss-Kojève debate in Leo Strauss, *On Tyranny* (Chicago: University Chicago Press, 2000), together with George Grant, *Technology and Empire* (Toronto: House of Anansi, 1969), pp. 81–109. For contemporary analyses, see Kenneth Waltz, *Theory of International Politics* (New York: McGraw Hill, 1979); John G. Ruggie "Continuity and Transformation in the World Polity," *World Politics* 35 (1983): 261–85; Christian Reus-Smit "The Constitutional Structure of International Society and the Nature of Fundamental Institutions," *International Organization* 51 (1997): 555–89; Alexander Wendt *Social Theory of International Politics* (Cambridge: Cambridge University Press, 2010); Louis Pauly and Edgar Grande, eds, *Complex Sovereignty: Reconstituting Political Authority in the 21st Century* (Toronto: University of Toronto Press, 2005).
47 Consider KSA 5, 79–81; *BGE*, 61.
48 *WP*, 874.
49 Plato *Republic*, 562a7–9.
50 *WP*, 128, 131; KSA 5, 182–3; *BGE*, 242.
51 *WP*, 130.
52 For a discussion about the problem of religious exaltation and the deliberate creation of the modern State as a situated remedy for the "theologico-political problem" of sixteenth-century Europe, see Pierre Manent. *An Intellectual History of Liberalism*, trans. Rebecca Balinski. (Princeton: Princeton University Press, 1994), pp. 3–9. See also Michael Allen Gillespie *The Theological Origins of Modernity* (Chicago University Chicago Press, 2009).
53 KSA 5, 145; *BGE*, 211.
54 See Hegel *Phenomenology of Spirit*, trans Miller (Oxford: Oxford University Press, 1977), Preface, sec. 5, together with Alexandre Kojève *Introduction to Reading of Hegel*, trans Nichols (Ithaca, New York: Cornell University of Press, 1969),

Ch. 4, pp. 75–99. The classical study exploring the intellectual-historical situation surrounding the Nietzschean friend-enemy connection with Hegelianism is Karl Lowith's *From Hegel to Nietzsche: The Revolution in Nineteenth-Century Thought*, trans. David Green (New York: Anchor Books, 1967).

55 KSA 3, 628–31; *GS*, 377. See Hegel, *Phenomenology of Spirit*, Preface, sec. 11, together with Leo Strauss, "Note on the Plan of Nietzsche's Beyond Good and Evil", in Laurence Lampert *Leo Strauss and Nietzsche* (Chicago: Chicago University Press, 1996), pp. 188–205.

56 Laurence Lampert, *Nietzsche's Task: An Interpretation of Beyond Good and Evil* (New Haven: Yale University Press, 2001), p. 119.

57 Cf. Jan Assman, *The Price of Monotheism*, trans. Robert Savage (Stanford: Stanford University Press, 2010).

58 Laurence Lampert, *Nietzsche's Teaching: An Interpretation of This Spoke Zarathustra* (New Haven: Yale University Press, 1986), p. 118. Consider also Leo Strauss *Natural Right and History* (Chicago: Chicago University Press, 1965), p. 15, towards the end.

59 KSA 5, 22, 27; *BGE*, 9, 13.

60 KSA 5, 232; *BGE*, 284.

61 For a discussion on the "sovereign individual" in Nietzsche, see Richard J. White *Nietzsche and the Problem of Sovereignty* (Chicago: University of Illinois Press, 1997), p. 75. White's text, however, lacks an analysis of the political implications of Nietzsche's insights on this regard; for a thoughtful study of a Nietzschean political philosophy, see Keith Ansell-Pearson *Nietzsche contra Rousseau: A Study of Nietzsche's Moral and Political Thought* (Cambridge: Cambridge University Press, 1991). For an intriguing allegory see Plato *Phaedrus* 245c-250b.

62 On Nietzsche as Socratic educator, see Ernst Bertram *Nietzsche: Essai de Mythologie*, Préface de Pierre Hadot (Paris: Editions du Felin, 1990), pp. 385–418.

63 Consider KSA 5, 233–4; *BGE* 288–9, together with Plato *Republic* 496d.

64 Michael Allen Gillespie, *The Theological Origins of Modernity*, pp. 81–92.

65 "The question as to whether or not a real friendship evolved between Nietzsche and Burckhardt has a significance that exceeds the merely biographical sphere." Martin Heidegger, *Nietzsche Vols I and II*, trans. David Farrell Krell (New York: Harper, 1984), p. 8. Heidegger also quotes Nietzsche's letter to Overbeck dated 7April 1884: "For the past few months I have been preoccupied with 'world history,' enchanted by it in spite of many hair-raising results. Did I ever show you Burckhardt's letter, the one which led me by the nose to 'world history'?" Heidegger, *Nietzsche*, p. 12.

66 *HL*, sec. 2.

67 *SE*, sec. 7.

68 *SE*, sec. 7; KSA 6, 298–301; *EH*, "Why I write such Good Books," sec. 1

69 A Nietzschean education in harmonious development would involve not only intellectual cultivation, but also individual considerations regarding "nutrition, place, climate, recreation, the whole casuistry of selfishness—[aspects which] are inconceivably more important than everything one has taken to be important so far. Precisely here one must begin to *relearn*." KSA 6, 295; *EH*, "Why I am so Clever", sec. 10. Hutter *Shaping the Future*, pp. 145–77.

70 Cf. Bertram *Nietzsche: Essai de Mythologie*, pp. 386–98.

71 Plato *Republic* 518d3-7.

72 *SE*, sec. 6.

73 Nevertheless consider KSA 79–81; *BGE*, 61.

74 Hutter, *Shaping the Future,* pp. 47–74.
75 Ibid., pp. 75–106.
76 Cf. KSA 5, 225–6; *BGE,* 270.
77 KSA 50–51, 144–5; *BGE* 32 with 211.Tracy B. Strong *Friedrich Nietzsche and the Politics of Transfiguration* (Berkeley: University of California Press, 1988), p. 293.

Translations used

Basic Writings of Nietzsche. Intro. by Peter Gay, Trans. Walter Kaufmann. New York: Modern Library, 2000.
The Gay Science. Trans. with Commentary by Walter Kaufmann. New York: Vintage, 1974.
The Will to Power. Trans. Walter Kaufmann and R. J. Hollingdale. New York: Vintage, 1967.
Thus Spoke Zarathustra. Trans. Graham Parkes. Oxford: Oxford University Press, 2008.
Untimely Meditations. Ed. Daniel Breazeale. Trans. R. J. Hollingdale. Cambridge: Cambridge University Press, 1997.

6

Nietzsche's Cruel Offerings: Friendship, Solitude, and the Bestowing Virtue in *Thus Spoke Zarathustra*

Willow Verkerk

In *Ecce Homo*, Nietzsche discusses retrospectively some of his personal struggles during the writing of *Thus Spoke Zarathustra*, one of which included a profound lack of understanding from his friends.[1] Nietzsche's protagonist, Zarathustra, a man of "great health,"[2] faces a similar experience during his narrative journey: he seeks companions who will understand and join him in agonistic interrelation, but instead finds only followers and disciples. Although Zarathustra hesitates to order his disciples toward one specific direction, he does accept the role of educator and offers his teachings to his prospective friends as a gift with which they may eventually do as they like.

In this article, I explore Nietzsche's treatment of friendship in *Zarathustra* as an extension of his own hope—a hope perhaps never fulfilled—that he might some day know other strivers, like-minded companions to share his ideas on the great health with. These are the individuals he calls free spirits (*freie Geister*)[3] and philosophers of the future, friends who would be worthy of his "truths," even if only after his death. Nietzsche employs Zarathustra as seducer and through him initiates his readers into the kind of self-questioning that one might ordinarily hesitate before, but suddenly finds oneself enmeshed in: a conversation with a cruel, but loving and provocative friend. In this respect, Nietzsche composes *Zarathustra* as a literary gift of friendship, a performance of hard generosity that champions the virtues of the warrior.

At first glance, what are most difficult to reconcile in *Zarathustra* on the topic of friendship are Zarathustra's seemingly contradictory claims: at one point, he advices generosity and rejoicing between friends, at another, he advocates enmity and competition. It is tempting to choose exclusively one approach over the other. Alternatively, we may assume that Nietzsche is strategically undermining our sociohistorical notions of friendship, only to show us that no such notions exist. This is certainly one thread that he follows in a number of different places in *Zarathustra*. For example, Nietzsche critiques our inability to be friends through our poor character traits, either being too slavish or too tyrannical[4]; elsewhere he attacks the Christian notion of neighborly love[5] for being merely a distraction from self-awareness, a kind of escapism from the self. In such instances, he is asserting that our modern notions of "friendship" bear very little resemblance to our lived interpersonal relationships. However, it is important not to therefore conclude he is also asserting that friendship should be altogether abandoned or that it is impossible. Rather, Nietzsche is taking it apart so that it can be rebuilt.

In the first part of *Zarathustra*, Nietzsche writes,

> I teach you the friend and his overfull heart. But one must know how to be a sponge if one would be loved by hearts that are overfull. I teach you the friend, in whom the world stands complete, a vessel of goodness—the creating friend, who always has a complete world to bestow.[6]

Zarathustra, and Nietzsche through him, is advocating the rebuilding of friendship, a new understanding of friendship that is connected to our own therapeutic self-overcoming and a striving toward the Overhuman. It may remain difficult to envision such a kind of friend, especially in light of what Zarathustra points out, namely, that we are in a state of lack. We may wonder, for example, how effective it is to replace former ideals with new ones, if we have failed so utterly in the past to live up to them. But, it is precisely such questioning, I would claim, that Nietzsche attempts to provoke in us through *Zarathustra*. The above quote is only one aspect of the polyvalent friend that Nietzsche gives to us. Through the narrative journey of *Zarathustra* and Zarathustra's teachings on these types, we may learn to influence the kind of relationships we have, to select and shape those relationships that are the healthiest.

As Nietzsche later proclaims in *Beyond Good and Evil,* his concept of friendship is difficult for his readers to understand, for it is situated within a framework unfamiliar to us.[7] According to Nietzsche, in modernity we have lost sight of the noble concept of suffering related to the tragic culture of Greek antiquity and with it a capacity for having human relationships that promote self-overcoming through contest, enmity, and hard generosity. We have collapsed a much richer notion of friendship in which spiritual cruelty was tolerated and even promoted, in favor of a notion that is definable and comfortable, but in doing so we have robbed friendship of its transformative powers. In fact, Nietzsche claims that many friendships that are worthwhile involve discomfort, competition, and even, at times, duplicity.

Rather than friendship, Nietzsche is often presumed to polemically advocate a radical individuality. However, careful attention to his texts show that this is not the case: we assume that he stands against friendship because we are limited by our own definitions of what friendship is, idealizing and oversimplifying it within the context of our modern paradigms of humanism, science, and Christianity. The modern conception of friendship is one that belies itself, according to Nietzsche, whereas his own understanding of friendship allows for a number of therapeutic possibilities, depending upon both the character of the person(s) in question and the stage that they are in their lives.

Still, we are left with a question mark. Between Nietzsche's biting remarks about erotic love and the herd, and a counseling to his disciples and free spirits to flee from others into solitude, it remains difficult to accept that he is proposing new kind(s) of friendship. Moreover, if Nietzsche associates creativity, self-overcoming, and his ultimate goal, the Overhuman, with solitude, what place does friendship have? It is tempting to conclude that Nietzsche's valuation of friendship is only secondary to his understanding of the self, in that he advocates the capacity of the great individual over and above any notion of "the good" between friends. Does he reject the traditional virtues of friendship and replace them with one of contest in which friends become merely means to another, higher end? In order to respond to such questions, the interplay between friendship and solitude and the role of the bestowing virtue in personal development and human relationships need to be examined in *Zarathustra*.

After some initial consideration of *Zarathustra*, we find two praiseworthy threads on friendship: one of the warrior of the agonistic, lion-hearted, and the other of the master, of the nobler type of self-affirming, bestowing person. These two threads do overlap and it can be difficult to decipher if they are actually separate types, or are just different aspects of a more complex understanding of friendship. The third and lower category of human relationships (which is also called friendship at times by Nietzsche) is allocated to usury, comradeship, and erotic love and involves relations of convenience, servitude, and tyranny. A fair amount of the provocative voice that Nietzsche employs in discussing friendship is for critiquing this third group. However, his provocative tone is also used to incite struggle between himself and his warrior spirited readers. In doing so, he hopes to foster friendships of loving cruelty between himself and his readers.

In the prologue, Zarathustra comes out of his many years of solitude in order to search out companions with whom he can share the wisdom he gained from spending time alone in contemplation. Here and throughout the narrative, Zarathustra is looking for friends to help him facilitate and ultimately fulfill the creative vision that he developed during his solitary days in the mountains. At the beginning of the second part of the book, Zarathustra proclaims,

> 'My Wild Wisdom became pregnant on lonely mountains; on roughest rocks she bore her young, her youngest. Now she runs foolishly through the harsh desert, and seeks and seeks for a soft greensward—my old Wild Wisdom! On the soft greensward of your hearts, my friends!—on your love she would like to bed down her dearest!'[8]

From this quote and others, Nietzsche expresses his view that, although wisdom and self-contemplation require solitude, friendship with one's equals[9] and the reflective gaze of the other,[10] are necessary parts of a healthy and creatively engaged life.

The idea that a good friend is a facilitator to one's own creative vision is essential to understanding Nietzsche's concept of friendship. It is not that friendship is at odds with solitude, but rather that there are times for both. Zarathustra portrays an attempt at the kind of self-awareness that is necessary for spiritual self-intelligence in that he moves in and out of solitude in the story, in order to assist his own self-overcoming and the self-overcoming of his disciple-friends.

For Nietzsche, being a facilitator does not only consist in the typical inclinations of kindness, generosity, or support that we might suppose. It more precisely has to do with the warrior friendship that is mentioned above, namely, one of *agon*, which mixes enmity with friendship and benefits itself most through openly combative relationships. Sometimes, being a good friend, according to Nietzsche, requires that we abandon the other, directly contradict him or force him to doubt his own suppositions (Zarathustra does all of these things and more with his companions).

We may provide a preliminary description of the type of character that is well-disposed toward warrior type friendships by examining Chapter 10 in the first part of *Zarathustra*, "On War and Warrior Peoples."[11] Here, Zarathustra describes the human characteristics of the people who will allow for the transformation of society through their agonistic natures. He underlines courage, honesty, strength, and respectful competition as the virtues of the warrior and claims that the contest of overcoming makes life and existence on earth more meaningful. Zarathustra not only empathizes with the warrior, he also expresses his affection for them through an attitude of brotherhood and cruel generosity: "I do not spare you; I love you from the ground up, my brothers in war!"[12]

The warrior represents a human type, or stage of development in the psychological disposition of the human being, that hungers for agonistic relationships. With those who are our "best enemies," our warrior friends, we should be truthful, even if it is cruel, according to Zarathustra. Zarathustra attempts to do precisely this with his disciple-friends, and Nietzsche with his readers. Zarathustra's advice to his warrior friends, who look for an enemy to strive against is: "You shall seek your enemy, you shall wage war—and for your own thoughts! And should you be defeated, your honesty shall still proclaim its triumph in that!"[13] Zarathustra exclaims that, if one cannot be a bestower of wisdom, then one should strive toward it and fight for it. He attempts to educate those with warrior-type personalities or those who are at the warrior-spirited lion stage of their life by proclaiming the heroic nature of their dispositions, praising their noble strength, and encouraging them toward spiritual and intellectual battle.

The warrior-spirited person is distinguished as living within the no-saying lion stage (as opposed to the camel or child).[14] He aspires toward greatness and is a knowledge-seeker, but is nevertheless angry, hateful, and envious of the "saints of understanding" (those capable of masterful friendships that have acquired greater wisdom). At their root, warriors lack in self-understanding and self-mastery: struggle and contest dominate their spirits, but they continue to strive on. Zarathustra urges these warriors of understanding to pursue their own path (not the one of the "Uni-form") and to seek out enemies, namely, those on whom they can test the adequacy of their own understanding.

In this chapter, Zarathustra states, "I am and have been of your kind." In stating this, not only does Zarathustra reassert that his warrior friends are his equals, he also suggests that the warrior type is a stage, a persona, or an aspect that one might reside or take part in, but that it should not generally be assumed as a complete picture of the self. It is fair to assume that the warrior friendship may also have a temporary quality, whether it is as a short-lived relationship that exists purely for the mutual facilitation of a particular goal, or as an aspect within a more complex relationship (which does mean that it can have an instrumental quality). Such a friendship may benefit from solitude in that the alone time allows for the integration of the new levels of reflection gained from the oppositional attitude of the agonistic friend. Thus, we return to the observation that friendship and solitude are not topics of tension or conflict within Nietzsche's work, but rather complimentary therapeutic devices that assist in self-intelligence and practical well-being.

The *First Book* of *Zarathustra*, "On the Friend" (Chapter 14) reasserts the necessity of *agon* in human relationships with an emphasis on the therapeutic powers of friendship, as well as its potential disadvantages. Zarathustra begins by addressing some of the challenges that the solitary person grapples with when it comes to relating to other people: for he already lives, at minimum, as a duality within himself.[15] Zarathustra contends that the contemplative and introverted nature of the solitary lends itself to internal conversation and strife. He lives as both a friend and an enemy with himself.[16]

The friend allows for an outside voice in the life of the solitary: for one can become lost and deluded in his conversation with himself, the friend provides a "third" voice. However, it is not certain that the friend will be helpful to the solitary, for in certain circumstances, "our belief in others betrays wherein we should like to believe in ourselves. Our yearning for a friend is our betrayer."[17] In other words, although the friend may provide another point of view that has the potential to be helpful, his perspective may also be deficient and/or have the potential of interrupting the solitary person's creative process and taking him away from his work.

Zarathustra proposes that one begins by requesting an enemy for intellectual combat, before presuming friendship, for in order to be a friend one must first be capable of being an enemy-friend. According to Zarathustra, one needs to be able to "honour even the enemy in one's friend." His suggestion for the avoidance of distracting and/or unhealthy relationships is to approach friendship with a sense of enmity, to consider the friend someone worth fighting with and subsequently worth fighting for. Characteristic of agonistic friendship, Zarathustra declares: "if one would have a friend, one must also want to wage war for him: and in order to wage war, one must *be able* to be an enemy." He adds, "In one's friend one should have one's best enemy. You should be closest to him in your heart when you strive against him."[18] Friendship has the potential of allowing for growth and change through mutual striving and competition, assuming that the friends are not too preoccupied by envy or jealousy of the other's characteristics.

Honesty may be a virtue of the warrior as well as the friend, but Zarathustra emphasizes that friendship is not about transparency. One must not attempt to disclose, or share everything about oneself with the friend, mutual respect demands some distance. "Whoever makes no secret of himself incenses others: you have that much reason to fear nakedness!"[19] For, in order to inspire another person, which is one of the greatest merits of friendship, you must be admirable. Although some disclosure is necessary to engage dialectically, too much creates an aura of weakness upon the other and encroaches upon the capacity for noble combat between equals.[20] As Zarathustra speaks, "You cannot adorn yourself well enough for your friend: for you shall be to him an arrow and yearning for the Overhuman."[21] In this respect, the friend who is esteemed makes for a respectable adversary.

Another commendable quality of friendship is that is allows for self-reflection and can assist one in the avoidance of self-deception and delusional behavior. Self-reflection can occur quite simply through spending time with the friend, for the face of our friend, "is your own face, in a rough and imperfect mirror."[22] Zarathustra teaches that the reactions of one friend to another has much to disclose about their interiority, their personal weaknesses and strengths, and through observance of this, friendship can assist self-understanding. Although the possibility that we are deceiving ourselves can never be completely eliminated, friendship which incorporates the cruel honesty of the warrior allows for another level of critical analysis to reflect on the possibility of delusion and self-deception.

Zarathustra may have just stressed that self-disclosure can be a vice in interpersonal relationships which attempt to nourish self-overcoming, but raw honesty, mediated by the particular needs of the friend in question, is deemed an integral characteristic of those friendships that he considers healthy.[23] As is apparent in the whole of Chapter 14, Zarathustra places a high value on the potentialities of friendship at the individual level for coping with self-deception, narcissism, and weakness of will. Yet, it is also apparent that Zarathustra is reluctant to make sure rules about friendship; he advices caution in many respects and emphasizes the development of particular character traits or virtues over prescriptive rules of behavior.

In Chapters 10 and 14, Zarathustra teaches his companions to look for relationships that cultivate the warrior virtues of strength, honesty, courage, and respectful competition between equals. In Chapter 16, "On Love of One's Neighbour," he maintains the import of these attributes for the development of self-love and healthy human relationships and then introduces another level of friendship, that of the bestower.[24] Here, Zarathustra offers his listeners a subtle and telling warning on the bestower and the challenges of being on the receptive side of such a person.[25] He speaks of the kind of friendship that implies the need for a sophisticated sense of vulnerability on the side of the giver and the receiver; he introduces an attitude toward reception, which seems quite different from the agonistic friendship of the warrior. At minimum, there is one common link between the virtues of the warrior friend and the bestower: both encourage striving for that which is higher through the admiration of the other, a striving above one's current reach.[26]

For Nietzsche, the bestowing or gift-giving virtue is expressed from a place of abundance, a healthy selfishness that out of its own fullness and self-mastery seeks others to express this fullness toward. As he writes in *Zarathustra*, being virtuous in the sense of the bestowing virtue specifies a particular approach toward both reception and offering.[27] Zarathustra exclaims that out of self-love, the one who masters the bestowing virtue offers his love to the world by affirming the earth (as opposed to the otherworldly) and sharing his wisdom without seeking a return. Thus, the action of giving itself is supposed to be motivated from a position without any expectation of calculated reward or benefit to the giver.

Zarathustra's last speech of the *First Part* occurs at the crossroads outside the town of The Motley Cow, where he has gained many followers. Zarathustra admits that he has aspired toward the highest virtue in his interactions with his companions, but has still not mastered it. As was the case in his speech on the warrior, Zarathustra attempts to gain the confidence of his disciple-friends through placing himself as a peer to them. He announces, "Verily, I divine you well, my disciples: you are striving, as I am, for the bestowing virtue."[28] Zarathustra states that he holds some knowledge about the bestowing virtue that his disciples are wanting for (which seems to undermine the notion that he is actually their peer) and he then proceeds to educate them on what the bestowing virtue consists in, what aspect of it they may already have, and how they can further come to bring it into their lives. Zarathustra proclaims that in order to give, one must first be overfull, and this fullness in turn must be nurtured by a healthy selfishness. He speaks to his listeners, as if they have already begun this process.[29]

Here, and very soon more openly, Zarathustra refers to the virtues of the warrior as foundational capacities that allow for one to become a bestower. The warrior spirited person is driven by a selfishness that squanders now to give later; he lives in *agon* and strives toward the building of his capacities for knowledge and understanding. This kind of "whole and holy" selfishness is distinguished from "a sick selfishness" or a "thieving greed" that is degenerate. Whereas the healthy selfishness of the striver is the enactment of a hunger for the accumulation of strength, wisdom, and self-love, the other kind of "skulking" selfishness attempts to steal, it takes from the bestowing spirit and thinks, "All is for me."[30]

Thus, Zarathustra qualifies the bestowing virtue as arising out of a healthy selfishness that stimulates creativity and self-love, which then has a need to express itself to others. But, progressively, as Zarathustra continues in his speech on the bestowing virtue, the wisdom of the bestower begins to catch a cruel light, like the virtues of truth and courage of the warrior: "When you despise what is pleasant and the soft bed, and cannot bed down far enough away from the soft-hearted: there lies the origin of your virtue." However, Zarathustra also distinguishes the virtue of the bestower from that of the warrior: "When you are elevated above praise and blame, and your will would command all things, as the will of a lover: there lies the origin of your virtue."[31]

In the case of his virtue, the bestower appears to be removed from relationships of competition (or at minimum, he is not invested in competitive relationships); although he may seek out inspiration from others and continue to strive toward greatness, he does not suffer from the same degree of envy or operate in the realm of *agon*. The bestower assists others in self-revelation indirectly in that he communicates allegorically (like the teachings of a sage), but also directly through commanding himself and others (not striving against or obeying others like the warrior). Thus, the bestower is distinguished from the warrior in that he has come to a place of self-mastery, because his inner life is not one of warring wills and strife, but has rather a master drive, set into a firm trajectory.[32]

With his words on power, the first section of "On the Bestowing Virtue" ends and Zarathustra becomes silent. Now he turns to his companions and speaks to them almost in a sentimental manner, imploring them to "Stay true to the earth" and repeats some of his earlier warnings against other-worldliness and escapism.[33] He underlines the import of seeking out knowledge and understanding and of healing oneself so that one can help to heal others. He speaks ambiguously of a new earth and a "new hope" and then draws himself into silence again, this time with greater pause.

When he speaks again, it is for the last time in the *First Part* and it is to bid farewell to his disciples. He announces that he goes into solitude and tells his disciples that they should do so also. His comportment shifts dramatically here, and we see an expression of the bestowing virtue that Zarathustra has not yet performed in his behavior with his disciples. Zarathustra names it later in the *Second Part* when he states that the most difficult task as a bestower is, "out of love to close the open hand and to preserve one's modesty, as a bestower."[34] Zarathustra leaves his disciple-friends and offers them a cruel expression of his love for them on his way out.

Zarathustra speaks provocatively to his followers, so that they will be forced to consider their own thoughts, not only the thoughts of Zarathustra. He recognizes that his disciples have become too loyal; Zarathustra is weary of his teachings being taken as dogma. As such he exclaims, "go away from me and guard yourself against Zarathustra! And better still: be ashamed of him! Perhaps he has deceived you."[35] Zarathustra is attempting to foster resistance in his companions, so that they will want to question the teaching of Zarathustra and consider the worth of it for themselves. Although Zarathustra recognizes a fraternity between himself and his companions, and even foresees a future community between them, he finds it imperative that they come to him from their own direction, not as "believers" of "Zarathustra." Thus, Zarathustra's abandonment is also a strategy of offering, an expression of love that is hurtful to both himself and his companions, yet concurrently in the interest of a higher goal: to facilitate overcoming. Behind Zarathustra, we can hear Nietzsche cautioning us not to become so enmeshed in the world of Zarathustra and the teachings of self-overcoming therein, that we forget ourselves: who we are and aim to be.

In what sense Zarathustra fully enacts or exemplifies the bestowing virtue is a matter of debate. It is questionable whether he (or Nietzsche as the originator of such a gift) is able to accomplish its most challenging tasks: to give without any calculated benefit. It seems that, if we consider *Zarathustra* as a literary gift of friendship to future philosophers from Nietzsche, or Zarathustra as himself (and his teachings) a performativity expression, or literary example of the bestowing virtue, one that concurrently requests dialectical involvement from the reader, then we are left with a number of questions. For instance, if Nietzsche is a provocative writer and Zarathustra himself is made to act to incite reaction, to both "wound and delight" the reader into self-questioning and self-overcoming, how can we claim that Zarathustra acts (or is made to act) without calculated benefit? If part of Zarathustra's generosity involves the teachings of eternal recurrence, *amor fati* and the Overhuman, is there not some expectation that his disciples, or his posthumous friends will learn, or engage with these teachings in a fashion that would be deemed noble by Nietzsche? It seems very problematic to make an offering that claims to lay the foundations for a new way of life, a "great noon," and a community of free spirits, yet concurrently to state that this gift requests no reciprocity from those who acquire it. Perhaps this is the case. However, I would argue that, when Zarathustra turns away from those that he loves and maintains his modesty as a bestower, he enacts the bestowing virtue in exactly this sense, namely, without expectation of return. After realizing he has nothing left to give, and he is in need of solitude to renew himself, Zarathustra departs. In this moment, Nietzsche's concept of friendship emerges as the radical expression of a healthy selfishness that overflows, yet does not request a return: a friendship that knows suffering, solitude, and agonistic relationships to be its most fruitful therapies.

In his relationships with his disciples and companions, Zarathustra ventures to act as both an agonistic and a bestowing friend, in order to facilitate them into self-questioning and self-overcoming. Perhaps his companions do not succeed in these tasks, but nevertheless we can recognize that through the speeches of Zarathustra, friendship is proposed as a meeting place from which modern individuals can attempt to, as Horst Hutter writes, "transcend their slavishness in a lasting manner."[36] In order to overcome weakness of will, narcissism, and self-delusion, free spirits need others of like minds, enemy-friends to strive against. Thus, what is suggested is a seeking out of companions who have shared goals: friends to come together for growth and then leave, once the period of growth is over (see the star friendship of GS 279; KSA 3, 523). It is in the same sense that Nietzsche wants us to read his text of *Zarathustra* as a book for self-overcoming: to accept it as a cruel offering of friendship, a bestowing which, through its teachings, offers us an alternate approach to relating to both ourselves and to the other.

Notes and references

1 "Solitude [*die Einsamkeit*] has seven skins; nothing penetrates them anymore. One comes to men, one greets friends—more desolation, no eyes offer a greeting. At best, a kind of revolt. Such revolts I experienced, very different in degree but from almost everybody that was close to me. It seems nothing offends more deeply than suddenly letting others feel a distance, those *noble* natures who do not know how to live without reverence are rare." EH TSZ 5; KSA 6, 342.

2 GS 382 and EH TSZ 2; KSA 3, 635 and KSA 6, 337.

3 See HAH 225; KSA 2, 189–90 for a description of the free spirit.

4 TSZ I: 14; KSA 4, 72.

5 TSZ I: 16; KSA 4, 77.

6 Ibid.; KSA 4, 78.

7 "The capacity for and the duty of, long gratitude and long revenge—both only among one's peers [*Gleichen*]—refinement in repaying, the sophisticated concept of friendship, a certain necessity for having enemies (as it were, as drainage ditches for the affects of envy, quarrelsomeness, exuberance—at bottom, in order to be capable of being good *friends*): all these are typical characteristics of the noble morality which, as suggested, is not the morality of 'modern ideas' and therefore is hard to empathize with today, also hard to dig up and uncover." BGE 260; KSA 5, 211.

8 TSZ II: 1; KSA 4, 107–8.

9 BGE 26 and 260; KSA 5, 44 and 211.

10 Nietzsche writes that your friend's face "is your own face, in a rough and imperfect mirror." TSZ I: 14; KSA 4, 72.

11 TSZ 1: 10; KSA 4, 58–60.

12 TSZ 1: 10; KSA 4, 60.

13 Ibid.; KSA 4, 58.

14 In TSZ I: 1 Zarathustra discusses the three transformations of the spirit that come to structure the process of self-overcoming that he teaches as well as his own development during the course of his journey (KSA 4, 29–31).

15 For a detailed analysis of Nietzsche's concept of the self as a "dividual," or a multiplicity of divides selves, see Horst Hutter *Shaping the Future: Nietzsche's New Regime of the Soul and Its Ascetic Practices* (Lanham: Lexington Books, 2006), 23: "Being human thus means to be alienated from a part of oneself, to be dividual and to bear the inevitable suffering entailed by self-division."

16 "'One person is always too many around me'—thus thinks the solitary. 'Always one times one—that yields in the long run two!' I and Me are always too zealous in conversation: how could it be endured if there were no friend? For the solitary the friend is always the third one: the third one is the cork that prevents the conversation of the two from sinking into the depths. Ah, there are too many depths for all solitaries. Therefore they long so much for a friend and for his height." TSZ I: 14; KSA 4, 71.

17 Ibid.

18 Ibid.; KSA 4, 71–2.

19 Ibid.; KSA 4, 72.

20 Nietzsche speaks of the necessity of hiding and masking oneself repeatedly. One such instance is in BGE 40; KSA 5, 57–8.

21 TSZ I: 14; KSA 4, 72.

22 Ibid.

23 "May your compassion be a divining: that you might first know whether your friend wants compassion. Perhaps he loves in you the unbroken eye and glance of eternity. May compassion for the friend conceal itself under a hard shell; you shall lose a tooth biting on it. Thus will it have its subtlety and sweetness. Are you pure air and solitude and bread and medicine for your friend? Many a one is unable to loosen his own chains and yet he is a redeemer for his friend." Ibid.

24 He foreshadows the bestower in Chapter 10 as the "saint of understanding" but does not explain: "And if you cannot be saints of understanding, then at least be for me its warriors." TSZ I: 10; KSA 4, 58.

25 "I teach you the friend and his overfull heart. But one must know how to be a sponge if one would be loved by hearts that are overfull." TSZ I: 16; KSA 4, 78. See also TSZ II: 3; KSA 4, 113–16.

26 "May the future and the farthest be the cause of your today: in your friend shall you love the Overhuman as your own cause." TSZ I: 16; KSA 4, 78. The differences between the warrior and bestowing friend are as follows: whereas the warrior friendship consists of a striving between peers and resembles the star friendship of *The Gay Science*, 279, the bestowing friend of the "overfull heart" seems to be already operating from a place of height where he must look below himself to find friendship. There are a number of comments from Zarathustra that suggest the friend cannot have the same significance for the bestower as the warrior: 1. the bestower gives to his "friend" without seeking reciprocity (TSZ I: 22:1; KSA 4, 97–8 and TSZ II: 5; KSA 4, 120–3); 2. the bestower has a greater sense of wisdom and strength than those who receive from him, and for this reason it is questionable whether he can accept those he gives to as his peers and thus his friends.

27 See TSZ II: 3; KSA 4, 114–16.

28 TSZ I: 22: 1; KSA 4, 97.

29 "'This is your thirst, to become sacrifices and bestowals yourselves: and therefore you thirst to pile up all riches in your souls. 'Insatiably your soul strives for treasures and jewels, because your virtue is insatiable in wanting to bestow.' 'You compel all things

towards you and into you, that they may flow back out of your wells as gifts of your love. Verily, a predator of all values must such a bestowing love become; but whole and holy do I call such selfishness.'" Ibid; KSA 4, 98.

30 Ibid.

31 Ibid; KSA 4, 99.

32 "'When you are willers of one will, and this turning of all need is for you called necessity: there lies the origin of your virtue. 'Power it is, this new virtue; a ruling thought it is, and around it a clever soul: a golden sun, and around it the serpent of knowledge.'" Ibid.

33 TSZ I: 22: 2; KSA 4, 99–101.

34 TSZ II: 1; KSA 4, 105.

35 TSZ I: 22: 3; KSA 4, 68.

36 Hutter, p. 76.

Selected bibliography

Alderman, Harold. *Nietzsche's Gift*. Athens: Ohio University Press, 1977.

Allison, David B. *Reading the New Nietzsche*. Lanham: Rowman & Littlefield Publishers, 2001.

— (ed.) *The New Nietzsche*. Cambridge: MIT Press, 1985; 1999.

Aloni, Nimrod. *Beyond Nihilism: Nietzsche's Healing and Edifying Philosophy*. Lanham: University Press of America, 1991.

Benson, Bruce Ellis. *Pious Nietzsche: Decadence and Dionysian Faith*. Bloomington: Indiana University Press, 2008.

Derrida, Jacques. *Given Time*, trans. Peggy Kamuf. Chicago: University of Chicago Press, 1992.

—. *Politics of Friendship*, trans. George Collins. London: Verso, 1997.

Deleuze, Gilles. *Nietzsche & Philosophy*, trans. Hugh Tomlinson. New York: Columbia University Press, 1983.

Daigle, Christine. "Nietzsche: Virtue Ethics . . . Virtue Politics?" *Journal of Nietzsche Studies* 32 (2006): 1–21.

Gooding-Williams, Robert. *Zarathustra's Dionysian Modernism*. Eds. Judith Butler and Frederick M. Dolan. Stanford: Standford University Press, 2001.

Hadot, Pierre. *Philosophy as a Way of Life*. Ed. Arnold Davidson, trans. Michael Chase. Oxford: Blackwell, 2000.

Hatab, Lawrence J. *Nietzsche's Life Sentence*. New York: Routledge, 2005.

Hunt, Lester H. *Nietzsche And The Origin of Virtue*. London and New York: Routledge, 1991.

Hutter, Horst. *Shaping the Future: Nietzsche's New Regime of the Soul and Its Ascetic Practices*. Landham: Lexington Books, 2006.

Lampert, Laurence. *Nietzsche's Teaching*. New Haven: Yale University Press, 1986.

Nehamas, Alexander. "For Whom the Sun Shines," in *Also sprach Zarathustra Herausgegeben von Volker Gerhardt*, Klassiker Auslegen, Bd. 14. Berlin: Akademie Verlage, 2000, 165–90.

Parkes, Graham. *Composing the Soul*. Chicago: The University of Chicago Press, 1994.

Pangle, Thomas L. "The 'Warrior Spirit' as an Inlet to the Political Philosophy of Nietzsche's Zarathustra." *Nietzsche-Studien: InternationalesJahrbuch für die Nietzsche-Forschung* 15 (1986): 140–79.

Pippin, Robert. "Irony and Affirmation in Nietzsche's *Thus Spoke Zarathustra*," in Michael Gillespie and Tracy Strong, (ed.), *Nietzsche's New Seas*. Chicago: University of Chicago Press, 1988, 45–71.

Van Tongeren, Paul. *Reinterpreting Modern Culture*. West Lafayette: Purdue University Press, 2000.

—. "On Friends in Nietzsche's Zarathustra." *New Nietzsche Studies* 5 (2003): 73–88.

—. "Politics, Friendship and Solitude in Nietzsche." *South African Journal of Philosophy* 19(3), (2000): 209–22.

7

The Advantages and Disadvantages of Nietzsche's Philosophy for Life

Bela Egyed

Nietzsche presents himself, behind the mask of Zarathustra, as the teacher of the Eternal Return,[1] and as the one who calls out for the Overman. As difficult as this project had turned out for his interpreters, nevertheless, he declares in the subtitle of *Thus Spoke Zarathustra* (Z) that it is a "book for everyone and no one." From this, one might conclude that anyone might elect oneself to be a student of that book. However, this impression is put under some strain by Zarathustra's constant reminder that he is speaking only to his disciples. He does not specify who would qualify as a disciple, but at one crucial point, the question of audience comes to the foreground. At the end of one the most important chapters of the book, "Of Redemption," Zarathustra is rebuked by the hunchback:

> "But why does Zarathustra speak to us differently than to his disciples?" Zarathustra answered:" What is surprising in that? One may well speak in hunchback manner to a hunchback!" "Very good" said the hunchback; and with pupils one may well tales out of school. But why does Zarathustra speak to his pupils differently than to himself?" (KGW VI, 178)

Presumably, the hunchback is the one who cannot, because he does not want to, hear Zarathustra's teachings. So, why is he there? Why is he listening? What about Zarathustra's disciples? Presumably, they want to hear. Still, even the hunchback notes that they do not hear what Zarathustra really wants to say. Is the hunchback resentful because he knows that Zarathustra does not really want him to hear what he teaches? If this is the case, then Z is not meant for everyone. And, if even his disciples cannot know what is on Zarathustra's mind, then who is Zarathustra really teaching? One easy answer might be that it is himself. But is this self-teaching of any use to disciples? Can anyone besides Zarathustra learn from his own self-teaching? In fact, what Zarathustra tells his disciples is that if they are to be good disciples, they must leave and teach themselves. His teaching is only a sign, pointing the way. From there on, everyone must make their own way.[2]

Nietzsche wrote Book II of *Zarathustra*, in which the chapter in question appears, in the early summer of 1883. At the same time, he is writing notes pertaining to apparently different matters.[3] Among these is a passage which might serve as beacon for evaluating Nietzsche's troubling references to the "crowd":

> Morality had up till now the limits that corresponded to that of the species: all past moralities were useful for the purpose of giving to the species, first of all, an absolute resistance: once this has been achieved, the aim could be placed higher.
>
> The first movement is unconditional – leveling of the species, great ant-buildings, etc. . . .
>
> The other movement: mine: is, conversely, the sharpening of all oppositions and widening of all gaps, to remove equality, the creation of over-powers.
>
> The first created the last man. Mine the Overman.
>
> It is absolutely not the aim to consider the last [Overman] as the masters of the first: rather: two types have to exist, one at the same time as the other – separated to the greatest possible extent: the one, like the gods of Epicurus, do not preoccupy themselves with the others. (KGW VII/1, 252 my translation.)

This passage is somewhat different in tone from other passages Nietzsche writes in which he calls for an "aristocracy" that would take an active role in "keeping down and keeping at a distance."[4] In those passages, he also calls for "*higher men*" to declare war on the masses.[5] Significantly, in the 1883 passage, Nietzsche mentions the "Overman" rather than the "higher men."[6] The distinction, as I see it, is between those human types who have incorporated the teaching of Eternal Return, and the one who enacts it.[7] Those who criticize Nietzsche for his "political perfectionism" miss his point. Nietzsche is an "elitist," an "aristocratic radical," as he likes to be called, but he is also an "a-political German." He has no political program to offer. However, those same critics who are wrong about condemning Nietzsche's political perfectionism are also wrong about praising his ethical perfectionism.[8] As the above passage shows—and there are many others that say the same thing—Nietzsche is not interested in educating the masses. He thinks that they are just fine as they are, with their morality and their religion. His main fear is that the higher types will be brought down to the same level. This must be avoided at all cost, even if it means causing pain and hardship.

If Nietzsche is neither a political nor an ethical perfectionist,[9] can his teaching offer any form of therapy? How can anyone benefit from his teaching? There are occasions when he admits that his writings can only hurt and cause distress.[10] But how can philosophy do otherwise? In the past, philosophers from Plato to Hegel have all declared war on commonly held opinions, but Nietzsche goes beyond them. It is not enough for him to reject beliefs held by the unenlightened masses. He believes that the whole structure of valuations and interpretation presumed by the philosophical tradition itself needs to be overturned: not just new values, not just new meanings, however "deep" they might be. Nietzsche wants new ways of valuing, new ways of living, new ways of sensing. The paradox of such an endeavor, and what makes it so daunting, is that in order to accomplish it one must first destroy, even if it means threatening the life that one has cherished, and has relied upon for nourishment, hitherto.

This, I think, is one of the clearest motives behind Nietzsche's doctrine of the Eternal Return. The realization that one's "sins" will not be redeemed in an afterlife—for, there is no "afterlife"—and that there are no absolute criteria for judging those who have harmed us, has the potential for crushing us. But then the realization that having given up the hope for redemption in an afterlife, or even the comfort of living within the framework of long established values, could give rise to a great sense of liberation. By incorporating the past, all of it not just what floats on the surface of our consciousness, we can become creators: to learn that however much we are children of our past, we can remain innocent in the face of our becoming. Usual strategies of survival will have to be replaced by uncharted experimentations. It is doubtful if any one of us can live without any strategies of survival, without any compromise with our past—only an Overman, the one beyond humanity and its exigencies could do that—but we can risk enough of our old selves to attain a measure of "critical freedom."[11]

So, if Nietzsche can offer medicine for our illness, it is bitter medicine, indeed. Curing ourselves involves risks. Still, he provides a context, one which could soothe the pains of self-overcoming. He tells us that there are forces active in us—he calls them "Will to Power"—which are far stronger then our conscious selves.[12] We need only to trust them, make them our friends. He also describes for us three possible ways of life: the one in which drives are in complete chaos, the one in which drives are consciously repressed, and one in which a great number of drives are organized as a unity. He invites those who are willing to make the experiment, to cultivate the last, the best. Ordinary human beings, such as ourselves, will strive cautiously to maintain an optimum balance of unity and diversity; taking care that we do not exceed the limits of what we are capable of. But, Nietzsche demands more of those who are to be the true therapist of culture: they must risk passing over the limits of what they can. In other words, they must, if they are to be true innovators, go to the limit without any precise notion of where that limit might be. What Nietzsche considers to be a healthy culture is one which has unity, in diversity. Once such a culture is achieved, it will be possible for its members[13] also to attain a healthy constitution. However, to achieve that, the "higher men" of today must be open to dangerous experiments with diversity even if they, themselves, break before attaining the required degree of unity.[14]

Nietzsche's highly laudatory remarks about Spinoza in his letter to Overbeck are well-known. What is perhaps less well known is that in his later[15] writings, he is sharply critical of Spinoza's doctrine of *conatus*—what he often calls, misleadingly, "the instinct of self-preservation." It is undeniable that there are deep affinities between their views on ontology (denial of transcendence, denial of teleology) and their ethics (denial of moral values, linking virtue and freedom to power). Consequently, one needs to pause at Nietzsche's hostility to Spinoza on this point.[16] He seems to interpret Spinoza's: "Each thing, as far as it can by its own power, strives to preserve in its existence"[17] as "each thing strives to conserve itself in the state that it actually finds itself." But this is not Spinoza's point. His point is a deeply ontological-ethical one. He wants to account for how *potentia*, the infinite power of the universe to be and to become (to act), is actualized in individual beings: to account for what constitutes their power to be and to act.[18] Given the ambiguities I have mentioned in connection with his own doctrine of "Will to Power," one would expect Nietzsche to be more accommodating on this point. Nevertheless, Nietzsche's insistence that Will to Power strives to be more, to exceed and to overcome, cannot be ignored. If Spinoza's *conatus* concept is to account for individuation, Nietzsche's Will to Power concept is to account, also, for dis-individuation. But, how is one to make sense of this, especially, in view of Nietzsche's claim that "The highest man would have the greatest multiplicity of drives, in the relatively greatest strength that can be endured?"[19] Does that not suggest a striving for unity, however much diversity one is able to tolerate? Elsewhere he calls the "greatest man, *the bow with the greatest tension.* (KGW VII/3, 238)

It would be tempting to dismiss Nietzsche's insistence that nothing in nature seeks to preserve itself, and that everything in nature strives to overreach itself, to overpower others, as a hasty scientific hypothesis. But, I think that the source of Nietzsche's "overpower" doctrine lies elsewhere. Already, in the famous Spinoza letter to Overbeck, Nietzsche notes that there are "tremendous divergences due more to difference in time, culture and science" (KGB III/1, 111). As I hinted earlier, I do not think that whatever Nietzsche might have learned about cosmology or biology would present serious problems for Spinoza's doctrine of *conatus*. Differences in time and culture are, on the other hand, significant. Take culture, for example. In spite of Nietzsche's preoccupation with the sciences of his day, his is basically an artistic culture. And while Spinoza flirts with the idea of loss of self-identity,[20] he does not consider how artistic creativity, or even the contemplation of works of art, might play a role in rearranging the internal structure of one's body-soul, or the external relation one's body-soul enjoys with others. However, by far the most significant source of difference in their divergent views on Power is the time in which they lived.

Why does Nietzsche, the great advocate for the revitalization of culture, accept that those whose task it is to carry out that task will be extremely vulnerable? Why does he warn that "Strange as it sounds, one always has to defend the strong against the weak; the fortunate against the unfortunate?" (KGW VIII/3, 96, 1888, WP 685). Or again, why does he believe that, "The richest and most complex forms – for the expression 'higher type' means no more than this – perish more easily?" (KGW VII/3, 109, WP 684). His answer is that this is so because "only the lowest preserve an apparent indestructibility" (ibid). There is a paradox here, how can Nietzsche, the advocate of life, have such a low opinion of the instinct of survival? How can he accept that his heroes, the champions of the future, be so extremely vulnerable? The answer, in my opinion, is that he is writing at the time when that modernity that Spinoza had championed has exhausted itself. Whereas Spinoza saw the great merit of democratic institutions in their contribution to social and political stability, for Nietzsche, the cost of this stability was too high. It led to mediocrity and to the debasing of culture. So, he cared less about the survival of individuals, even of the exceptional ones, than he cared about breathing new life into culture. The exceptional ones, the creators whom Nietzsche also calls "legislators," will have to make the highest sacrifice for their creation: their own survival.[21] This, in turn, will inspire others to cultivate new experiments in thinking and sensing and to encouraging them to take risks with new forms of life and new forms of expression.[22]

The conclusion is unavoidable: Nietzsche attaches a higher value to life lived intensely than to a life lived within the comfort and security of hitherto existing norms. He warns those who feel themselves superior to the present to avoid contact with those values that dominate at present. They should not seek to change the values sustaining life as it is lived at present, and certainly, they should avoid using those values as "devices of leadership": "The values of the weak prevail because the strong have taken them over as devices of leadership."[23] Much of Nietzsche's harsh language can be explained by this. He considered the instinct of survival, the will to deprive life of its tragic joy, as a curse. He saw this as a great danger to culture and to those who had the potential to give it a new energy. His great fear, and love, was for them, and for their task. He feared that they abandon, and betray, the calling which was theirs: to make life, here on earth, in its tragic beauty a source of joy, once more.[24]

If we now come back to the question "of what use is Nietzsche's philosophy for life?" The answer I offer in this paper is that it is harmful for the life as we now live it. But, it promises another life, not an after-life, but one which we can live on this earth, in the time that is allowed to us. As beings thrown into this world we can "throw" ourselves further, once again. Is everyone today ready for this new life? Certainly not! But no one is prevented from taking a first step in its direction, if they so will. And, by taking this first step one might, if circumstances are favorable, allow for as much diversity as one's nature, and those circumstances—their cultural surroundings—permit. But there needs to be those who embrace this new life fully, regardless of the immediate dangers it involves. These will be the ones to create a newly revived culture, and, perhaps—along the way—those who are willing to join them.

Notes

1 The idea of Eternal Return is first introduced in the penultimate section of Book Four of *Gay Science* (GS 341), which is immediately followed by the section entitled: *Incipit Tragoedia*, ushering in Zarathustra.

2 The question of audience in Nietzsche's writings is an important one. For example, Z can easily be misread if one loses sight of who speaks, and to whom. In other works, too, it is important to know to whom Nietzsche is speaking, and in what voice. Who is his audience in *The Birth of Tragedy*? Is it Wagner? Is it the philological community? Or in the *Second Untimely Meditations*, is it his philologist critics? Is it the youth of his time? Each of his work is addressed to some specific audience, and what that is, provides a clue as to what is at stake for Nietzsche in that work. In my view, in his later writings, both published and unpublished, Nietzsche addresses an increasingly narrow audience, including himself.

3 These are the manuscripts M III 4b (7[1]-[274], of the Colli-Montinari edition. They treat of questions of morality making reference to earlier works and anticipating later ones. This passage does not occur in *Will to Power*, (WP) an arbitrary selection (and re-arrangement) of passages, made by Nietzsche's sister after his death. By now, thanks to the work of Colli and Montinari, we have a reliable edition of Nietzsche's unpublished writings. And, while I do not share Heidegger's view that they represent Nietzsche's essential thought, I find them to be valuable indicators of the way his thinking had developed.

4 See, for example, *Beyond Good and Evil*, (BG) 257 and 211. In BG 211 (KGW VI/2, 148) he says: "*Genuine philosophers . . . are commanders and legislators*" (Nietzsche's italics).

5 "A declaration of war on the masses by *higher man* is needed!" (KGW VII/2, 56) 1884; (WP: 861).

6 In Z IV "higher man" has a rather pejorative connotation, which it does not have in later writings. But, even then, the distinction between "Overman" and "higher man" is made clearer, than it seems to be in this passage.

7 The "dice throw" as it is presented by Deleuze helps to illustrate this point. In a sense, even the higher men risk being bad "gamblers," that is, they bring a little of their conscious memories, fears, and expectations into their actions and decisions: their "throws." They also forget at times that they are thrown by necessity themselves. And, when they "throw" themselves unselfconsciously, they risk destruction. It is only the Overman that can act completely freely by affirming all of necessity: being destroyed and re-created eternally. That is why throwing oneself freely is to throw oneself beyond the human condition. Great historical figures, in great historical moments, can attain, but only for a moment, the highest form of freedom. These are the ones Nietzsche sees as true creators of new worlds, new values. What shocks us in Nietzsche is the human sacrifices he is prepared to tolerate in order to attain such men, in such moments: see, for example, "a good and healthy aristocracy . . . [should accept] with a good conscience the sacrifice of untold human beings who for its sake, must be reduced and lowered to incomplete human beings, to slaves, to instruments." (BG 258: KGW VI/2, 216).

8 Richard Rorty is a prime example of such critic. See, for example, his "Moral Identity and Private Autonomy," in *Essays on Heidegger and Others*, p. 194.

9 In spite of a number of vague references to the need for strong aristocratic individuals who would rule over society, there is ample evidence that, upon clear reflection, by "rule," Nietzsche could not have meant "political rule." He thinks that however "boring" democratic institutions may be, they are both useful and unavoidable (WS 289). Also, he thinks that any involvement in actual politics is bound to demean higher spirits (15 [79] 1888]. The reason he cannot be called an "ethical perfectionist" is that his aim is not the increase human happiness. His aim is to create the spiritual conditions for an intensified human existence.

10 See, for example, GS 325.

11 I owe this term to Paul Patton. He distinguishes between "positive freedom" as autonomy and "critical freedom" as the freedom to change. See his *Deleuze & the Political* (London: Routledge: 2000), pp. 83–5. In the same context, Patton introduces the distinction between "relative" and "absolute" deterritorialization. This distinction corresponds to what the "higher man" and what the Overman is capable of.

12 "Will to Power" is best seen as a direct, and unconscious, expression of power in action (what Spinoza understands by *potentia)*; and not as a, conscious, wish to attain power under one of its representations (as a *potestas*, again in Spinoza's terminology). In spite of his numerous attacks on teleology, there are times when Nietzsche speaks of power as if it were a goal sought by the *will*. In other words, in his many discussions of "Will to Power," the distinction between power as *potentia* and power as *potestas* is not always clear. His most problematic comments on "Will to Power" occur in passages where he flirts with political aristocratism. See BGE 257 and 259, for example.

13 At this point, the question of whether the "crowd" will also be transformed in a revitalized (tragic) culture has to be addressed. From the passage I quoted earlier (KGW VII/1,252), it follows that Nietzsche thinks that morality will not cease to be normative for the crowd in any cultural context. Yet, it is difficult to accept that a revitalized culture would have no effect on the lives of all citizens. The way to avoid a possible tension here would be to say, that in a tragic culture the crowd will still

follow moral norms, but it would recognize their contingency. These norms would still be "imposed" on it—but now only conditionally—by the example of those who have spiritual-cultural authority, and not simply by political power.

14 Some have suggested that Nietzsche made that experiment himself, and broke (down) in the process.

15 The letter to Overbeck is dated July 30 1881. There are criticisms of Spinoza already in notes written around the same time. See, for example KGW V/2, 415. However, the virulence of Nietzsche's attacks on *conatus* does not appear till years later. It is possible that as time went on he began to assimilate Spinoza's views to Darwin's (or, more accurately to Spencer's), thereby distorting it.

16 Some of Nietzsche's comments on Spinoza verge on the abusive.

17 *Ethics* Part III, Proposition 6.

18 Although he does not say so, it is possible that Nietzsche's aversion to the notion of "infinite force," stated several times in the notes, written also in the summer of 1881, might also have extended to Spinoza's notion of "infinite substance." This question will be relevant to a more serious confrontation of the two philosophers than I am willing to enter into here.

19 KGW VII/2, 289, 1884, (WP: 966). See also BG 212.

20 See, for example, his story about a Spanish poet who lost all memory of his previous self, and Spinoza's conjecture that one might be persuaded that one is not the same person one was as a child. *Ethics* Part IV, Proposition 39.

21 Schopenhauer's vivid description of the cost to the artist involved in creating a work of art (at the end of Book III of *The World as Will and Representation,* Vol. I, p. 267) was, I think, a decisive factor in determining Nietzsche's conception of those who needed to be protected, both from themselves, and from the "herd."

22 In short, the difference between Spinoza and Nietzsche is that the first warns his best readers to be aware of their limits, whereas the second urges his best readers to transgress them. That is the reason why Spinoza is primarily a teacher of ethics: how to seek the good life; whereas Nietzsche is not. He does not teach how to be happy, he teaches how to become other, how to acquire a new sensibility.

23 KGW VIII/3, 249, 1888, WP: 863. It is significant that at the beginning of this note Nietzsche writes "NB NB" emphasizing its importance. I know of no other example where he does this.

24 *The Birth of Tragedy* would fit the description of "monumental history." Notwithstanding the fact it, as well as the work introducing the concept of "monumental history": *The Advantages and Disadvantages of History for Life,* are relatively early (1870–73); the "classic age of the Greeks" continued to be a key point of reference for Nietzsche's thinking about cultural revival. He looked to it, and wanted his disciples to look to it, for inspiration.

8

Nietzsche's Agonistic Rhetoric and its Therapeutic Affects

Yunus Tuncel

Nietzsche's writing style is often characterized as bellicose, with its abundance of phrases borrowed from war terminology, such as *Streitschrift* and *Streifzüge*, for subtitles or chapter headings of his books. His texts are strewn with aggressive words and phrases, and there is almost no historical figure of importance—of those who appear in his writings—whom Nietzsche does not attack. Even Heraclitus gets a punch, albeit a rare occurrence, in *Twilight of the Idols*. Many readers, including some of his contemporaries, have found his style unpleasant or perhaps vulgar, without asking some fundamental questions as to why and in what spirit Nietzsche attacks and what the contexts for his attacks are.

There are at least two important areas that play a significant role in the development of Nietzsche's bellicose style from its earlier stages: Greek rhetoric and Greek agonistics. For Nietzsche, rhetoric,[1] that art of persuasion and embellished speech, is autochthonously related to language, not simply because language is its medium, but mostly because rhetoric, just like language, is an interpretive and a *fictional* scheme. Therefore, rhetoric is effective insofar as it *uses* the basic elements of language and language-making. In his lectures, Nietzsche presents these basic elements as *tropes* of speech. Since the domain of rhetoric is public, and for Nietzsche to be public ought to mean to be agonistic, rhetoric is almost always conceived as agonistic by him.[2] In this article, I will examine Nietzsche's agonistic rhetorical[3] tactics, including how he attacks, whom he attacks, his motives for his attacks, and his position in the games of agon that he plays. Before doing so, I will briefly discuss some of the building blocks of Nietzsche's agonistic spirit, as influenced by his studies of ancient Greece, and his conception of agonistic power and the will to power. Moreover, as I shall show, there are healing aspects of agonistic practices, not only at the level of direct engagement with an opponent, but also in their other dimensions such as training and dietary regimes. I will show how and why Nietzsche may have considered agonistics as a therapeutic cultural formation.

Nietzsche's agonistics: An introduction

Most of Nietzsche's knowledge of agonistics comes from ancient Greek authors and his older contemporaries such as Jacob Burckhardt and Ernst Curtius. It is necessary to briefly present the basic elements of Greek agon,[4] before I discuss in the later part of the chapter how these elements appear in his texts or in their subtexts.

Agon and myth.[5] The *agonal* age of ancient Greece was a mythic age. The spirit of agon trickled down from gods to mortals. At the top of the hierarchy are the gods who oversaw contest games in their own sacred precincts (Zeus and Hera at Olympia, for instance); these gods themselves were agonistic and competed among each other. Among these, one can count the contest between Apollo and Hermes in footrace and wrestling and the contest for the golden apple between Hera, Athena, and Aphrodite; there are many fights among gods, but not all fights can be said to be agonistic in the narrow sense of the word, or as the Greeks understood it in their *agonal* age. Then there were heroes from older times who had achieved great deeds, like Pelops and Heracles. Each major contest site is associated with a hero and his cult; according to one thesis, contest games originated from the cult of the dead hero and the games organized to his honor, as in the funeral games for Patroclus. Another possible origin that has its roots in the Homeric literature is that agon is a part of a social event as in marriage rites and wedding ceremonies. A third possibility has to do with fertility rites. Poets of ancient Greece not only transmitted these agon sagas (like Homer and Hesiod), but later on became integral elements of the actual contest games, as they developed *epinikea*, a poetic genre that is dedicated to the victor (like Simonides, Bacchylides, and Pindar). Nietzsche had an intimate and in-depth knowledge of the agonistic nature of Greek mythology.

On the sacred in agon. Contest games in ancient Greece were organized as religious festivals. The rituals of these festivals revolved around the sacred (that which heals) and included offerings and animal sacrifices to appease local gods and heroes. There were holy persons (priests and religious functionaries) who monitored the sites and organized the necessary rituals. Neither the role of the sacred nor the role of sacrificial rites in agon can be underestimated. All contestants, *by way of a symbolic connection*, considered themselves to be both sacred and the sacrifices for their gods and heroes and were thereby disposed toward death. Violence, injuries, blood-spilling, and readiness for death while fighting in these contest games can thus be explained. Therefore, both winning and losing were already modulated according to a sacrificial disposition. Losing, however painful and shameful for a contestant, could be understood from this standpoint.

Violence, cruelty, and destruction. Contest games in ancient Greece were public events (often in the form of festivals) for trained and selected contestants to compete with their approximate equals in their fields under agreed-upon norms. These games were violent and often resulted in injuries and death. As such, they were outlets for violence and destruction. Nietzsche frequently discusses the necessity for a culture to have such outlets. Contest releases all the destructive forces of the individual who, in contest, is governed by feelings of envy, hatred, and ambition; however, the individual is also restrained within the framework of the contest. Therefore, his ambition has to be reciprocally balanced directly by his enemies and limited indirectly by the other forces of agon. As Nietzsche observes, "contest releases the individual, and at the same time, it binds the individual according to eternal laws."[6] Here lies the poetic/philosophical genius of ancient Greece in transforming the bad Eris (Strife) into the good Eris, a point Nietzsche makes in "Homer's Contest," and repeats elsewhere in his notes: "The poet overcomes the struggle for existence by idealizing it into a free contest." (KSA 7, 16 [15])

Transfiguration of war. Nietzsche considers agon a transfiguration of war and discusses this theme by way of Hesiod and Heraclitus in his early works. The philosopher, like Heraclitus, transfigures war into a playful contest as he sees the world as play (KSA 7, 16 [17]). Consequently, the poetic genius of idealization (as in Homer or Hesiod) and the philosophical genius of transfiguration (as in Heraclitus) coincide in the culture of *agon*. Many of Nietzsche's tropes of war are, in fact, derived from the culture of competition. Why Nietzsche uses tropes of war when he means contest can be explained by way of the proximity between agon and war in antiquity. However, this proximity should not be read as sameness. The culture of agon stood by itself, with its own rituals, institutions, and sites in ancient Greece.

Agonal feelings. There are certain feelings in the culture of competition that are vital for striving and fighting; these are envy, hate, and ambition. No doubt, these feelings must have their own context and be expressed in their proper doses. Nietzsche considers these feelings *necessary* for any contest. Contestants must envy the prize of contest, victory, and all others things that are emblematic of agon, such as athletic heroes. They must hate their enemies (or opponents), who are their equals, but not despise them (as Zarathustra teaches his disciples in "On War and Warriors"). Finally, contestants must have ambition to struggle and to win the game.

Agonal justice. Contests in ancient Greece were highly formal and defined by rules and rituals. It was important that all contestants abided by these rules and competed fairly. Now, the spirit of fairness had to be established and sustained by some agency; this fell on the *Hellanodikai*, the judges of Greece. It is reasonable to presume that they were former contestants. The judges at Olympia, the Elisian judges, became famous all throughout antiquity for always upholding fairness—though no doubt, there could have been exceptions. These judges had the capacity to oversee contests, hold the opposing contestants together in a fair fight, be strong enough to bear the violence of the fight, flog the fouling contestant to bring him back into fair fight, and at the end, pass a fair judgment for the winner and honor the victor. In this affirmation of life forces among the judges of agon, Nietzsche must have detected a sense of justice (an "active justice" which he discusses in GM II) that is different than our traditional form of justice, which is based on revenge and retribution. The former is based on the judgment of the strong, the latter that of the weak.

Training and education. A contestant started his integral training at a young age in a gymnasium or a palaestra with an emphasis on a special field that conformed with his *physis*, which could mean "temperament," "character," and "growth" (which implies a capacity for change toward higher states). Greek education was not only based on natural talent, but it was also an individualized education. There was an intimate bond between the trainer and his pupil; through this bond and in the interaction with other pupils, the pupil learned his craft and how to be strong. Moreover, bodily education was central to this holistic education; this is why it is common to find many philosophers and politicians in ancient Greece who were also accomplished athletes. Nietzsche was cognizant of the agonistic nature of Greek training and education: "Every talent must unfold itself in fight: that is the command of Hellenic popular pedagogy . . . And just as the youths were educated through contests, their educators were also engaged in contests with each other . . ."[7] And he lamented the absence of agonistic education in his age.

From the agonistic hero to the Overhuman. One important antecedent for Nietzsche's conception of Overhuman is the Greek contestant. To put it simply, the Overhuman is Nietzsche's interpretation of the Greek agonistic hero within the context of nineteenth century Europe. Just as the older (Homeric) Greek hero crystallized into the later athletic hero through the functions of heroization in the *agonal* age, all the tendencies and struggles for overcoming and striving for higher states were transfigured into the Overhuman by Nietzsche. Although the historical contexts are different, there are many parallels between the two at the symbolic level. They both symbolize struggle and self-transformation through toil and rigorous training. They both entail a sculpting of the self through the regimes of the soul and the body. They both accept or even embrace suffering and affirm life forces. Finally, they both exist (can exist) in an openly acknowledged hierarchical world. A Greek athlete, like Nietzsche's Overhuman, knows how to look up (to his trainers, judges, heroes, and gods), down (those who are less than him), and also sideways (*inter pares*).

Spectacle and festival of contests. One important aspect of Greek agon was that it was public to a large extent, and contest games were organized as part of a festival (festivals were opening up of cults to public with different degrees of openness). In fact, many Greek authors use words that mean "festival" as the synecdoches of the whole event. Many people came from different parts of the Greek world (they were not, however, open to all) to watch the games and become part of the festival, which included, in addition to the games, many communal activities and religious services. In some period of the history of Olympic games, philosophers, historians, and poets were said to have visited Olympia to become famous, since they had the best possible audience from the Greek world. Both Burckhardt and Nietzsche were drawn to such ancient festivals where communal functions were infused with a noble sentiment and art and religion could coexist in their heightened states as they reinforced one another. Finally, the spectators formed the collective unconscious for the public fights of contestants. In this way, the culture of agon rejuvenated itself in spectacles and festivals that were accompanied by music.

Finally, the culture of agon has, at least, two other symbolic elements: the first is *agon*[8] in the broad sense which is the symbolic assembly space, or sometimes the physical place, of the competing forces. The second symbolic element has to do with contests in which the agonists contend for a prize or for victory, which the ancient Greeks called *athlos*, from the verb *athleuein*, which is the root of the word "athlete." While the former refers to the whole economy of the agonistic forces and underlies the *process* of the struggle and the *process* of producing the agonistic subject in struggle including its pedagogy, the latter refers to the outcome-driven competition. Nietzsche emphasizes the former without dismissing the latter; in fact, he places the *athlos* within the larger context of agon.

Agonistic power

Nietzsche's later development of his conception of power is, in many ways, prefigured in the agonistic philosophy of his early works. I do not suggest here that power is only agonistic for Nietzsche, but agonistic power is pervasive in his philosophy of power and can be seen in many of his reflections on power and in the many formulations of the will to power. Below I will present some aspects of Nietzsche's agonistic conception of power.

First of all, what Zarathustra learns from life on power (TSZ II, "Self-Overcoming") is that power is about obeying and commanding; that is, it is about a hierarchy whether it is within the individual or within a community. It is important to remember here that *agon* takes place in a highly hierarchical world although the contest itself occurs among more or less equals. Even if there is less of a hierarchy among the contestants, one can still talk about a relation of obeying and commanding among them as one contestant is ahead of the other in the game and commands in this way.

The second agonistic teaching of life has to do with the desire to be master; in the contest, this is the desire to be the victor. In winning the contest, the victor has gained mastery over his or her weaknesses and also over the weaker contestants. Third, the weak have to serve the strong; the losing contestants must accept their defeat and look up to the strong. Here the mythic hierarchy facilitates the acceptance of defeat since all contestants, the strong or the weak, look up to their gods and heroes as exemplary models of strength. The fourth teaching has to do with self-overcoming (TSZ II, "Self-Overcoming") Life is overcoming: man is something that has to be overcome toward the Overhuman (*Übermensch*). In contest, one is always striving to be higher than what one already is at least until the end of the actual contest. The idea of transforming oneself as one strives higher, which is one meaning of the Overhuman, is already an agonistic idea. The fifth teaching of life is that it is oppositional: "Whatever I create and however much I love it—soon I must oppose it and my love; thus my will wills it." Opposition is the fuel for self-overcoming; the contestant opposes not only his enemies in strife but also the prize itself if he becomes the victor. He gives up the prize for his polis and her gods. He cannot remain as the permanent victor. On the one hand, the victor can always be displaced in the round; on the other hand, because of this possibility of loss, the victor is compelled to continue with his discipline and training. In this way, contest renews itself; so do the contestants. Here lies the importance of competition as a process of renewal, a process in which power flows and power dynamics are constantly shifting.

Moreover, one of Nietzsche's concerns in his philosophy of power is how individuals, given their uniqueness, can find their place in the chain of power relations within in their historical contexts. One already detects this in *Daybreak* perhaps in his first insightful observations on power where he problematizes both impotence and lust for power and searches for a golden mean in power (Aphorism 23). In the first appearance of the term "will to power" in Nietzsche's *Nachlass*, he brings up exactly this power problematic:

> The main element of ambition is to come to the feeling of its power. The joy of power is not to trace back onto that which we rejoice, to remain admired in the opinion of others. Praise and blame, love and hate are the same for the ambition seeker (the ambitious) who wills power.
>
> Fear of power (negative) and will to power (positive) explain our strong regard for the opinion of human beings.
>
> Power lust—the lust for power can be explained by the dislike (or disgust) of dependence or powerlessness, experienced in a hundred (thousand) ways. (KSA 8, p. 351, translation is mine)

Fear of power and lust for power are equally problematic. And it is not even sufficient to say in an Apollinian way "know your power in a given hierarchy," because power relations are always shifting. Nonetheless, what is at stake for Nietzsche is to find one's *own* place in power relations, as individuals, as collective bodies, and most importantly, as an epoch. I believe that Nietzsche sees in *agon* the function of a power arbiter, since *agonal* dynamics place the struggling individuals on the horizontal and vertical structures of power relations according to their strengths and weaknesses within the context of the struggle. Individual struggle under the same conditions determines who the strong contestant is in a specific constellation.

Furthermore, the will to power is an agonistic concept in the following ways: on the one hand, it refers to the competing forces as in lateral power relations and, on the other hand, it is what holds the competing forces together and as such symbolizes the hierarchical, that is, vertical power relations (this is the relationship between the stronger and the weaker); it is, at the same time, the agonistic individual force and the agonistic unity. The competing forces expand, appropriate, assimilate, and resist; these are the qualitative functions of the forces that are fighting, which are also quantitative. "The will to power can manifest itself only against resistances; therefore it seeks that which resists it . . . Appropriation and assimilation are above all a desire to overwhelm, a forming, shaping and reshaping, until at length that which has been overwhelmed has entirely gone over into the power domain of the aggressor and has increased the same . . ." (WP 656) Pleasure and displeasure are, among others, feelings that underlie these forces: expansion of power, victory, and mastery as being pleasurable, and defeat or inability to resist as being unpleasurable (WP 703). I want to emphasize here that, for Nietzsche, pleasure and displeasure are not detached from one another, as cut by a razor blade.[9] On the contrary, fighting itself is full of suffering, and the state of displeasure is not lacking in the economy of the feeling of the agonist even if he becomes the victor. Agon, moreover, as an institution and a structure, is a manifestation of this mastery, where "man becomes master over the forces of nature, master over his own savagery and licentiousness . . .—man, in comparison with a pre-man—represents a tremendous quantum of *power*. . ." (WP 704)

Deleuze, in *Nietzsche & Philosophy*, also highlights this double aspect of the will to power: "We should not be surprised by the double aspect of the will to power: from the standpoint of the genesis or production of forces it determines the relation between forces, but, from the standpoint of its own manifestations, it is determined by relating forces."[10] The former applies to the agonistic unity that holds all competing forces together, the latter to the competing forces themselves. In this way, the will to power is determining (it creates the structure, the rules, in which the agonists compete) and is determined (this is how all the contestants affect the sum total of that agon in a particular context). Agon then presents itself as a fluid, protean formation that is affected and affecting, or to use Deleuze's terms, that is qualified and qualifying. According to Nietzsche, this would be one cultural formation that approximates life itself, its vitality amid the cycle of creation, growth, and destruction. This is what, in another work[11] and within the context of Nietzsche's early works, I called "the cycle of agon" through which the agonistic microcosmos (mythology, polis, the structure of agon) and the agonistic individual reciprocally enhance one another.

Agonistic *Askesis* and its therapeutic aspects

One may ask oneself how attacking and being attacked can have any therapeutic effect on the individual. This way of approaching the subject, however, not only sidesteps the larger world of agon, which I tried to illustrate above in summary, but also undermines the dynamics of agon at its microlevel. There are many forms of healing, which are at the disposal of a culture and which its members can use depending on their individual type and constitution. Agonism can be construed as a form of healing. In what follows, I will try to show in several points how agonistic practices can have functions of healing both for an individual and for a culture.

Discharge of cruelty and aggression within the bounds of a cult defined by myth. Freud, in his *Civilization and its Discontents*, diagnoses *thanatos* as a major impediment to culture[12] and sees it as the seat of all aggression and destruction. Nietzsche, on the other hand, considers it, though in his own terms, a challenge toward higher forms of creation. Both thinkers accept aggression as a fundamental human condition that must be reckoned with, although they would not agree on the ways of reckoning. Nietzsche, for instance, would not accept that aggression can be talked away in psychotherapy or that bodily regimes can be replaced by soul regimes. Aggression must have its own externalization in its own appropriate outlet depending on the type, the degree, and the dose of aggression; for instance, combat sports and those of track and field would not be on the same level of aggressivity. Expression of aggressive forces in culturally acceptable forms will have their own therapeutic effect both for the individual and the culture.

Rechanneling of destructive forces from war into agon. One central aspect of agon that was attractive to the young Nietzsche was the transformation of war into contest, whether that was in myth and poetry as in Hesiod's Eris or in Heraclitus' wisdom of transfiguration. War and agon have one thing in common: they are both expressions of the cycle of destruction. However, while agon recognizes the endless playfulness of conflicting forces, war ends it and as such relies on teleological view of existence. This is not to say that the agonist does not erect any goals on the way, but this goal-setting does not marginalize or eradicate the playful process; the agonist, unlike the warrior, wants his opponent to live so that he can keep playing. There is no therapy in war for the individual player; it may be the end of all therapy for him.

Thumotics of feeling.[13] Agonistic practices call for a specific arrangement of human feelings: an open hatred and love of the enemy; envy of the victor and striving for victory; love among contestants or what can be called "athletic erotics"; and *Machtgefühl* (sense of power). Two points on healing can be raised here: first, the necessity for the discharge of such intense emotions as hate, envy, and ambition within culturally accepted formations and second, the need to learn how to exercise power within lateral and vertical structures. Nietzsche himself did not bring agon and power together since the former appears mostly in his early writings while the latter mostly in his late writings. An agonistic conception of power and its therapeutic effects, however, can be elicited out of Nietzsche's works.

Active justice. Agonistic practices call for an active justice that is based on strength and the demands and aspirations for being strong. This is how the Greek judges of contest games assessed competitions and how the rites and rituals of these games expected all participants to abide by the demands of active justice. Nietzsche's notion of active justice, which he reconstructs (to a large extent in GM I and II) in opposition to our customary reactive, retributive justice, was shaped by such an agonistic practice of active justice.

Regimes of exercise. Agonism promotes bodily regimes; after all, a major portion of agonistic games in ancient Greece were athletic games. The nonathletic games, as in drama, music, and signing, did not necessarily exclude bodily practices either. Therefore, the agonist had to train his body for the contest games and follow a strict diet, as he was prepared in other fields that were necessary for his overall upbringing. Here we must not forget the erotic practices of Greek athletes and trainers; such practices also belong to bodily regimes. An active body is already self-therapeutic. Nietzsche's discussion of *askesis* in *On the Genealogy of Morals* does not preclude all forms of *askesis*, but only those exercises that deny, in any form, bodily functions in their multiple aspects, as in ascetic idealism. As Horst Hutter states,[14] Nietzsche himself is calling for a new regime of *askesis*, which, to a large extent, is informed by ancient Greek agonistic practices.

Struggle for higher states, learning how to be strong and how to exercise power. Because agon can exist only in a highly hierarchical world—as our age refuses to understand—an agonist learns the dynamic, the polysemic, and the multidirectional forms of power. Therefore, an agonist can look up and down as much as he can look sideways. He knows his place in the vertical and horizontal power relations, but this place is never a static place. He rises or falls with his struggles, changing his position in the world of agon. But why and how can being adept in the exercise of power be therapeutic? As

Nietzsche and recent thinkers of power like Foucault and Deleuze have shown, power exercise is pervasive to our basic human condition. Many of our social ills stem from shunning power and not developing healthy forms and exercises of power. An agonist shuns neither and accepts to face his approximately equal enemy (in an open, lateral power relation) and the end-result of the game received by the judge and the agonistic community (in an open, vertical power relation).

Community. In ancient Greece, agonistic practices took place in communal forms in which all of the participants from priests and judges to athletes and spectators came together to observe the rituals of contest games. They were festive and spectacular events, which bound the competitive forces together in an ecstatic communion at at least three different strata of community-building: (a) they helped create a community around the gymnasium/palaestra within the *polis*; (b) they fostered communal bonds among different *poleis*, despite on-going hostilities among some of them; and (c) a spirit of community evolved out of the forces of competition. Nietzsche's attraction to Greek agon cannot be understood solely because of his ideas on great individualism and the *Übermensch*, but also because the *agonal* culture of ancient Greece offered a different paradigm of communal assembly, a paradigm that helps heal the soul of individuals and culture at the same time.

Agonistic praxis and attacks

What interests me the most in this regard is how Nietzsche himself practices *agon* and how he exercises agonistic power as a writer and as a thinker. I will first start with general principles that Nietzsche lays forth and then speculate on the symbolism and functionality of his attacks.[15] In *Ecce Homo*,[16] he presents four propositions as his war-praxis, which, in fact, is his *agon-praxis*; briefly, they are:

1. To attack victorious causes (which means, to attack those who have established themselves as strong);
2. To attack alone with no allies since agon is an individual strife (in the spirit of Olympic Greeks Nietzsche does not consider group contests);
3. Not to attack persons (or out of personal reasons, grudges, etc.) but to attack for the sake of greatness in culture;
4. To attack out of good will, even out of gratitude (not out of revenge or *ressentiment*).

It is not only that Nietzsche *wants* to have enemies whom he can attack; his conception of life itself is agonistic, as one senses it *consistently* in his texts. ". . . life itself is *essentially* appropriation, injury, overpowering of the strange and the weaker, suppression, severity, imposition of one's own forms, incorporation, and, at the least and mildest, exploitation . . ." (BGE 259). Although many weak-hearted readers may shudder at these qualifiers, for Nietzsche, contest always occurs in a context, and they describe agonistic struggles and states. Later in *On the Genealogy of Morals*, he writes of nobles who adventure, expand, and attack; it is the nature of their agonistic power. In what follows, I will make some observations on how Nietzsche attacks and what he considers the function of agonistic attacks to be.

How does Nietzsche attack? The following can be some indications for this: fast tempo; indication of movement—an attack intensifies when the attacker is on the move, like the Asiatics of the steppe who shot arrows on horseback; fast blood circulation; excitement; anxiety of victory or defeat with an acknowledgment of one or the other; and anxiety of public performance before an adversary (note that Nietzsche is most aggressive in his published or to be published writings); plunging unto the unknown; and finally fear of death. The following are some examples—and many others exist—for how Nietzsche attacks and his state of mind before, during, and after his attacks:

1. *Dancing around the opponent and a punch or a series of punches*. Nietzsche's attacks against Socrates in BT and TI can be cited here; Socrates must have known close quarter fighting to be able to serve in the army and his ugly nose may have been the result of a blow. In BT, Nietzsche warms up with Euripides before Socrates shows up in the ring; and even then he dances for a while (sec.11 and beginning of sec.12) before he starts throwing his punches (the first big blow comes at the end of sec.12). Dancing around Socrates, he keeps boxing. In TI, on the other hand, there is not much dancing, but a series of blows. Twelve blows altogether— is Socrates knocked out? We shall never know; at least, not yet, not now, not in this age of nihilism.
2. *A direct strong punch and a quick withdraw, sometimes followed by more quick punches.* For example, in the *Twilight of the Idols* against writers Renan, Sainte Beuve, Eliot, Sand, Carlyle et al. What characterizes these attacks is that they are short, some of them are made for a knockout—whether his opponents receive them or not or how they receive them is a different matter. Here is a list of Nietzsche's blows: For Renan, "nobody can equal him when it comes to adoring in a manner of endangering life itself"; for Sainte Beuve, "nothing of virility"; for Eliot "little moralistic females à la Eliot"; for Sand, "cold . . . like all the romantics"; and lastly for Carlyle "a constant passionate dishonesty against himself . . ."[17]
3. *Plunging head and shoulders to grasp, lift, and throw down the opponent as in wrestling*. With Plato, for instance; most likely Nietzsche knew that Plato was a wrestler[18] and competed at Isthmus. Plato, "the most beautiful growth of antiquity,"[19] cannot be disfigured with blows, but one can engage in a wrestling match with his oily body. When Nietzsche attacks Plato, he often uses terms of refinement for him (the noble youth who is corrupted or Plato's way of thinking as noble[20]); he attacks Plato, but he touches and grasps him before doing so.
4. *A cavalry charge*[21] *with a sword or a javelin in hand*. Here we see a continuous attack that lasts for a while, until he believes he has subdued the enemy via encirclement. Nietzsche's attack against David Strauss in the first of the *Untimely Meditations* is symbolic of a cavalry charge for several reasons (for this fight to be a contest, Strauss must too be mounted on a horse waiting to combat Nietzsche): first, it comes as a surprise, almost out of nowhere; allegedly, Strauss himself had expressed how surprised he was. Second, once the stage is set in the first two sections, there is a barrage of attacks for the next ten. Such a dense attack in a short span of time is difficult to achieve on foot.
5. *An arrow*[22] *shot from a distance, often directed at the readers*. Here Nietzsche knows that he is mostly protected, perhaps by hiding behind the bushes, but he must be aware that some readers may also be armed with a bow and be good

shooters like the disciples of Artemis. Forty-four arrows are shot at the reader in the first section of the *Twilight of the Idols*. The best way to protect oneself against arrows is to have a good shield and to know how to use it; the second best is to have a thick hide. Those who have neither will perish under Nietzsche's arrows.

6. *Fencing and the attempt to plunge with and without success.* [and Nietzsche also gets wounded several times.] Many of Nietzsche's attacks on Schopenhauer and Wagner, especially in his late writings, invoke images of fencing. Out of all the sports listed, fencing is the only sport where the instinct to kill is sublimated (or where one is very close to killing); one wants to kill, but yet one does not kill. Nietzsche darts at his adversary with a sword to kill, but does not kill.

Agonistic rhetorical tactics

In this final section of the chapter, I would like to entertain the following questions in Nietzsche's war or agon praxis: what are Nietzsche's agonistic rhetorical devices? Who or what types of figures does he attack and how does he attack them? Now we do not have an assembly place where we can watch Nietzsche's contest with his enemies; his type of contest is not in athletics. Therefore, it is symbolic, and many of the forces of agon, such as gods, judges, and the prizes of victory, are absent or only implicitly present in the text. All of these factors make it difficult to fully bring out Nietzsche's symbolic contests to the surface.

Despite the difficulty, I have extrapolated three types of symbolic contests from Nietzsche's works, the shifting dynamics of which I will explore below in a sketchy way: (1) Nietzsche's contest with the "workers of the spirit," what Nietzsche calls "physicians of culture" or "value-creators"; (2) Zarathustra's contest as a judge and a contestant; and (3) Nietzsche's contest with his readers as a judge and as a contestant.

(1) Nietzsche's contest with value-creators

In this form of contest, Nietzsche chooses his more or less equals when he attacks; more often than not he seeks stronger enemies, figures who are well established in history or culture. The most recurring figures for Nietzsche's attacks, such as Socrates, Plato, Schopenhauer, and Wagner testify to this statement. In this respect, Nietzsche can be said to be agonistic although he is taking on stronger, "already victorious" enemies. Two questions, however, arise here: the first one points to a hermeneutic problem: how is Nietzsche's opponent present in the contest? We cannot expect Nietzsche to re-present his opponent; he can only call him to fight. Otherwise, it will not be an agon. How can I be a contestant and stand for my enemy at the same time? Therefore, the burden here falls on the reader who, as the spectator, if not the judge of agon, has to make Nietzsche's enemy present to the contest. This may be a challenge for the reader especially if there is a predisposition toward Nietzsche on his or her part, which may cause a mis- or an under-representation of Nietzsche's opponent. Briefly stated, one cannot *experience* Nietzsche's agon with his enemies fully unless one knows the talents and the prowess of his enemies. One cannot silence the enemy at the outset and expect this to be a contest. Being a philologist himself, one can surmise that Nietzsche would expect his readers to be familiar with those figures that he attacks; therefore, he ends up upholding the spirit of competition. As for being a judge in his contests, only time and the unfolding of history will show if Nietzsche is the victor in his agon with the other value-creators whom he perpetually attacks.

The second problem has more to do with Nietzsche and understanding his dispositions in his attacks. Here we may be guided by what motives, hopes, and feelings underlie the spirit of agon: *respect* for one's enemy even if the enemy is to be *hated*; not to see oneself as a permanent victor; not to turn the victory into hubris; to be governed by hate, envy, and ambition but in their appropriate doses; to fight under the norms of the contest and to remove every personal grudge from the spirit of competition. Every feeling that is based on weakness, such as pity, revenge (especially the mediated type), and *ressentiment*, is removed from the spirit of contest. Pity occurs in a problematic exercise of power where it is sly and manipulative; the one who invokes pity pretends to be powerless and attempts to exercise power by manipulating the other's weak sentiments and relationship to suffering. The spirit of contest calls for suffering and open power relations; weak sentiments are not promoted here. Revenge, especially the mediated type, on the other hand, is the desire of the weak to undo the strong by any means; it is a pretension of the weak to be equal to the strong. It is the most powerful weapon of the masses against strong individuals. Such a relationship is already not agonistic. Finally, *ressentiment* is reactive and rejects that which is different at the outset (GM I, sec.10) and would not, therefore, allow for a struggle with equal enemies. Those who would be enemies are already despised at the outset, not hated. In such a value-scheme, there would not be any contest, but only one ultimate ruler in whom all power is concentrated. And we have come a full circle, back to the question of the victor in *agon* and why and how, in terms of feelings, a permanent or an ultimate victor is not accepted or not desired in the culture of competition.

(2) Zarathustra's contest

Analogous to Homer, Nietzsche makes Zarathustra create the spirit of competition among his disciples as he urges them to compete. He is the judge of agon and the prize set for the victor is the achievement of an overhumanly *status* that he is teaching. I say the status, because Overhuman is not something that can be possessed but is an ongoing state. In TSZ, one senses many traces of Zarathustra's spirit of competition; in the following paragraphs I will highlight four areas based on the text.

In "On War and Warriors" (Part I), Zarathustra sets the mood of contest for his disciples. At the outset, he declares himself to be the *commander* of the warriors: he will tell them the truth of fighting. Their work should be a struggle; while others seek peace, they should fight and seek victory; they can hate their enemies but not despise them, because their success is measured on the success of their enemies; and finally, they should be great enough to have hatred and envy in their hearts. Hate and envy, as shown earlier, are two feelings that drive the spirit of competition. However, they have to manifest themselves within an agonistic context and be of the *right* (i.e., moderate) dose; excessive hate and envy will (and usually does) end the spirit of agonism. These two feelings, moreover, will propel them to fight and overcome themselves toward the Overhuman, which is given to them as a command by Zarathustra. In this particular section of the book, Zarathustra is clearly a war-like spirit, but for Zarathustra (and for Nietzsche), it is not any war or any kind of war that is waged here. What matters is that the symbolism of war is akin to that of agon, which consists of struggle, enmity, feelings that underlie them (such as hate and envy), the idea of *inter pares* (i.e., respect for the enemy), and so on. That Zarathustra is war-like does not negate the fact that he is also a *commander* with love although he *loves* in his own way; therefore, he appears to be an Empedoclean figure in this context.

A second trace of agonism can be seen in "On Free Death" where Zarathustra throws a golden ball at his disciples who are his heirs; here the golden ball, like the golden apple, is a symbol for the prize of victory. It is important to die at the right time and not to keep the prize of victory always to oneself and always to know when to step aside so that the agonistic spirit can live on. Zarathustra says: "More than anything, I like to see you, my friends, throwing the golden ball . . ."[23] More importantly, however, agon is about death; it is throwing oneself unto death in struggle without necessarily dying, an ecstatic leap into the game of the unknown. "He that consummates his life dies his death victoriously."[24] To consummate, one must *act*, and competing is a form of *acting*. "To die thus is best; second to this, however, is to die fighting and to squander a great soul . . ." In agonistic strife, one consumes oneself and dies only to be reborn in a new spirit. This is the "free death" that Zarathustra praises, because it is the death that comes to him because he wants it; it is not a death dictated by cowardice or by the preachers of slow death. In free death, one has one's individual goal and one's heir; one strives toward something higher and thus leaves a legacy behind.

Finally, Zarathustra provokes his disciples to guess the riddles he presents to them; one such scene is in "On the Vision and the Riddle": "Guess me this riddle that I saw then, interpret me the vision of the loneliest."[25] Since guessing a riddle is an individual effort to bring out the insight buried in it, all the sailors must struggle individually to unravel it. The one who guesses the riddle with the most profound insight wins the contest. Moreover, in the narration of the riddle much about the symbolism of agon is present: the high and the low (Zarathustra's height and the weight of the dwarf that pulls him down), courage (courage that attacks, playfulness of attack, courage as the best slayer), and the teaching of eternal recurrence (the mythic time of the contestant).

(3) Nietzsche's contest with his readers

Another complicated area in Nietzsche's contest is in his relationship with his readers. That Nietzsche calls for agonistic readers either implicitly or explicitly goes without saying. What I want to explore are some specific tactics Nietzsche uses vis-à-vis his readers. Here we can consider Nietzsche as a judge or as a contestant.

Nietzsche as a judge of agon. Nietzsche is more like a judge when he presents his visions and riddles, like Zarathustra, to the readers to solve. Here he is in his prophetic mood and wants to say to the reader: "I have a vision, I will present it as a riddle. Try to unravel it and you will understand my vision." Now the readers who are provoked by this vision will strive to unravel it, and the prize will be the individual understanding of the vision itself that Nietzsche is holding above the readers. Nietzsche has run the course, has become a victor, and is now assuming the role of an *agondikast*.[26] Textual examples are too many to cite, but I will mention some aphorisms to illustrate this point:

In GS 283, Nietzsche calls for "preparatory human beings" who will set the stage for a new, war-like age as he presents its agonistic building blocks, or the "norms of the contest," such as heroism, courage, victory, festivity, fighting among equals, and dangerous living. In GS 285, Nietzsche explains the path of the agonists and the process of their struggle in symbolic terms; there is nothing ultimate in this path, there are no friends and guardians as the agonist struggles alone, no resting place, and no ultimate peace. The *excelsior* as the agonist shall will the eternal recurrence of war and peace, which is the mythic, nonteleological, and nonlinear *time* of competition in the *agonal* age.[27] In GS 289, Nietzsche gives the start signal to the agonistic philosophers to discover another world that is antipodal to this moral world. A new world is needed in which the exceptional human being is no longer pitied, forced to confess or forgiven, a world in which this type of human being simply is and finds his place in the sacred order of all beings. Only the agonistic philosophers can create this new world, because they can fight and they can say "No": they are the antipodes. Finally, GS 316 is a declaration of what it means to be prophetic, what it means to be *above* others, an *agondikast*, and there are two primary, interrelated ingredients in it: suffering and being an animal (which means having open senses and a *natural* capacity to suffer). The writer's tone of voice in relation to the reader and the way he addresses him indicate that he is *looking down* on the reader: ". . . *You* have no feeling for the fact that prophetic human beings are afflicted with a great deal of suffering . . ."[28]

Nietzsche as a contestant. On the other hand, when Nietzsche makes psychological observations on human character and attacks the reader with his insights and sarcasm, he is seeking contestants who will fight back with other ideas or new insights on the same subject matter. One finds this prominently in his aphorisms[29] where he is shooting arrows at the reader. Now if the reader is strong enough, he or she may dodge the arrow or be shot, but also shoot back at Nietzsche; if not, the reader will perish or will turn bitter or will promise never to read him again. I am not suggesting here that all the strong readers of Nietzsche are Nietzsche's equals in general.

On the other hand, a strong reader may have an equally strong insight as Nietzsche on a given topic in which a contest with him can be possible. This idea of reader as a kindred and therefore agonistic spirit is suggested by Nietzsche in the opening line of the Preface to the second edition of GS when he says "this book may need more than one preface, and in the end there would still remain room for doubt whether anyone who had never lived through similar experiences could be brought closer to the *experience* of this book by means of prefaces."[30]

Epilogue

There is hardly a book written by Nietzsche published by him or intended for publication, which is not *polemical* and which does not include attacks on some historical figures, schools, or movements. Why a writer attacks and how he attacks are no doubt important, but in Nietzsche's case, it is doubly important, because for him a bellicose style in rhetoric is indicative of an agonistic practice with the underlying premise of its healing powers. Nietzsche considers contest to be a cultural agency that plays a crucial role in the production of greatness—toward heightened states such as the Overhuman—within a public arena, without which a culture would be emaciated and deprived of its basic vital function. While attempting to revive an agonistic culture,

Nietzsche also tried to revitalize the oral traditions of the past in which the eloquent speech of the speaker had an *organic* resonance in the audience, as the former was tightly bound to the latter. The speaker used a variety of agonistic functions to leave an impact on his listeners and thereby engage them in the speech. However, Nietzsche's double challenge in the revival of this oral tradition[31] and its agonism may miss our ears, and we may be doubly duped.

Notes

1 Nietzsche discusses ancient Greek rhetoric extensively in the lectures he gave at Basel on ancient rhetoric, translated into English as *Friedrich Nietzsche on Rhetoric and Language*, edited and translated by S. L. Gilman, C. Blair, and D. J. Parent (Oxford: Oxford University Press, 1989). The influence of ancient rhetoric on Nietzsche is undeniable; he uses many of the techniques of ancient rhetoric in his writings as he tries to transplant an archaic method into a modern context (with many challenges). As a result, Nietzsche's language smells ancient with a modern aura.

2 "Therefore, what is typical is broken down first by means of transference into the *cultured* domain of language, and second, through the general requisite of the 'embellishment' of speech. This is to be explained from the ancients' *agonale* [competitive] tendency—all public appearance of the individual is contest: however, not only strong weapons, but also *brilliant* ones, are suited to the combatant. One must handle the weapons not just suitably, but also beautifully; to win 'elegantly,' not to just to be victorious, is required among a people with a sense of competition" (Ibid., p. 37). As Nietzsche frequently does in his early works, here too he brings artistic creation and contest together. They are integrally interwoven; this is how it was with the Greeks and this is how it is for Nietzsche.

3 Nietzsche is not the first to use a bellicose rhetorical style in modern age. Schopenhauer's acerbic style and Marx's polemical attacks can be cited as examples from the nineteenth century. However, Nietzsche's style is distinctly imbued with the spirit of agonism.

4 The author dealt with this subject at length in an essay entitled "Agon Symbolism in Nietzsche" which appeared in Nikephoros, Volume XXII. A more comprehensive study by the author on the same subject, which engages with ancient Greek works and Nietzsche's texts appeared in *Agon in Nietzsche*, (Milwaukee: Marquette University Press, 2013).

5 I. Weiler discusses agon myths of ancient Greece extensively in his work, *Agon in Mythos* (Darmstadt: Wissenschaftliche Gesellschaft, 1974).

6 KSA 7, 16 [22].

7 "Homer's Contest," in *Portable Nietzsche*, trans. by Walter Kaufmann (New York: Penguin Books, 1968), p. 37.

8 The term "agon" was used in many different ways in ancient Greek literature from Homer to Pausanias: assembly, game, contest, and court case were some of the usages of the term.

9 For this topic, see WP 695–7, 699–704.

10 *Nietzsche & Philosophy*, trans. by Hugh Tomlinson (New York: Columbia University Press, 1983), p. 62.

11 I dealt with this issue in my doctoral dissertation, "The Principle of Agon in Nietzsche's (Ann Arbor: UMI Dissertation Services, Bell & Howell Company, 2000).

12 See *Civilization and its Discontents*, trans by Peter Gay (New York: W. W. Norton, 1961).

13 On this topic, I have benefited much from my conversations with Dr Horst Hutter.
14 *Shaping the Future: Nietzsche's New Regime of the Soul and Its Ascetic Practices* (New York: Lexington Books, 2006), p. 9.
15 The term "attack" appears profusely in Nietzsche's works, either in the substantive (*Angriff*) or the verb (*angreifen*) form. It may have originated from wrestling or close-quarter fighting because of its root *greifen*, which means to grip.
16 "Why I am So Wise," Sec.7.
17 *The Portable Nietzsche*, pp. 513–21.
18 It may be due to this and his earlier training that wrestling imagery and symbolism appears frequently in Plato's texts, more frequently than any other Greek sport. On this topic, see C. D. Corcoran, "Wrestling and the Fair Fight", *Nikephoros* 16 (2003): XVI.
19 BGE, Preface. *Basic Writings of Nietzsche*, p. 193.
20 Ibid., p. 212.
21 Nietzsche knew how to ride a horse, but his horse-riding activities were cut short due to an accident in March 1868 when he was serving in the Prussian army stationed in Naumburg. Horse race and chariot race were fields of contest in ancient Greece, but not a sword fight on horse. The closest contest game to the one described above is medieval jostling.
22 Nietzsche uses the symbolism of archery frequently in his writings, perhaps more than any other sport. Ironically, ancient Greeks did not compete in archery in their panhellenic sites, but it is a field of competition in Homer (in the funeral games for Patroclus in the *Iliad*) and was a contest game in some local festivals. As far as it is known, Nietzsche was not an archer.
23 TSZ, p.186.
24 Ibid., p. 184.
25 Ibid., p. 268.
26 Nietzsche had much knowledge of the role of the judge in Greek contests from his studies of Greek literature, and there are frequent appearances of the term "judge" or "umpire"—he often uses the German word "Richter"—in his writings. I also claim that this Greek institution and praxis of justice in agon played a significant role in Nietzsche's understanding of active justice.
27 This is the first appearance of the eternal recurrence of the same in Nietzsche's published writings. And it is presented within an agonistic context since, for Nietzsche, war means agon, destruction and its cycle; agon is the transfiguration of this cycle into a cultural formation. The eternal recurrence is the expression of the unity of creation and destruction, life and death, the cyclical aspect of all that is, as the archaic societies lived it and as the agonist Greeks understood it. Agon too is the unity of the forces of life (a heightened body, sensuality, and vitality are present in agon) and the forces of death (agonists struggle onto death and there show humility both in victory and defeat).
28 GS, p. 251. (Emphasis mine).
29 As Jill Marsden correctly observes, ". . . the maxim aggresses against our ingrained philosophical instincts which favor doctrine over declamation and expansiveness over brevity." "Nietzsche and the Art of Aphorism," in *A Companion to Nietzsche* (Oxford: Wiley-Blackwell, 2007), Ch. 2, p. 22. An attack jolts us from our current position, just as an aphorism may provoke us to think.
30 GS, p. 32.
31 Horst Hutter traces this emphasis on oral tradition to Nietzsche's desire to found a school or a communion of free spirits and also in his desire to have disciples. *Shaping the Future*, pp. 38–9.

9

True to the Earth: Nietzsche's Epicurean Care of Self and World[1]

Keith Ansell-Pearson

Epicurus has been alive in all ages and he lives now, unknown to those who called and call themselves Epicureans, and without a reputation amongst the philosophers. He too forgot his own name: it was the heaviest burden he ever cast off (WS 227)

Epicurus relates to the Stoics as beauty does to sublimity; but one would have to be a Stoic at the very least to catch sight of this beauty at all! To be able to be jealous of it!

(Nietzsche 1883, KSA 10, 7 [151])

That Nietzsche is concerned with forms or modes of philosophical therapy which will promote human flourishing is, I think, evident from the concerns of his earliest writings, such as his conception of the philosopher as the physician of culture. Here my focus is on the Epicurean-inspired therapy we find put to work in the middle period writings. Although the late Nietzsche has problems with Epicurus, in his middle period writings, he writes in praise of him and draws upon his philosophy as a way of promoting what I would like to call an Epicurean-inspired care of self. At the start, we can note the following: Epicurus becomes a significant and inspiring figure for Nietzsche at the time of his free spirit middle period (1878–82); by the time of the late writings (1886–8), he is a more ambivalent figure for Nietzsche, still celebrated for waging war against Christianity in its preexistent form but also said to be a typical decadent (A 30). With the return of the Dionysian in his thinking, which on the surface seems to disappear in his middle period writings, we get the fundamental contrast between "Epicurean delight" (*Vergnügen*) and "Dionysian joy" (*Lust*): "I have presented such terrible images to knowledge that any 'Epicurean delight' is out of the question. Only Dionysian joy is sufficient: *I have been the first to discover the tragic*" (KSA 11, 25 [95]: WP 1029). In this chapter, I do not wish to subject this later contrast to analysis. Instead, I want to show how Nietzsche draws on Epicurus in his middle period writings and deploys Epicurean ideas as a way of promoting a care of self and world.

In Nietzsche's middle period writings, we encounter a significant portrait of Epicurus as the inventor of a specific and unique mode of philosophizing. For

Nietzsche, Epicurus's teaching can show us how to quieten our being and so help to temper a human mind that is prone to neurosis. Nietzsche confesses to having dwelled like Odysseus in the underworld and says that he will often be found there again. As a "sacrificer" who sacrifices so as to talk to the dead, he states that there are four pairs of thinkers from whom he will accept judgment, and Epicurus and Montaigne make up the first pair he mentions (AOM 408).[2] Epicurus, along with the Stoic Epictetus, is revered as a thinker in whom wisdom assumes bodily form (AOM 224). Indeed, Nietzsche admits at this time to being inspired by the example of Epicurus whom he calls one of the greatest human beings to have ever graced the earth and the inventor of a "heroic-idyllic mode of philosophizing" (WS 295).[3]

It is heroic, then, because conquering the fear of death is involved and the human being has the potential to walk on the earth as a god, living a blessed life, and idyllic because Epicurus philosophized, calmly and serenely, and away from the crowd, in a garden.[4] In *Human, all too Human* Nietzsche writes of a "*refined heroism*" "which disdains to offer itself to the veneration of the great masses . . . and goes silently through the world and out of the world" (HH 291). This is deeply Epicurean in inspiration: Epicurus taught that one should die as if one had never lived. I think this Epicurean philosophy, which so inspired Nietzsche in his middle period, is highly relevant to our concerns today regarding the care of the planet and I will seek to indicate this in more detail in the final main section of the chapter.

Nietzsche and Epicurus

Catherine Wilson neatly lays out the central tenets of the Epicurean system in her recent study, *Epicureanism at the Origins of Modernity*. They include: the denial of supernatural agency engaged in the design and maintenance of the world; the view that self-moving, subvisible particles acting blindly bring about all growth, change, and decline; and the insistence that the goal of ethical self-discipline, which involves asceticism, is the minimization of mental and physical suffering.[5] There is much here that accords with what Nietzsche found appealing in Epicurus. However, it is also the case that Nietzsche's reception of Epicurus has quite specific features. For example, he shows little interest in the ontological status of atomism and the problems of the theory of knowledge and much more interest in Epicurean cosmology, such as its distinction between world and universe. As one commentator has noted, this focus on the world and distrust of the idea of *the* universe, including the idea of the sum of all possible worlds, "allowed Nietzsche to collect the themes of Epicurean divinity, blessedness, friendship and philosophical regimen around the focus of the ancient science of this world of 'meteorology.'"[6] As Liba Taub has put it, the Epicurean aim "was to demonstrate that the universe and various distant phenomena can be explained without reference to anything outside nature, or extraordinary."[7] Informing Epicurean views on cosmology and meteorology was the desire to eliminate fear and anxiety, especially about the intervention of the gods in the world. Epicurus thus developed a strict materialist philosophy that was designed to provide natural explanations of phenomena that were often seen as due to the activities of supernatural powers.[8]

Although acknowledging the existence of an infinite number of worlds (*cosmoi*), Epicurus sought to account for the *meteōra*, such as the phenomenon of the sky and earthquakes, in terms of the natural workings of our local cosmos. Thus, the fundamental Epicurean aims, such as the alleviation of anxiety, are at the heart of their cosmological and meteorological explanations. In the middle period, Nietzsche is inspired by Epicurus's focus on the world, his redemption of nature from human projection and teleology, and his conception of philosophy as the art of living in which one lives the philosophical life and does not engage merely in theoretical discourses.

In Nietzsche's time, there was something of a revival of interest in Epicurus and Epicureanism, and Nietzsche's texts, especially *Dawn*, can be seen as part of this development and the attempt to retrieve the resources of ancient materialism. Writing in 1878, the French naturalist philosopher, Jean-Marie Guyau, hailed at the time as the "Spinoza of France," portrayed Epicurus as the original free spirit, "Still today it is the spirit of old Epicurus who, combined with new doctrines, works away at and undermines Christianity."[9] In Germany, Friedrich Albert Lange's *History of Materialism* of 1866, a text that deeply impressed the young Nietzsche, was largely responsible for the revival of interest in Epicurus. Lange devoted a chapter to Epicurus and a separate chapter to Lucretius's poem, *On the Nature of the Universe* (*De Rerum Natura*).[10] The aim of the explanation of nature sought by Epicurus "is to free us from fear and anxiety."[11] As Lange notes, in Epicurus, physics is placed in the service of ethics: "The mere historical knowledge of natural events, without a knowledge of causes, is valueless; for it does not free us from fear nor lift us upon superstition. The more causes of change we have discovered, the more we shall attain the calmness of contemplation; and it cannot be supposed that this inquiry can be without result upon our happiness."[12] If events can be explained in accordance with universal laws, with effects attributable to natural causes, an important goal of philosophy can be attained and secured, chiefly liberation from fear and anxiety. Moreover, if peace of soul and freedom from pain are the only enduring pleasures, then these constitute the true aim of existence, including the philosophical endeavor. For Lange, Greek philosophy, properly understood, begins with the Ionian natural philosophers and terminates with Epicurus and his school: the further developments in it belong to the natural sciences while speculative philosophy—notably in the form of neo-Platonism—is a "thoroughly degenerate" expression of philosophy.[13] Epicurus is to be praised not so much for his system as for the "general Materialistic principles" which underlie it.[14] Finally, Lange notes the "quietistic and contemplative" character of Epicureanism, and it's this character that appeals to the Nietzsche of the middle period[15] (the late Nietzsche is quite different on this point).

In his book *Nietzsche and Modern Times*, Laurence Lampert notes that the portrait of Epicurus that can be drawn from Nietzsche's scattered reflections provides us with an important component in understanding his genealogy of philosophy. He rightly notes, however, that Nietzsche provides his readers only with "fragmentary glimpses" of his interpretation of Epicurus even though it forms a major element in his reworking of the history of philosophy.[16] Nietzsche writes in 1882 that he is proud of the fact that he experiences the character of Epicurus differently from perhaps everybody else: "Whatever I hear or read of him, I enjoy the happiness of the afternoon of antiquity"

(GS 45). Lampert claims that Nietzsche's "recovery" of Epicurus forms a key component in his new history of philosophy, providing a point of access to its all-important themes such as the philosophical and scientific tradition prior to Socrates—typically demoted in the history of philosophy to the status of mere *pre-Socratic* thought—that Epicurus sought to preserve.[17] He further argues that Nietzsche experienced Epicurus in a way different to everybody else because he was able to experience him as an heir to what was best in Greek science.[18] However, this cannot be right since, as we have just seen, it is precisely in these terms that Lange writes in praise of him. Much better, I think, is when Lampert claims that Nietzsche located a peculiar happiness in Epicurus's life and teaching. He notes that the happiness of Epicurus does not stem from Epicurean *ataraxia*, conceived as an indifference to all passions, but that it arises *from a passion*, from a *Wollust* "grown modest and transformed into the observing eye that watched the sun set out on the magnificence of antiquity."[19]

As Lampert's appreciation indicates, Nietzsche is capable of arresting psychological insight into Epicurus. In 1882, he writes, for example:

> I see his eyes gaze upon a wide, white sea, across rocks at the shore that are bathed in sunlight, while large and small animals are playing in this light, as secure and calm as the light and his eyes. Such happiness could be invented only by a man who was suffering continually. It is the happiness of eyes that have seen the sea of existence become calm, and now they can never weary of the surface and of the many hues of this tender, shuddering skin of the sea. Never before has voluptuousness (*Wollust*) been so modest (GS 45).

As Monika Langer has recently noted in her interpretation of this aphorism, although clearly a paean of sorts to Epicurus, Nietzsche does not elaborate on the origin or nature of his happiness and suffering, but rather tacitly encourages the reader to consider various possibilities. In the end, she argues that Nietzsche is reading Epicurus as a figure who while standing securely on firm ground, gazes at the sea and is able to enjoy the possibility of uncertainty it offers. She writes, "Literally and figuratively he can float on the sea."[20] Epicurus is depicted as the antithesis of modernity's shipwrecked man since such is his liberation and serenity he can "chart his course or simply set sail and let the wind determine his way."[21] Although he might suffer shipwreck and drown or survive he does not live in fear of dangers and hazards: "In taking to the sea he might lose his bearings and even his mind." In contrast to modern man who is keen to leave behind the insecurity of the sea for the safety of dry land, "Epicurus delights in the ever present possibility of leaving that secure land for the perils of the sea."[22]

I think this interpretation is too strong and misses the essential insight Nietzsche is developing into Epicurus in the aphorism. Rather than suggesting that the sea calls for further and continued exploration, hiding seductive dangers that Epicurus would not be afraid of, Nietzsche seems to hold to the view that Epicurus is the seasoned traveler of the soul who has no desire to travel anymore and for whom the meaning of the sea has changed. Rather than serving as a means of transportation or something that beckons us toward other shores, the sea has become an object of contemplation in the here and now. It is something to be looked at for its own sake and in a way that discloses its infinite nuances and colors. One might describe this in Heidegger's terms, with its mode of being changed from the ready-to-hand (either threatening or alluring, but in both cases on the background of a form of instrumentalization, such as exploration) to something more akin to the present-at-hand, except that here the disclosing attitude is not one of theoretical detachment but a sensitivity that entails a special receptivity that is hard to attain and maintain.[23] One might even invoke *Gelassenheit* to define the experience. This interpretation is in accord with the stress Nietzsche places in his middle period writings on the joyful riches, calm and serene, to be had from the *vita contemplativa* (see D 440; GS 329). Nietzsche even discovers what one might call a materialist sublime in the contemplation of nature:

> One day, and probably soon, we need some recognition of what above all is lacking in our big cities: quiet and wide, expansive places for reflection. Places with long, high-ceilinged cloisters for bad or all too sunny weather where no shouting or noise of carriages can reach and where good manners would prohibit even priests from praying aloud – buildings and sites that would altogether give expression to the sublimity (*Erhabenheit*) of thoughtfulness and of stepping aside. The time is past when the church possessed a monopoly on reflection, when the *vita contemplativa* had to be first all a *vita religiosa*; and everything built by the church gives expression to that idea. I do not see how we could remain content with such buildings even if they were stripped of their churchly purposes. The language spoken by these buildings is far too rhetorical and unfree, reminding us that they are houses of God and ostentatious monuments of some supramundane intercourse; we who are godless could not think *our thoughts* in such surroundings. We wish to see *ourselves* translated into stones and plants, we want to take walks *in ourselves* when we stroll around these buildings and gardens (GS 280).

In short, for the middle period Nietzsche, Epicurus is a figure who has liberated himself from the fear and anxiety of existence and is capable of spiritual joyfulness that consists, in part, in the serene contemplation of the beauty and sublimity of things and a cultivation of simple, modest pleasures. Epicurus is a figure who was "true to the earth," abandoning all hubristic conceptions of human significance, including exceptionalism, and who taught that one should die as if one had never lived. As Nietzsche astutely noted, never in the history of thought has such a voluptuous appreciation of existence been so modest.

Nietzsche on Epicurus in the middle period

With respect to the middle period Epicurus is important to any appreciation of Nietzsche's sources and influences because it is primarily from him that he gets the inspiration to detach from the first and last things and to devote attention to the closest things—and, moreover, to learn to know and accept, even embrace, the mortal conditions of human existence. These are some of the major concerns Nietzsche has in his middle period. What appeals to Nietzsche about Epicurus is the emphasis on a refined egoism, the teaching on mortality, and the general attempt to liberate the mind from unjustified fears and anxieties. One of the earliest references to Epicureanism is an incidental remark in *Schopenhauer as Educator* where Nietzsche says that to write today in favor of an education that sets goals beyond money and acquisition, that takes a great deal of time, and also encourages solitude, is likely to be disparaged as "refined egoism" and "immoral cultural Epicureanism" (SE 6). Epicurus does not become an important component in Nietzsche's philosophy until around 1879, and it is in these terms—refined egoism—that he draws on him again and becomes inspired by certain Epicurean notions and ideals. Indeed, at this time, he was inspired by Epicurus's conception of friendship and the ideal of withdrawing from society and cultivating one's own garden. In a letter to Peter Gast of 1883, Nietzsche writes that Epicurus "is the best negative argument in favour of my challenge to all rare spirits to isolate themselves from the mass of their fellows" (KGB III, 1, 418). Like Epicurus, Nietzsche's philosophical therapy is in search of pupils and disciples: "What I envy in Epicurus are the *disciples* in his garden; in *such circumstances* one could certainly forget noble Greece and more certainly still ignoble Germany!"[24]

If, as Pierre Hadot has suggested, philosophical therapeutics is centered on a concern with the healing of our own lives so as to return us to the joy of existing,[25] then in the texts of his middle period Nietzsche can be seen to be an heir to this ancient tradition. Indeed, if there is one crucial component to Nietzsche's philosophical therapeutics in the texts of his middle period that he keeps returning to again and again it is the need for spiritual joyfulness and the task of cultivating in ourselves, after centuries of training by morality and religion, the joy in existing. In the final aphorism of *The Wanderer and his Shadow*, Nietzsche writes, for example:

> Only the *ennobled human being may be given freedom of spirit;* to him alone does *alleviation of life* draw near and salve his wounds; only he may say that he lives for the sake of *joy* (*Freudigkeit*) and for the sake of no further goal . . . (WS 350)

The difference from Epicurus is that he is developing a therapy for the sicknesses of the soul under modern conditions of social control and discipline. Nevertheless, it is the case that Nietzsche at this time is seeking to revive an ancient conception of philosophy. In a note from 1881, he states that he considers the various moral schools of antiquity to be "experimental laboratories" containing a number of recipes for the art of living and holds that these experiments now belong to us as our legitimate property: "we shall not hesitate to adopt a Stoic recipe just because we have profited in the past from Epicurean recipes" (KSA 9, 15 [59]). Nietzsche recognizes in Epicurus what he calls in one note a "refined heroism," and here the thought seems to center on conquering the fear of death, of which Nietzsche says he has little of it (KSA 8, 28 [15]). For Epicurus, the study of nature should make human beings modest and self-sufficient, taking pride in the good that lies in themselves, not in their estate, and as opposed to the display of learning coveted by the rabble.[26] Indeed, Nietzsche admires Epicurus for cultivating a modest existence and in two respects: first, in having "spiritual joyfulness (*Freudigkeit*) in place of frequent indulgence in single pleasures" (KSA 8, 41 [48]), and, second, in withdrawing from social ambition and living in a garden as opposed to living publicly in the market-place.[27] As Nietzsche stresses, "A little garden, figs, little cheeses and in addition three or four good friends – these were the sensual pleasures of Epicurus" (WS 192).[28] Nietzsche is appreciative of what one commentator has called the "refined asceticism" we find in Epicurus, which consists in the enjoyment of the smallest pleasures and the disposal of a diverse and delicate range of sensations.[29]

In the middle period, then, Epicurus is an attractive figure for Nietzsche because of the emphasis on a modest lifestyle, the attention given to the care of self, and also because he conceives philosophy not as a theoretical discourse but one that, first and foremost, is a kind of practical activity aimed at the attainment of eudemonia or the flourishing life.[30] Nietzsche wants free spirits to take pleasure in existence, involving taking pleasure in themselves and in friendship, and in simple and modest living.

Nietzsche, then, is keen to encourage human beings to cultivate an attitude toward existence in which they accept their mortality and attain serenity about their dwelling on the earth, to conquer unjustified fears, and to reinstitute the role played by chance and chance events in the world and in human existence (D 13, 33, 36).[31] As Pierre Hadot notes, for the Epicurean sage, the world is the product of chance, not divine intervention, and this brings with it pleasure and peace of mind, freeing him from an unreasonable fear of the gods and allowing him to consider each moment as an unexpected miracle. Each moment of existence can be greeted with immense gratitude.[32] Indeed, as Graham Parkes has noted, Nietzsche expresses in his writings, especially *Thus Spoke Zarathustra*, a kind of gratitude with respect to life that is "reminiscent of Epicurus," with meditation cultivating "a keen appreciation of the 'once-only' character of existence in a radically contingent universe."[33] Parkes cites from section 5 of "Old and New Law-Tablets" in *Zarathustra*: "Thus does the nature of noble souls wish it: they want to have nothing for free, and least of all life. Whoever is of the rabble wants to live for free: we others, however, to whom life has given itself – we are always wondering *what* we can best give *in return*!"

Epicurus's teaching is that gratitude should be our primary attitude toward life and a result of our acceptance and recognition of life's essentially finite character. We are to accord value to the slightest moment of existence.[34] As Hadot has pointed out, Epicurus's teaching seeks to transform our relationship to time, in which we become focused on the present moment, and this transformation presupposes a quite specific conception of pleasure, "according to which the quality of pleasure depends neither on the quantity of desires it satisfies, nor on the length of time it lasts."[35] As Guyau notes, true pleasure bears its infinity within itself, and as Nietzsche teaches the time of the moment is "eternity," an eternity reclaimed "for the fair earth," as Herbert Marcuse put it.[36] According to Hadot, the secret of Epicurean joy and serenity is to live each instant as if it were the last, but also as if it were the first. In this way we, "experience the same grateful astonishment when we accept the instant as though it were unexpected, or by greeting it as entirely new . . ."[37] (225). Metrodorus memorably expressed the wisdom one might acquire by living the Epicurean life: "Remember that, born a mortal, with a limited life-span, you have risen up in soul to eternity and the infinity of things, and that you have seen all that has been and all that shall be."[38]

In *The Wanderer and his Shadow*, Nietzsche describes Epicurus as "the soul-soother (*Seelen-Beschwichtiger*) of later antiquity." He had the "wonderful insight" that to quieten our being it is not necessary to have resolved the ultimate and outermost theoretical questions (WS 7). To those who are tormented by the fear of the gods, one points out that if the gods exist, they do not concern themselves with us and that it is unnecessary to engage in "fruitless disputation" over the ultimate question as to whether they exist or not. Furthermore, in response to the consideration of a hypothesis, half belonging to physics and half to ethics, and that may cast gloom over our spirits, it is wise to refrain from refuting the hypothesis and instead offer a rival hypothesis, even a multiplicity of hypotheses. To someone who wishes to offer consolation—for example, to the unfortunate, to ill-doers, to hypochondriacs, and so on—one can call to mind two pacifying formulae of Epicurus that are capable of being applied to many questions: "firstly, if that is how things are they do not concern us; secondly, things may be thus but they may also be otherwise" (WS 7).

In the middle period, then, Epicurus is one of Nietzsche's chief inspirations in his effort to liberate himself from the metaphysical need, to find serenity within his own existence, and to aid humanity in its need to now cure its neuroses. Epicureanism, along with science in general, serves to make us "colder and more sceptical," helping to cool down "the fiery stream of belief in ultimate definitive truths," a stream that has grown so turbulent through Christianity (HH 244). The task, Nietzsche says, is to live in terms of "a constant spiritual joyfulness (*Freudigkeit*)" (HH 292) and to prize "the three good things": greatness, repose, and sunlight, in which these things answer to thoughts that elevate, thoughts that quieten, thoughts that enlighten, and, finally, "to thoughts which participate in all three qualities, in which everything earthly comes to transfiguration: it is the kingdom where there reigns the great *trinity of joy* (*Freude*)" (WS 332).

Care of self

It is also from Epicurus that Nietzsche gets the inspiration to give up on what he calls the first and last things, the questions of a theologically inspired metaphysics, and devote attention to the closest things. Nietzsche has made this decision in 1878–9, and it provides the context for much of what it follows in the free spirit works of the middle period. Let me outline some of its features. Before I do, let me simply note that I think in making this decision Nietzsche is, in fact, reviving the antique conception of ethics as centered on a care of self. Foucault contends that in Greek ethics we find a focus on moral conduct, on relations to oneself and others, rather than a focus on religious problems such as what is our fate after death? What are the gods and do they intervene in life or not? For the Greeks, Foucault argues, these were not significant problems and not directly related to conduct. What they were concerned about was to constitute an ethics that was an "aesthetics of existence."[39]

In modern culture we can detect, Nietzsche writes, a "feigned disrespect for all the things which human beings in fact take most seriously, *for all the things closest to them*" (WS 5). As Ruth Abbey notes, in devaluing the small, worldly matters Christian and post-Christian sensibility, "puts people at war with themselves and forbids a close study of which forms of care of the self would be most conducive to individual flourishing."[40]

As Nietzsche notes, most people see the closest things badly and rarely pay heed to them, while "*almost all the physical and psychical frailties* of the individual derive from this lack . . . being *unknowledgeable in the smallest and everyday things* and failing to keep an eye on them - this it is that transforms the earth for so many into a 'vale of tears'" (WS 6). Our understanding of existence is diverted away from the smallest and closest things:

> Priests and teachers, and the sublime lust for power of idealists of every description . . . hammer even into children that what matters is something quite different: the salvation of the soul, the service of the state, the advancement of science, or the accumulation of reputation and possessions, all as the means of doing service to mankind as a whole; while the requirements of the individual, his great and small needs within the twenty four hours of the day, are to be regarded as something contemptible or a matter of indifference. (WS 6)

Nietzsche notes that our greatness does not crumble away all at once but through continual neglect:

> . . . the little vegetation that grows in between everything and understands how to cling everywhere, this is what ruins what is great in us – the quotidian, hourly pitifulness of our environment that goes overlooked, the thousand tiny tendrils of this or that small and small-minded feeling growing out of our neighborhood, our job, the company we keep, the division of our day. If we allow these small weeds to grow unwittingly, then unwittingly they will destroy us! (D 435)

The closest things are those things which are overlooked or even disparaged by priests and metaphysicians who devote all their time and energy to the care of the soul. They include things like eating and diet, housing, clothing, and social intercourse. These should all be made the object of constant impartial and general reflection and reform. Nietzsche argues: "Our continual offences against the most elementary laws of the body and the spirit reduce us all . . . to a disgraceful dependence and bondage . . . on physicians, teachers and curers of soul who lie like a burden on the whole of society" (WS 5). All the physical and psychical frailties of the individual derive from a lack of knowledge about the smallest and most everyday things, such as what is beneficial to us and what is harmful to us in the institution of our mode of life, in the division of the day, eating, sleeping, and reflecting, and so on (WS 6).

Nietzsche insists that we do not require certainties with regard to the first and last things—what he calls "the furthest horizon"—in order to live a "full and excellent human life" (WS 16). He proposes a fundamental rupture be affected with regard to customary habits of thinking. In the face of questions such as, what is the purpose of man? What is his fate after death? How can man be reconciled with God? It should not be felt necessary to develop knowledge against faith; rather we should practice an indifference toward faith and supposed knowledge in the domains of metaphysics and religion. From this Epicurean-inspired demotion of metaphysics, he proposes the following as a principle of the new life: "life should be ordered on the basis of what is most certain and most demonstrable, not as hitherto on that what is most remote, indefinite, and no more than a cloud on the horizon" (WS 310). This concern with the small things and "casuistry of selfishness" continues well into the late Nietzsche, with Nietzsche writing in *Ecce Homo* that "nutrition, place, climate, recreation" are "inconceivably more important than everything one has taken to be important to date," and here it is necessary to relearn (EH II: 10).

An Epicurean attachment to life

It is important that we appreciate the distinctive character the enjoyment of life has for the Epicurean. This is what I want to focus on in this section of the chapter.

In the letter to Menoeceus, Epicurus seeks to identify what the study of philosophy can do for the health of the soul and on the premise that, "pleasure is the starting-point and goal of living blessedly."[41] Epicurus stresses that he does not mean the pleasures of the profligate or of consumption; rather, the task is to become accustomed to simple, nonextravagant ways of living. Although Epicurus regards *voluptas* as the highest good, in which we can take delight in all that nature has provided to stimulate pleasure, it is an error to suppose that for him happiness is to be found "simply in eating, drinking, gambling, wenching, and other such pastimes."[42] Nietzsche seems to have fully appreciated this point. The key goal for Epicurus is to liberate the body from pain and remove disturbances from the soul. Central to his counsel is the thought that we need to accustom ourselves to believing that death is nothing to us; our longing for immortality needs to be removed: ". . . there is nothing fearful in life for one who has grasped that there is nothing fearful in the absence of life."[43] What appears to be the most frightening of bad things should be nothing to us, "since when we exist, death is not yet present, and when death is present, then we do not exist."[44] The wise human being "neither rejects life nor fears death. For living does not offend him, nor does he believe not living to be something bad."[45] If, as Epicurus supposes, everything good and bad consists in sense-experience, then death is simply the privation of sense-experience. The goal of philosophical training, then, is freedom from disturbance and anxiety in which we reach a state of *ataraxia* or psychic tranquility: the body is free from pain and the soul is liberated from distress.

But is Epicureanism a philosophy of life-affirmation, or does it simply depict a universe of atoms and the void that is indifferent to life and in which freedom consists in little more than attaining a contemplative tranquility with respect to this fact? As James Porter notes, life has no intrinsic value for Epicurus, but does this mean that life is an indifferent for him?[46] When viewed from a third-person point of view, that is, the cosmological one (of atoms and the void), then life has no claim on us; rather, it discloses to us that "we are nothing more than physical entities, mere fortuitous combinations of matter which reduce to their elements upon disbanding."[47] From the viewpoint of nature, then, life is an indifferent. The matter changes, Porter argues, when we view things from a first-person perspective on life, that is, the world of sensations, desires, and needs, or of nature in its human aspect. Here we find that life by definition is not indifferent but a meaningful source of value. As Porter puts it, the issue facing the Epicurean philosopher "is to decide just what this value is and where it lies."[48] The argument is that life is a source of human pleasure and thus of moral happiness, involving a strong attachment. Porter argues that once we connect pleasure to life, it is possible to show that Epicurus has a philosophy of life in addition to a philosophy of death and that, in fact, it is this emphasis on life and not death that dominates his writings.

Porter goes on to note that the "apparent pessimism" of the doctrine "clashes with the joy and even fascination with life" that are found in the Epicurean perception of the world.[49] The task is to account for this disparity and the question to focus on is that of what makes creatures cling to life and remain attached to it. We can rule out, he thinks, the fear of death since such a fear produces phantasms of life (such as ideas of the afterlife) and does not prolong or propagate life itself. He thinks that love of life, in the form of an attachment to life, precedes the fear of death, operating at a primitive level of psychic attachment, and may even precede what he takes to be the most primitive root fear present in the fear of death, that of the fear of the blank void or *horror vacui*. Furthermore, it cannot be supposed that what makes us cling to life is constant novelty since this seems to be a consequence of the love of life and not its cause. The Epicurean affirmation of life, the practice of its love, consists in attending to and enjoying the present feelings or sensations of life, that is, living in the here and now without desire and expectation and in a condition of gratitude. As Porter puts it, "To love life is to be in an unqualified state of affirmation about what lies most immediately to hand: it is the pleasure, the unalloyed passion, and even thrill, of living itself."[50] For Epicurus, then, a correct understanding of our mortality is one that should lead to the enjoyment of this mortal life. The Epicurean love of life "*is a love of mortal life* and not a love of life abstracted from death, much less of immortal life."[51] Moreover, this Epicurean love of life is not a longing for life, but "rather an immediate expression of what is dear about life, what is most life worthy in life," and which makes it something fragile and easily ruptured.[52]

We are perhaps now in a position perhaps to grasp something of the special nature of Epicurean pleasure. As Porter states, "what an Epicurean enjoys is not some pleasure that is distinct from life, but life *qua* pleasure."[53] Epicurus does not, then "disdain life" and has little truck with the pessimist who maintains, as he puts it in his letter to Menoeceus, it is good not to be born and once born to pass through the gates of Hades as quickly as possible.[54] A key point to appreciate is that pleasure is not simply bound up with moral hedonism but also with an epistemology: "as a criterion of truth, as one of the *pathê* by which we feel our way through the world."[55] In contrast to pain, which causes us to shrink back from the world, pleasure draws us to it: it is both congenital and congenial.[56] The Epicurean state of mind (ataraxy) is best described as one of "stable (*katastematic*) pleasure," and, furthermore, as the "basal experience of pleasure" on account of it being the criterion of all pleasure. In this sense, then, it is more than a condition of simple or mere happiness: "it seems to operate as life's internal formal principle, as that which gives moral sense and shape to a life that is lived . . ."[57]

As Porter incisively brings out, the theory of pleasure we find in Epicurus is minimalist in that the highest kind of pleasure consists not in seeking out a range of pleasures but rather focusing on a single kind of pleasure and that presents the fewest possible requirements, and hence his theory of autarky or self-sufficiency. Moreover, experiencing this stable or static pleasure is not a matter of "the defection of pain" (of having painless sensory pleasures), as this would amount to a solely negative definition.[58] As Porter puts it, it is rather the case that "pleasure is the removal, by subtraction, of pain . . . and then the discovery of what is left once that removal has been made."[59] He maintains that what is left is a positive pleasure in its own right and that does not amount to a merely painless sensory pleasure but is a purer and higher form of pleasure. He adds that this discovery "may bring joy and delight, but these are contingent pleasures of a kinetic kind, caused by an underlying pleasure of a stable kind, which is ataraxic and valuable in and of itself."[60] Bliss or ataraxy, then, involves a rediscovery of this primary form of pleasure and it is what is perceived once all pain has been removed: it is life experienced in a moment of special intensity. In its higher form, then, pleasure is not a desire, and curiously perhaps, not a desire for pleasure: to want pleasure is to perceive a lack, but in the experience of tranquility one lacks nothing.[61]

What does it mean to live well for Epicurus? Porter answers this question exquisitely, so let me cite him:

> Its lesson is simple and basic: it is that we ought to cultivate an attentiveness to ourselves and to the world, which is to say to redirect our bodies and minds away from pain, not so much in the direction of pleasure as in a direction *away from pain*, with this redirection constituting our pleasure. The redescription of pain as painless or indifferent, achieved pragmatically through intense mental focusing, disposes us . . . to the Epicurean virtues: to pleasure, happiness, justice, piety, and friendship . . . To be virtuous just is to experience a precious attachment to the world and to its highest reality.[62]

Before we move back to Nietzsche, a final point is worth making and this concerns Epicurus's so-called hedonism. As Porter points out, Epicurus comes to value pleasure owing to his affirmative philosophy of life. Hedonism is Epicurus's "wager that life on balance will prove more attractive than death," and it is for this reason that pleasure resides at the center of his thinking: "it would be a mistake to say that Epicurus entertains the value of life to the extent he does just because he is a hedonist. The truth is the other way round: Epicurus is a hedonist just because he believes at some level in the moral value of living. What Epicurus enjoys is not some pleasure that is distinct from life, but life *qua* pleasure."[63]

Nietzsche appreciated the special quality of Epicurean pleasure. In *The Wanderer and his Shadow*, he depicts an idyllic scene entitled "*Et in Arcadia ego*," involving looking down "over waves of hills, through fir-trees and spruce trees grave with age, towards a milky green lake" (WS 295). While cattle graze on their own and gather in groups, the narrator of the aphorism experiences "everything at peace in the contentment of evening." While looking upon the herders in the field, he witnesses mountain slopes and snowfields to the left and, high above him, to the right two gigantic ice-covered peaks that seem to float in a veil of sunlit vapor: "everything big, still and bright" (ibid.). The beauty of the whole scene induces in him an experience of the sublime, "a sense of awe and of adoration of the moment of its revelation"; involuntarily, as if completely natural, he inserts "into this pure, clear world of light," free of desire and expectation, with no looking before or behind, Hellenic heroes, and he compares the feeling to that of Poussin and his pupil (probably Claude Lorrain), at one and the same time heroic and idyllic, noting to himself that some human beings have actually *lived* in accordance with this experience, having "enduringly *felt* they existed in the world and the world existed in them" (ibid.).[64] Epicurus is singled out for special mention. As one commentator notes, for Nietzsche, the idyll is not in any inaccessible celestial heavens but belongs in this world and is within our reach, and what takes place after death does not concern us anymore.[65] Nietzsche writes: "An unspeakable blessing . . . and once again, Epicurus triumphs!" (D 72)

Nietzsche finds in Epicurus a victory over pessimism in which "death becomes the last celebration of a life which is constantly embellished"[66] (Roos 2000: 299). This last of the Greek philosophers "teaches the joy of living in the midst of a world in decay and where all moral doctrines preach suffering."[67] As Roos puts it, "The example of Epicurus teaches that a life filled with pain and renunciation prepares one to savour the little joys of the everyday better. Relinquishing Dionysian intoxication, Nietzsche becomes a student of this master of moderate pleasures and careful dosages."[68] Roos asks what I think is the decisive question concerning this appropriation of Epicurus: can this teaching fill the void left by the loss of faith, the abandonment of Schopenhauer, and the renunciation of Dionysian music? His answer to the question is incisive: "he clings to Epicurus and his consolations with a vigour proportional to the violence of the Christian temptation."[69] In Epicurus, Nietzsche discovers what Roos calls aptly an "irresistible power" and a rare strength of spirit and quotes Nietzsche from 1880: "I found strength in the very places one does not look for it, in simple, gentle and helpful men . . . powerful natures dominate, that is a necessity, even if those men do not move one finger. And they bury themselves, in their lifetime, in a pavilion in their garden" (KSA 9, 6 [206]).[70]

An ecological Nietzsche?

I think that an appreciation of Nietzsche's Epicurean care of self (and world) is relevant to engaging with the debates on Nietzsche and ecology. There has been a lively set of debates in the literature concerning Nietzsche's credentials as an ecological thinker with those in favor arguing that both his lifestyle and his naturalistic way of thinking make him a forerunner of ecological ideas, and with skeptics insisting that his focus is on aristocratic self-cultivation, not the fate of the planet. I do not want to enter directly into this debate here but would argue instead that we need to follow an Epicurean lead. We need to discover this Epicurean-inspired Nietzsche for ourselves and in part as a way of contesting Heidegger's reading of Nietzsche which focuses on the late writings, mostly the *Nachlass*, and construes all the major concepts of the late period, notably the will to power and the overman, as indicating that Nietzsche is the "technological" thinker of our age.[71] In an essay on Nietzsche and ecology, Michael Zimmerman follows Heidegger in focusing on the late Nietzsche and argues that he does not share the anti-anthropocentrism and asceticism of the environmentalist movement and that his main concern is "how to avoid degeneration and *nihilism*, not how to avoid environmental destruction and *ecocide*."[72] Furthermore, he thinks that Heidegger offers "a plausible, though controversial, reading of Nietzsche's Overman as heralding the culmination of 2,500 years of metaphysics, which takes the form of technological domination of the planet."[73]

My view is that we need a much more subtle and nuanced appreciation of Nietzsche than this Heideggerian reading permits, and one way to develop this is to focus on the neglected middle period of Nietzsche's writings. It is here, I believe, that we find rich resources for recognizing a Nietzschean commitment to ecology. The historian of ancient ecological thought J. Donald Hughes has argued that Epicurean philosophy, especially evident in the work of Lucretius, asked questions that are now regarded as ecological, including alluding to air pollution due to mining and the disappearance of forests, as well as arguing that human beings are not radically distinct from animals.[74] The Epicurean philosophy of nature, with its principle of conservation—nothing is created by divine power out of nothing and nature never reduces anything to nothing—thus tends toward an ecological mode of thinking.[75] Let me make clear that I think it is anachronistic to state that Nietzsche is, as Laurence Lampert has claimed, following Max Hallman, a "deep ecologist."[76] Moreover, there is no, as we might put it, "politics" of ecology to be found in Nietzsche. If anything Nietzsche recommends at this time, social withdrawal, even isolation, and on this point, he adheres to Epicurean principles (see GS 338).[77] We have to acknowledge that there are limits to any use we can make of Nietzsche for the ends of an ecological-centered politics: his thinking is too complex and contradictory to serve as the basis for a programmatic ecological philosophy.[78] Nevertheless, I think there is to be found within the writings what one might call an "ecological" conscience and this conscience informs his new appreciation of nature, a nature that has been de-deified and that requires the "naturalization" of humanity (GS 109).

Let me list what I see as some of Nietzsche's principal "ecological" concerns in his middle period writings:

- A critique of commercial society and an emerging consumer culture.
- A commitment to stable pleasures and mental equilibrium over the need for *constant* change.
- An attempt to live free of the delusions of human exceptionalism, and free from the gods, especially the fear of the gods.
- An emphasis on a therapy of slowness and the *vita contemplativa*, including a tempering of the human mind in order to liberate it from moral and religious fanaticism.
- The search for a simpler and cleaner existence purified of the metaphysical need with an attention to the importance of the closest things.
- A care of self that is intended to be coextensive with the whole of life, suggesting an ecological rather than atomistic approach to the art of living.

My contention, then, is that if Nietzsche is to be claimed for ecological thinking, it can be done wisely on the basis of his Epicurean attachments and inspirations.

Conclusion

The evaluation of Epicurus we find in the late Nietzsche stands in marked contrast to the appreciation we find in his free spirit period. In Nietzsche's late writings, from *Beyond Good and Evil* onward, Epicurus becomes a much more ambivalent figure for Nietzsche. In *Beyond Good and Evil*, he refers to both Epicureanism and Christianity as offering a medicine that tranquilizes (BGE 200), while in the *Genealogy*, he refers to the super cool but "suffering Epicurus" as one who may have been hypnotized by the "feeling of nothingness" and the "repose of deepest sleep," that is, the promise of the absence of suffering (GM III. 17). In the middle period, however, Epicurus is deployed, at least in part, as a way of breaking with fanatical enthusiasms and intoxications, including quite possibly Nietzsche's own early Dionysian ones. The serene teaching of Epicurus provides Nietzsche with one way of shedding his previous skin, that of *The Birth of Tragedy*, and now conducting the patient labor of self-analysis and self-cultivation as a therapy of body and soul. For the middle period Nietzsche, Epicurus is the philosopher who affirms the moment, having neither resentment toward the past nor fear of the future.[79] Moreover, he teaches us the value of self-sufficiency and his cultivation of a refined egoism greatly appeals to Nietzsche. The late Nietzsche is marked by the explicit return of Dionysus in his thinking and this seems to influence his reception of Epicurus, giving rise to the contrast between "Epicurean delight" and "Dionysian joy."[80]

In his middle period, Nietzsche portrays an Epicurus that represents an alternative model to his later configuration of Dionysian joy, the importance of which perhaps the extreme pathos of his last years blinded him to. In the middle period, Epicurus is prized as one of those rare souls who remain true to the earth by demythologizing nature, embracing human mortality, and accepting human nonexceptionalism. What Nietzsche does seem ambivalent about in the course of his writings is the kind of "happiness" symbolized by Epicurean delight. Sometime he depicts this, as in GS 45, as a happiness that is hard-won, conscious of its precarious character, and inseparable from suffering: the sea of existence has become calm but, as one commentator has put it, "its continued calmness cannot be guaranteed, and the 'shuddering skin of the sea' is a constant reminder of the turmoil that may return."[81] At other times, especially in his late writings, he depicts it as a form of tranquility, a kind of Schopenhauerian release from the turmoil of existence and the cravings of the will. When he reads it in these terms, it is viewed as an expression of decadence.

Let me end by returning to the portrait of Epicurus we encounter in the beautiful aphorism from *The Gay Science*. The scene Nietzsche depicts is one of Epicurean illumination or enlightenment: Epicurus is not estranged from nature and recognizes his kinship with animals and the elements of nature. Rather than deploying his contemplation of the sea to bolster his own ego (thinking of his own safety or taking pride in fearlessness), Epicurus abandons his sense of self altogether so that he can open himself up to the sea of existence, and perhaps here we find an alternative to Dionysian ecstasy, entailing a more peaceful and less grandiose loss of the self into the *Ur-Eine*. Unlike Christ, Epicurus does not walk on the water but floats serenely on the sea, buoyed up by it and even cradled by it, happy with the gifts life has to offer, and existing beyond fear and anxiety even though he is opening himself up to troubling realities, such as the approach of death and his personal extinction: "We are born once and cannot be born twice, but we must be no more for all time."[82]

Notes

1 This chapter has been greatly inspired by the work of Horst Hutter and Michael Ure, and I am indebted to both. For comments and feedback that enabled me to improve this chapter, I am indebted to Daniel W. Conway, Beatrice Han-Pile, Rainer J. Hanshe, Lawrence J. Hatab, and Michael Ure. Thanks also to Andreas Urs-Sommer for supplying me with references to Nietzsche on Epicurus in the German and French scholarship, and to Frank Chouraqui for assisting me with the translations of the chapter from French version written by Richard Roos.

2 The other three pairs are: Goethe and Spinoza, Plato and Rousseau, and Pascal and Schopenhauer.

3 According to Julian Young *WS* "is impregnated by Epicurean philosophy," *Friedrich Nietzsche. A Philosophical Biography* (Cambridge: Cambridge University Press, 2010), 281.

4 On philosophy and the heroic, see also *GS* 324.

5 Catherine Wilson, *Epicureanism at the Origins of Modernity* (Oxford: New York, Oxford University Press, 2008), p. 37.

6 Howard Caygill, "Under the Epicurean Skies," *Angelaki* II(3), (2006): 107–115, 107.

7 Liba Taub, "Cosmology and meteorology," in James Warren (ed.), *The Cambridge Companion to Epicureanism* (Cambridge: Cambridge University Press, 2009), pp. 105–24, 124.

8 Ibid., p. 105.

9 Jean-Marie Guyau, *La Morale D'Epicure* (Paris: Librairie Gemer Baillière, 1878), p. 280.

10 See Nietzsche's letter to Carl von Gersdorff of enf of August 1866, in Christopher Middleton (ed.), *Selected Letters of Friedrich Nietzsche* (Indianapolis: Hackett, 1996), pp. 18–19.

11 F. A. Lange, *The History of Materialism* (London: Kegan Paul, 1925), First Book, 103.

12 Ibid., p. 102. See also Lucretius, *On the Nature of the Universe*, trans. R. E. Latham (Middlesex; Penguin, 1994), p. 39: "All life is a struggle in the dark . . . This dread and darkness of the mind cannot be dispelled by the sunbeams, and the shining shafts of day, but only by an understanding of the outward form and inner workings of nature."

13 Ibid.,p. 112.

14 Lange notes, astutely I think, that Epicurus's reverence for the gods is not a case of hypocrisy; it is, rather, that they, as "careless and painless" ones, represent "an incarnated ideal of his philosophy," namely, being in a condition free from pain (ibid., p. 101). There is thus no real contradiction between his reverence for the gods and his general attack on the fears and superstitions of the mind. As Lange puts it: "Thus Epikuros could at once impart a flavour of piety to his life, and still make the central point of his philosophy the effort to win that calmness of the soul which finds its only immovable foundation in deliverance from foolish superstitions" (ibid.).

15 Ibid., p. 121.

16 Laurence Lampert, *Nietzsche and Modern Times: A Study of Bacon, Descartes, and Nietzsche* (New Haven: Yale University Press, 1993), p. 423.
17 Ibid., p. 427.
18 Ibid., p. 426.
19 Ibid., p. 423.
20 Monika M. Langer, *Nietzsche's Gay Science: Dancing Coherence* (Basingstoke: Palgrave Macmillan, 2010), p. 67.
21 Ibid.
22 Ibid.
23 See Martin Heidegger, *Being and Time*, trans. John Macquarrie and Edward Robinson (Oxford: Basil Blackwell, 1980), pp. 99–103. I am grateful to Beatrice Han-Pile for suggesting this use of Heidegger to illuminate the section.
24 See letter to Peter Gast, August 26, 1883, in Oscar Levy (ed.), *Friedrich Nietzsche: Selected Letters*, trans. A. N. Ludovici (London: Soho Book Company, 1985), p. 164.
25 Pierre Hadot, *Philosophy as a Way of Life*, trans. Michael Chase (Oxford: Basil Blackwell, 1995), p. 87.
26 Epicurus, "Vatican Sayings," no. 45.
27 See Julian Young, *Friedrich Nietzsche. A Philosophical Biography* (Cambridge: Cambridge University Press, 2010), p. 279.
28 Young describes the asceticism advocated by Epicurus as a "eudaemonic asceticism," which is clearly very different to ascetic practices of world denial and self-denial. Young, 2010, p. 279.
29 Richard Roos, "Nietzsche et Épicure: l'idylle héroique," in Jean-François Balaudé and Patrick Wotling (eds), *Lectures de Nietzsche* (Paris: Librairie Générale Française, 2000), pp. 283–350, 298.
30 For further insight, see Young, 2010, pp. 279–81.
31 On Epicurus on fear and chance, see Hadot, 1995, 87, 223, and 252. See also A. A. Long, "Chance and laws of nature in Epicureanism," in Long, *From Epicurus to Epictetus: Studies in Hellenistic and Roman Philosophy* (Oxford: Oxford University Press, 2006), pp. 157–78.
32 Hadot, 1995, p. 252.
33 Graham Parkes, "Nature and the human 'redivinised': Mahāyāna Buddhist themes in *Thus Spoke Zarathustra*," in John Lippitt and James Urpeth (eds), *Nietzsche and the Divine* (Manchester: Clinamen Press, 2000), pp. 181–99, 195.
34 Hadot, 1995, p. 222.
35 Ibid., p. 223.
36 Marcuse, 1987, p. 123.
37 Hadot, 1995, p. 225.
38 Ibid., p. 226.
39 Michel Foucault, "On The Genealogy of Ethics: An Overview of work in progress", in Foucault, *Ethics: The essential works 1*, ed. Paul Rabinow, trans. Robert Hurley & others (Harmondsworth, Penguin 1997), p. 255.
40 Ruth Abbey, *Nietzsche's Middle Period* (Oxford: Oxford University Press, 2000), p. 99.
41 Epicurus, in Brad Inwood and L. P. Gerson (eds), *The Epicurus Reader* (Indianapolis: Hackett, 1994), p. 30.
42 Howard Jones, *The Epicurean Tradition* (London: Routledge,1989), p. 152.
43 *The Epicurus Reader*, p. 29.
44 Ibid.
45 Ibid.

46 James I. Porter, "Epicurean Attachments: Life, Pleasure, Beauty, Friendship, and Piety," *Cronache Ercolanesi* 33(2003): 205–27, 206.
47 Ibid., p. 207.
48 Ibid.
49 Ibid., p. 211.
50 Ibid., p. 212.
51 Ibid.
52 Ibid.
53 Ibid., p. 213.
54 Epicurus, *The Epicurus Reader*, p. 29.
55 Porter, 2003, p. 214.
56 Ibid.
57 Ibid., pp. 214 and 218.
58 Ibid., p. 216.
59 Ibid.
60 Ibid. On the distinction between katastematic (stable) and kinetic (transient and episodic) pleasures, see Raphael Woolf, "Pleasure and desire," in Warren, 2009, pp. 158–78, 170–7. On the status of "joy" (*khara*) in Epicurus's account of the emotions, see David Konstan, *A Life Worthy of the Gods: The Materialist Psychology of Epicurus* (Las Vegas: Parmenides Publishing, 2008), chapter one, especially 13–18. According to Konstan, it is best not to confuse *khara* with the goal of philosophy, which is described as either as *hêdonê* (the absence of feeling pain in the body or disturbance in the soul) or as *ataraxia* (freedom from perturbation), and with the former being a kinetic activity, the latter a katastematic pleasure.
61 Ibid., p. 217.
62 Ibid., p. 225.
63 Ibid., p. 226.
64 One might even see in this contemplation of nature, where all is peace and calm and where we have moved beyond "desire and expectation," something of Schopenhauer's ideas on art, including the release from the subjectivity of the will and the attainment of "objectivity" or pure perception. Schopenhauer, in fact, depicted such a state in Epicurean terms: "Then all at once the peace, always sought but always escaping us on that first path of willing, comes to us of its own accord, and all is well with us. It is the painless state, prized by Epicurus as the highest good and as the state of the gods; for that moment we are delivered from the miserable pressure of the will." Schopenhauer, *The World as Will and Representation*, in two volumes, trans. E. F. J. Payne (New York: Dover Press, 1966), volume one, section 38, 196. See also Schopenhauer on the "aesthetic delight" to be had from the experience of light: "Light is most pleasant and delightful; it has become the symbol of all that is good and salutary," 199. For further insight into Nietzsche's "Epicurus" as mediated by Schopenhauer, see Fritz Bornmann, "Nietzsches Epikur," *Nietzsche-Studien* 13 (1984); and Andrea Christian Bertino, "Nietzsche und die hellenistische Philosophie: Der Übermensch und der Weise," *Nietzsche-Studien* 36 (2007). See also Roos 2000, p. 293. Roos also notes the influence of Montaigne and Jacob Burckhardt on Nietzsche's appreciation of Epicurus.
65 Roos 2000, p. 322.
66 Ibid., p. 299.
67 Ibid., p. 301.
68 Ibid., 309.

69 Ibid., p. 333.
70 Ibid., p. 300.
71 Martin Heidegger, "The Word of Nietzsche: 'God is Dead'," in Heidegger (ed.), *The Question Concerning Technology & Other Essays*, trans. William Lovitt (New York: Harper & Row, 1977), pp. 53–112, especially 83–4, 96–101. For Heidegger Nietzsche's philosophy of the will to power and overman is part of the history of metaphysics conceived as the history of subjectness. He thus writes in his reflection on the word of Nietzsche: "Man, within the subjectness belonging to whatever is, rises up into the subjectivity of his essence . . . The world changes into object. In this revolutionary objectifying of everything that is, the earth, that which first of all must be put at the disposal of representing and setting forth, moves into the midst of human positing and analyzing. The earth itself can show itself only as the object of an assault, an assault that, in human willing, establishes itself as unconditional objectification. Nature appears everywhere – because willed from out of the essence of Being – as the object of technology" (100).
72 Michael E. Zimmerman, "Nietzsche and Ecology: A Critical Inquiry," in Steven V. Hicks and Alan Rosenberg (eds), *Reading Nietzsche at the Margins* (West Lafayette: Purdue University Press, 2008), pp. 165–86, 167.
73 Ibid.
74 See J. Donald Hughes, *Pan's Travail: Environmental Problems of the Ancient Greeks and Romans* (Baltmore: John Hopkins University Press, 1994). Cited in John Bellamy Foster, *Marx's Ecology: Materialism and Nature* (New York: Monthly Review Press, 2000), p. 37.
75 See Foster, *Marx's Ecology*, pp. 35, 37.
76 Lampert 1993, p. 279. See Max O. Hallman, "Nietzsche's Environmental Ethics," *Environmental Ethics* 13 (1991): 99–125. For a critique of Hallman, see Ralph R. Acampora, "Using and Abusing Nietzsche for Environmental Ethics," *Environmental Ethics* 16 (1994): 186-94. For a response to Acampora see Graham Parkes, "Nietzsche's Environmental Philosophy: A Trans-European Perspective, " *Environmental Ethics* 27(1), (2005): 77–91. Inspired by Lampert, Parkes has written that Nietzsche's philosophy of nature "qualifies him as one of the most powerful ecological thinkers of the modern period." See Parkes, "Staying Loyal to the Earth: Nietzsche as an Ecological Thinker," in John Lippitt (ed.), *Nietzsche's Futures* (Basingstoke: Macmillan, 1998), pp. 167–88, 167.
77 On the Epicurean avoidance of political activity, see Eric Brown, "Politics and Society," in James Warren (ed.), *The Cambridge Companion to Epicureanism* (Cambridge: Cambridge University Press, 2009), pp. 179–97, especially 180–2.
78 This is a point noted by Lane and Clark in their consideration of *Rousseau's* importance for deep ecology. See Joseph H. Lane and Rebecca R. Clark, "The Solitary Walker in the Political World: The Paradoxes of Rousseau and Deep Ecology," *Political* Theory 34(1), (2006): 62–94, 83.
79 Howard Caygill, "The Consolation of Philosophy; or neither Dionysus nor the Crucified," *Journal of Nietzsche Studies* 7(1994): 131–51, 144.
80 For insight into the disappearance and reappearance of Dionysus in Nietzsche's writings, see Adrian Del Caro, "Nietzschean self-transformation and the transformation of the Dionysian", in Salim Kemal, Ivan Gaskell and Daniel W. Conway (eds), *Nietzsche, philosophy, and the arts* (Cambridge: Cambridge University Press, 1998), pp. 70–92. He maintains that a transformed Dionysian surfaces around the time of *Dawn* and gains in concreteness throughout the 1880s, "closely associated

with Nietzsche's disavowal of metaphysics, and with his articulation of the major tenets of life-affirmation . . ." (73). Furthermore, "No longer an artistic deity or an aesthetic principle by 1880, the Dionysian became a hypostatization for the life-affirming individual, and it transformed as Nietzsche himself transformed" (83).

81 Richard Bett, "Nietzsche, the Greeks, and Happiness (with special reference to Aristotle and Epicurus)," *Philosophical Topics* 33(2), (2005): 45–70, 63.

82 Epicurus, "Vatican Sayings,"p. 14.

Editions of Nietzsche used

A *The Anti-Christ*, trans. Judith Norman (Cambridge: Cambridge University Press, 2005).

AOM *Assorted Opinions and Maxims*, trans. R. J. Hollingdale (Cambridge: Cambridge University Press, 1986).

BGE *Beyond Good and Evil*, trans. Marion Faber (Oxford: Oxford University Press, 1998).

BT *The Birth of Tragedy*, trans. Ronald Speirs (Cambridge: Cambridge University Press, 1999).

D *Dawn: Thoughts on the Presumptions of Morality*, trans. Brittain Smith (Stanford: Stanford University Press, 2011).

EH *Ecce Homo*, trans. Duncan Large (Oxford: Oxford University Press, 2007).

GM *On the Genealogy of Morality*, trans. Carol Diethe (Cambridge: Cambridge University Press, 2006).

GS *The Gay Science*, trans. Walter Kaufmann (New York: Random House, 1974).

HH *Human, all too Human*, volume one, trans. Gary Handwerk (Stanford: Stanford University Press, 1995).

KGB *Nietzsche Briefwechsel: Kritische Gesamtausabe*. Eds. G. Colli and M. Montinari (Berlin and New York: Walter de Gruyter, 1981).

KSA *Friedrich Nietzsche: Sämtliche Werke. Kritische Studienausgabe*, Eds. G. Colli and M. Montinari (Berlin and New York/Munich: dtv and Walter de Gruyter, 1967–77 and 1998).

WP *The Will to Power*, trans. Walter Kaufmann and R. J. Hollingdale (New York: Random House, 1968).

WS *The Wanderer and His Shadow*, trans. R. J. Hollingdale (Cambridge: Cambridge University Press, 1986).

10

Nietzsche's "View from Above"[1]

Michael Ure

In the past decade, there has been a renaissance of scholarly interest in Nietzsche's relationship to Darwinism and other contemporary evolutionary theories.[2] This scholarship demonstrates that in the late 1870s and early 1880s, Nietzsche attempted to make contemporary naturalism the basis of a new method of historical inquiry and a new style of moral criticism and experimentation. Arguably this scholarship has successfully challenged Martin Heidegger's attempt to purge Nietzsche of the "alleged biologism," which early critics and commentators had associated with his philosophy.[3] In the recent debate, most commentators agree that Nietzsche is a naturalist of one stripe or another, and the main interest lies in identifying his interpretation of nineteenth-century naturalism.[4]

Yet this period also marks the highpoint of Nietzsche's engagement with the Hellenistic model of philosophy. [5]In the middle period, Nietzsche is attracted by the general Hellenistic notion of philosophy as a practice or way of life. He explicitly conceives the moral schools of antiquity as "experimental laboratories" whose arts of living "we" might freely use to attain equanimity.[6] "What engages Nietzsche" as Julian Young observes of *The Wanderer and his Shadow* "are ideas common to all ancient philosophies."[7] One of the common ancient ideas that attracted Nietzsche in this period was the idea of surveying human life, as if from above.[8] This perspective then fits well with his whole overall approach of his reasoning in terms of a medical diagnosis and therapeutic suggestions.

In this chapter, I argue that we can develop a fuller appreciation of Nietzsche's therapeutic philosophy by seeing how he sought to renovate the ancient model of philosophy in light of the new naturalisms. He sought to retain the Hellenistic notion that a global evaluation of life follows from "physics," or a systematic view of nature.[9] Hellenistic philosophers conceived the elevation of the soul as the principle justification of "physics."[10] In this philosophical framework, physics was inseparable from the understanding and realization of the good life. In the late 1870s and early 1880s, I argue, Nietzsche attempts to refract the new naturalistic theories through the ancient model of philosophy and its "spiritual exercises." This chapter shows that Nietzsche's philosophy stands at the intersection of two very different naturalistic traditions: classical and Hellenistic naturalisms that conceived physics as part of a philosophical therapy, and nineteenth-century evolutionary naturalism that focused on empirically grounded, causal explanations of natural phenomena. I suggest that Nietzsche attempts to use the ancient model of philosophy to "incorporate" these new naturalisms. Nietzsche emulates the ancients by trying to make science "therapeutic" or "liberating" and does so partly by drawing on ancient spiritual exercises.

In particular, I argue that Nietzsche hinges one particular ancient spiritual exercise—the "view from above"—to the new naturalisms. It is partly for this reason that, despite his naturalistic commitment to formulating causal explanations compatible with scientific findings, his texts look, as Janaway rightly observes "starkly unlike scientific literature."[11] In line with that Hellenistic tradition, Nietzsche frames nature to achieve a fundamental value conversion from ordinary emotions to the philosophical passion of joy. In this way, Nietzsche's philosophy sharply diverges from modern naturalism. This chapter charts his shifting analysis of the relationship between his conceptions of nature or "physics" and his "ethics" conceived as a basic evaluative orientation or philosophical passion. It suggests that in *Human, All Too Human*, Nietzsche tries to convert his newly discovered positivist value neutrality into an ethical stance, which we might call the "stoicism of the intellect." In *Daybreak*, he oscillates between an Olympian and a Stoic "view from above," both of which enable free spirits to take joy in nature.

Nietzsche's Dilemma: Positivism or Classicism?

In the late 1870s, Nietzsche evinces ambivalence about the classical model of philosophy as a transformative practice that enables its practitioners to achieve the good life. On the one hand, he recognizes that the classical and Hellenistic attempt to make "physics" the basis of ethics necessarily carried with it epistemic dangers. If philosophy is predominantly considered an art of living, then it is easy to see how and why unpalatable truths might be sacrificed for the sake of flourishing or happiness.[12] On the other hand, Nietzsche seems reluctant to simply jettison this philosophical framework and rest content with the positivist program. He is just as concerned with addressing or ameliorating the potentially "tragic" consequences of pursuing knowledge or science at any cost.

Nietzsche then identifies the following dilemma: adopt the Hellenistic schools' stance of making physics a handmaiden to human flourishing with its associated epistemic risks, or adopt positivism but only at the "tragic" cost of a certain kind of disenchantment or despair. The dilemma turns on the idea that truth and flourishing might be incompatible. In *Human, All Too Human*, Nietzsche nominated as his *fundamental insight* the claim that there is no *necessary* connection or preestablished harmony between truth and flourishing.[13] We cannot, so he claims, reasonably assume the utility or value of truth for life, for "truth" may prove inimical to life. Worse still, so Nietzsche claimed, we can only discover this incompatibility between life and truth *ex post facto*. According to Nietzsche, if we adopt the new positivist approach, we cannot avert the dangers it carries because we cannot know about them in advance. In the case of the consequence or impact of knowledge on life, the Owl of Minerva spreads its wings only with the falling of dusk. On Nietzsche's analysis, then, if the classical model carries epistemic dangers (the sacrifice of truth), the new positivism carries "existential" dangers (the sacrifice of flourishing or "happiness"). This led Nietzsche to formulate the following question: "Can we (consciously) live in 'untruth' in order to survive and flourish or can we somehow incorporate science?"[14]

One of his main responses to this dilemma, so I shall argue, was to draw on the ancient schools' spiritual exercises (or *askesis*), especially the "view from above," to incorporate the discoveries of the new naturalisms. In this sense, then, Nietzsche was unwilling to relinquish the classical notion that the role of philosophy is to facilitate human flourishing. Even in his so-called "positivist" period, he sought to maintain and revive the ancient idea of philosophy as a way of life or practice that shapes or transforms its practitioner's basic "ethos" or disposition. It is indicative of this commitment that Nietzsche was never content simply to report or develop "scientific" discoveries; he always remained equally concerned, indeed often more concerned, with the effects and "after-effects of knowledge."[15] Nietzsche did not simply draw on contemporary naturalistic explanatory models or attempt to formulate his own causal accounts of moral phenomena. He also sought to identify both the emotional effects of such knowledge and to find ways of making it the basis of a positive ethical conversion. Like the classical philosophers, Nietzsche remained vitally concerned with how physics or science might fold back onto and transform agents. In the following sections, I examine how Nietzsche deploys the view from above to resolve the dilemma of "life" versus "truth."

Human, All Too Human: Free Spirit as Stoic of the Intellect

In conceiving philosophy as an art of living that enables individuals to overcome various malaises and in doing so to achieve a fully flourishing life, Nietzsche made himself an epigone of the Hellenistic philosophical tradition. In the middle period especially, Nietzsche seems committed to reviving philosophy as a therapeutic practice aimed at achieving *eudaimonia*. This is particularly evident in the way he makes frequent use of the famous Hellenistic analogy between philosophy and medicine, the philosopher and the physician.[16] Nietzsche believes that a philosophy worthy of the name is a practice that aims to cure disease and restore full health.

Yet at the same time that he seeks to reclaim philosophy's practical-therapeutic character with its eudaimonistic orientation, Nietzsche also entertains a general concern about the dangers of a philosophical orientation that gives priority to the issue of "happiness" or "well-being." He worries that once philosophy constitutes itself as a practice that aims to transform the lives of individuals so that they can achieve *ataraxia* and *autarkeia*, it must part company with science. In *Human, All Too Human*, Nietzsche crystallizes this problem in his pointed criticism of the Socratic schools. Their eudaimonistic orientation, he argues, only serves to restrict scientific inquiry.[17] This observation pinpoints one of his ongoing anxieties about practical philosophy: it purchases serenity only at the price of disturbing scientific investigation.

However, while Nietzsche recognizes the epistemic shortcomings of these classical and Hellenistic philosophies, he also acknowledges that contemporary sciences generate a range of "existential" or "ethical" difficulties. Science's explanations, he claims, destroy metaphysical and other prescientific views that hitherto provided the species with moral guidance or action-orientation. "(O)ur mode of thinking," as he explains, threatens to become "inimical to life" insofar as it annihilates both "religion" and "morality."[18] "Science," as Habermas glosses Nietzsche's point, "is not emancipatory, but nihilistic."[19] In *Daybreak*, Nietzsche elaborates how scientific causal explanation undermines morality as an action orienting interpretation of the world:

> In the same measure as the sense of causality increases, the extent of the domain of morality decreases; for each time one has understood the necessary effects and has learned how to segregate them from all the accidental effects and incidental consequences (post hoc), one has destroyed a countless number of *imaginary causalities* hitherto believed as the foundations of customs – the real world is much smaller than the imaginary – and each time a piece of anxiety and constraint has vanished from the world, each time too a piece of respect for the authority of custom: morality as a whole has suffered a diminution. [20]

Nietzsche's concern is that causal analysis demonstrates that our "motives" have been based on "errors."[21] "With each step of scientific development," as Habermas explains this point, "archaic world views, religious outlooks and philosophical interpretations lose ground. Cosmologies, as well as all pre-scientific interpretations of the world that make possible action orientation and the justification of norms, lose their credibility to the degree that an objectified nature becomes known in its causal connections and subjected to the power of technical control."[22]

We encounter here a fundamental tension in Nietzsche's philosophy between his positivistic commitment to scientific explanation and his commitment to philosophy as a practice integral to human flourishing. On the one hand, Nietzsche appears to concede a monopoly of knowledge to modern science, and in doing so rejects metaphysical claims. On the other hand, from the point of view of "practical" or "therapeutic" philosophy, scientific knowledge itself is necessarily problematic because it dispenses with metaphysics' innate connection with practice or life.[23]

The difficulty Nietzsche faces is how to retain a commitment to science, and the positivist notion that only empirically verified hypotheses count as knowledge, *without* losing this connection to the classical ideal of philosophy as a way of life. Science threatens to leave the human species without any value orientation or "meaning," and yet, as Nietzsche acknowledges, this need for "meaning" or "purpose" has become one of its newly acquired and unique needs.[24] Nietzsche, Habermas remarks, recognizes that the positivistic sciences' dissolution of dogmas "produces not liberation, but indifference."[25]

Yet it might be more accurate to say that Nietzsche's first response to this dilemma is to conceive positivist neutrality or indifference *as* liberation. Nietzsche's attempt to find a silver lining in positivism stands somewhat at odds with his "official" position that the question of the value or utility of science is beyond the scope of legitimate philosophical discussion. Like all other natural phenomena, he argues, science is not designed for a purpose. In *Human, All Too Human* 38, Nietzsche draws an analogy between nature's nonteleological achievement of perfect organic adaptations (i.e., the Darwinian perspective) and science's accidental contribution to the welfare of the human species. Later, in *Daybreak*, Nietzsche concedes as a matter of principle that the natural history of metaphysics may have less utility or value for the species than the metaphysical speculations it supplants. In his postmetaphysical incarnation, he assumes that scientific inquiry, including his own history of morality, does not embody or express a teleological purpose or final end that necessarily conforms to the interests of human welfare. In other words, he believes that it is a matter of contingency whether or not his natural history of morality proves a blessing or a curse for the general welfare or individual happiness. Nietzsche expresses his point in the form of a rhetorical question: "(W)hat have [known truths] in common with the inner states of suffering, stunted, sick human beings that they must necessarily be of use to them?"[26] If we accept a Darwinian or nonteleological notion of nature, then we must accept that, like any random variation, scientific inquiry only produces things or outcomes that prove useful to humanity as a matter of pure contingency, not because it is informed or guided by any final purpose or *telos*.[27] Whether or not scientific discoveries serve human life is just as contingent as whether or not a particular plant has medicinal properties. In both cases, it is a matter of contingency, not design. While we might hope that science is only capable of producing salutary results, we could only justify this wish, so he argues, on the basis of a fundamental metaphysical "error": *viz.*, the teleological belief that humankind is the goal of nature.[28] Until recently, we may have expected and indeed received consolation from metaphysical errors, but we have no reasons for believing that scientific inquiry will deliver consolation or cure.

For this reason, Nietzsche holds that, strictly speaking, we should bracket the question of science's value. Yet, although he wants to bracket this question, he also observes that science will require mitigation insofar as it is currently proving itself inimical to life. If we follow science in recognizing the "goallessness" of the species, he concedes in *Human, All Too Human* 33, "our philosophy" is in danger of becoming "tragedy."[29] It is modern sciences' destruction of all teleological accounts of the species' evolution, he suggests, that makes the question of science's value such a pressing issue.

What mitigates the tragedy of science's assault on the teleological view of nature and the corresponding notion of objective values and purposes? Nietzsche claims that our distress and contempt for life might gradually wane once we relinquish the great passions that hinged on belief in objective judgments or values. Once these passions dissipate, he suggests, free spirits can become akin to stoics who take "joy" [*Freude*] in contemplating nature from a standpoint of evaluative indifference.[30] Nietzsche conceives this indifference as science's positive aftereffect. Free spirits disinterestedly contemplate the spectacle of nature:

> Under the influence of purifying knowledge one would live among men and with oneself as in *nature*, without praising, blaming, contending, gazing contentedly, as though at a spectacle.[31]

Since free spirits recognize that natural events are necessities not governed by any purpose, they also understand that it is meaningless to judge them as "successes" or "failures" or to offer "praise" or "blame." Such judgments rest on belief in objective values, purposes, or intentions. Since science shows that the values we have projected or implanted in things are metaphysical illusions, free spirits, as long as they reside in truth, must content themselves with hovering above life. They are purified insofar as they are free of the tumultuous passions, particularly the so-called "moral" emotions that hitherto arose from such metaphysical illusions.

Clearly Nietzsche's concern is not simply with natural science's discoveries, or the application of its methods to moral and cultural phenomena, but also and crucially with how new scientific knowledge shapes or transforms agents. Like Schopenhauer, Nietzsche conceives knowledge as a mechanism that *purifies* individuals of their will or passions.[32] Science, he maintains, purifies us of passions or value-feelings that were hitherto anchored in our beliefs in objective purposes and values and in doing so leaves us in a state of indifference. We discover that values do not have any objective existence even though our passions make it appear that the world contains such properties.[33] Liberated from these value errors, Nietzsche suggests, free spirits can observe nature without will or passion. We might say then that Nietzsche's free spirits become "stoical" insofar as they live without making value-judgments. In *Human, All Too Human*, Nietzsche advocates what he will call "intellectual" stoicism. In a later autobiographical passage, Nietzsche uses this former concept to criticize the kind of contemplative indifference he had supported in *Human, All Too Human*:

> Perhaps I am all too familiar with . . . that stoicism of the intellect that finally forbids itself a 'no' just as strictly as a 'yes'; that wanting to halt before the factual, the *factum brutum* . . . that renunciation of all interpretation (of doing violence, pressing into orderly form, abridging, omitting, padding, fabricating, falsifying and whatever else belongs to the *essence* of all interpreting) . . . .[34]

The grounds of Nietzsche's postmetaphysical, positivistic indifference in *Human, All Too Human* are distinct from the grounds of what we might call cosmological Stoicism. The cosmological Stoic achieves *ataraxia* through both a rejection of the passions as false judgments *and* a cosmological view of the universe as embodied reason.[35] Nietzsche's antiteleological conceptualization of nature, which in *Human, All Too Human* he tends to conceive in terms of a purposeless "squandering" of energy, runs contrary to the cosmological Stoicism's conception of a providential universe. Science, Nietzsche averred in *Human, All Too Human*, does not support this ancient providential cosmology; if anything it supports a *naturalized* Schopenhauerian view of the cosmos as eternally repeating, purposeless chain of events.

Nietzsche later rejected the "stoicism of the intellect" that characterized his ethical stance in *Human, All Too Human*. Yet even in this text, he only half-heartedly celebrates intellectual stoicism. If positivism engenders a kind of contemplative neutrality, he implies, it is worth only "two cheers": it may free the species of grand moral commitments and passions based on errors (e.g., guilt, sinfulness, remorse) and contribute to the amelioration of material existence, but it does not satisfy those metaphysical needs religion satisfied, particularly the need for belief that existence has a purpose or *telos*. That is to say, while the scientific assault on metaphysical beliefs and presuppositions liberates free spirits from the burdens of responsibility, guilt, and sin, its attack on teleological commitments also leaves them without grounds for the belief that individual or collective endeavors have a final end or purpose. Positivistic skepticism therefore generates a new sense of innocence ("irresponsibility"), but only by eliminating the metaphysical presuppositions that underpinned both moral passions and future oriented passions like "hope." Without these teleological commitments, he claims, the free spirit must "pour mockery and contempt on the passions which reach out to the future and promise happiness in it."[36]

In this case, "a free, fearless hovering above men, customs, laws and traditional evaluations of things must *suffice* him as the condition he considers most desirable."[37] While Nietzsche suggests that free spirits take "joy" in this view from above, he also concedes that the fact free spirits can communicate nothing more than this state of indifference counts as "one more privation and renunciation."[38] Though he does not state it explicitly, presumably Nietzsche conceives their first privation as merely hovering above existence they believe is devoid of purpose or goal, rather than engaging passionately in events that they believe realize a higher purpose. "(A) man who lives only to know better" he remarks "must forgo almost everything upon which other men place value."[39] Most notably, free spirits renounce those moral passions and judgments that turn on the belief that nature expresses or embodies a metaphysical purpose that conforms to human wishes for redemption from suffering at the end of time or history. Nietzsche implies that a passionate life is tied to a belief in objective moral values and final ends and that, measured against this life, the free spirit's stoicism of the intellect must seem like a renunciation or living death. Nietzsche suggests that the free spirits' *second* privation consists in having nothing more to communicate to others than their "joy in this condition" of passionless contemplation.[40] Their "glad tidings" are nothing more than a disengaged hovering above existence. In *Human, All Too Human*, Nietzsche's joyful science is a curiously joyless affair.

In *The Wanderer and his Shadow*, Nietzsche returns to the issue of how to frame the scientific insight into nature's purposelessness in a way that inspires or warrants joy. His first response is to use the ancient model of the "view from above" as a device for cognitively reframing nature. This philosophical "elevation" dramatically transforms the reception of nature as a nonteleological chain of events that cause humanity "purposeless" suffering. Nietzsche conceives it as an exercise that makes it possible for free spirits to take pleasure in mocking humanity and liberate themselves from taking its sorrows and sufferings seriously. It is an antidote to a certain form of compassion. He shows how a certain kind of philosophical joy might derive from ascending to a higher perspective.

We can see this move in *The Wanderer and his Shadow* 14 "*Man, the comedian of the world.*" Here he conceives the view from above as an exercise that makes human suffering a source of amusement or comedy. It enables the philosopher to laugh at humanity's grandiose belief that it is the *telos* of existence:

> Let us hope there really are more spiritual beings than men are, so that all the humour shall not go to waste that lies in the fact that man regards himself as the goal and purpose of the existence of the whole universe and that mankind will not seriously rest satisfied with itself as anything less than the accomplisher of a universal mission.[41]

Nietzsche uses the view from above to deflate the seriousness that accompanies the metaphysical belief shared by Kantian and post-Kantian philosophers that humanity is the goal or "meaning of creation . . . the solution of the cosmic riddle, the mighty ruler over nature and the despiser of it, the creature which calls *its* history *world history*! – *Vanitas vanitatum homo*!"[42] Nietzsche explains the teleological conception of nature as a symptom of vanity or "cosmic narcissism": humans believe in their species' metaphysical import in order to avoid the pain of recognizing the cosmic insignificance of existence. As Nietzsche succinctly puts it later: "What truly enrages people about suffering is not the suffering itself, but the meaninglessness of suffering."[43] Teleological conceptions of nature serve to justify or give meaning to the "evil" of suffering. Nietzsche claims that humanity "would never have come into existence" without metaphysical errors: for example, the error of freedom of the will and the error that it is the goal or purpose of creation.[44] The fundamental human feeling, he suggests, remains "metaphysical" or a feeling based on the belief that humanity has a metaphysical significance or purpose.

Once we bracket the Kantian and Hegelian metaphysical "conceit," he claims, we must recognize that the human species history is no more significant than the history of any other species. From the point of view of Nietzsche's postmetaphysical, nonteleological conception of nature, the Kantian and Hegelian notion of humanity's metaphysical *telos* is analogous to "the ant in the forest" imagining that "it is the goal and objective of the forest."[45] However, thanks to Kantian and Hegelian metaphysicians, Nietzsche suggests, humanity now suffers from cosmic narcissism: the erroneous belief that its realization or completion is the ultimate goal of the whole universe.[46] Any challenge to this metaphysical teleology therefore comes at the price of wounded narcissism and undermines what has hitherto been the basis of humanity's fundamental feeling. Humanity imagines that its destruction would also mean the end of the universe.[47]

Nietzsche uses a cosmic (or astronomical) perspective to imply that biological life itself is a contingent eruption devoid of any metaphysical import. From this cosmic perspective, the destruction of biological life or humankind has no significance; nothing special or unique is lost. The genesis and demise of biological "life" is merely one natural process among others, despite humanity's vain belief that it is the ultimate objective or purpose of existence. Nietzsche then imagines a hypothetical creation story:

> If a god created the world then he created men as the *apes of god*, so as always to have on hand something to cheer him up in his all too protracted eternities. The music of the spheres encompassing the earth would then no doubt be the mocking laughter of the all other creatures encompassing man. That bored immortal tickles his favourite animal with pain, so as to take pleasure in the proud and tragic way this vainest of all creatures displays and interprets his sufferings and in his spiritual inventiveness in general – as the inventor of this inventor.[48]

What would amuse such a god about his favorite animal is the vanity and pride of this insignificant creature interpreting its sufferings as if they carried the most profound cosmic or metaphysical significance. Nietzsche replaces the harmonious music of the spheres with mocking laughter at humanity's absurd vanity. This god-like perspective humiliates humanity. From this "Olympian" view, humanity's metaphysical self-delusion is risible: humanity takes its redemption from suffering as the final purpose or goal of existence when its suffering is merely a means for a god's amusement.[49]

Yet as Bernard Williams observes, the mere idea that the species' suffering is an amusing spectacle for the gods cannot *alone* serve to make these sufferings bearable for individuals. On the contrary, the idea that the gods amuse themselves by tickling the species with pain might serve to justify ontological *ressentiment*.[50] What joy could there be in recognizing oneself as the plaything of a malevolent god who delights in one's suffering (*Schadenfreude*)? One possibility here is that human actors and sufferers identify themselves with these gods. This is what Nietzsche proposes in *The Wanderer and his Shadow* when he hopes that there are more spiritual beings than men who can enjoy the comic spectacle of human suffering in the manner of the gods who view them from the heights of Olympus.

Daybreak: Free Spirit as Olympian or Sage

In *Daybreak*, the "view from above" is central to Nietzsche's account of the new "dawn" that he hopes will bring to a close the species' metaphysical "night." We can see this in two important claims he makes in this text. Nietzsche claims that science is motivated by the "exaltation" or "elevation" that free spirits derive from sacrificing humanity on the altar of knowledge. Knowledge, he asserts, is a prize that justifies this sacrifice. In this sense, he believes that the passion for knowledge entails an Olympian attitude toward humanity: free-spirited philosophers delight in the suffering they cause by pursuing their passion for knowledge. Second, Nietzsche praises their intellectual courage to assume the sage's view from above and see nature without metaphysical and moral illusions. In this context, he explicitly draws on the ancient sage's "view from above" as a "spiritual exercise" or cognitive device for reframing nature as an object that elicits and warrants "joy." By adopting the sage's view from above, he suggests, they take a "generous" view of nature, affirming it as a whole rather than morally condemning it on the basis of the sufferings of its parts.

In *Daybreak*, then Nietzsche attempts to resolve the tension between truth and life. This resolution takes the following form: science or truth might prove fatal for those whose ethical and existential orientation is anchored in metaphysical convictions and hopes, but free spirits can make the pursuit of truth a passion that elevates them above distress so that they can enjoy nature as a spectacle. In other words, he recognizes science as a fatality for those wedded to metaphysical errors and illusions (e.g., teleology), but as the pathway to reclaiming joy in the spectacle of nature for the free spirit.[51] Yet clearly Nietzsche cannot derive this philosophical joy in nature simply from identifying or reporting new scientific explanations of natural phenomena. Science *alone* cannot transform the naturalist's emotional or affective orientation toward life. In *Human, All Too Human*, as we have seen, Nietzsche claims that the postmetaphysical, "disenchanted" view of nature might liberate free spirits from the burden of the prospective passions of desire and fear. However, this salutary transformation, he observes, hinges on a person's "temperament."[52]

In *Daybreak*, he now emends and develops his account of science and its relationship to philosophical passions. Nietzsche emends this claim by suggesting that science not only liberates free spirits *from* certain passions, but also that it satisfies certain kinds of passions, particularly a certain kind of joy or delight. Nietzsche develops this account by showing more clearly how science or "physics" only facilitates this transformation if it is mediated by certain kinds of spiritual exercises. It is not merely free spirits' temperament that determines the impact of science on their emotional order, but also these exercises. In *Daybreak*, Nietzsche implies that an Olympian or sage-like "view from above" is required to take joy in nature.

Here his conception of this "view from above" wavers between Stoicism's untroubled, serene spectatorship based on the judgment that nature's "cruelty" is a necessary or fated part of the whole, and the Olympian view of suffering as a delightful, entertaining spectacle. From the heights of Olympus, the gods enjoy the spectacle of human strife and suffering; from their cosmic view from above, Stoics conceive nature as a rational whole that justifies its parts. Olympian gods maliciously yet serenely enjoy the tragic drama of human existence from the vantage point of immunity granted by their immortality; Stoics enjoy the universe's perfect lawfulness by identifying themselves with nature as a whole. We can distinguish these two "views from above" in terms of different types of laughter. We might call Stoic laughter "*euthumiē*" and Olympian laughter *Schadenfreude*.[53] The former expresses Stoics' peace of mind and cheerfulness based on a view from above that generates a rationalist cosmology; the latter expresses an Olympian delight in the spectacle of human striving and conflict. The Olympian gods are emotionally absorbed in the agonistic drama of human *agon* hence their fluctuating affections for their mortal heroes and favorites. Yet, as Halliwell suggests, the Olympians can maintain their delight in this spectacle because they are immune from its terrible consequences and they alone have the option of divine withdrawal and detachment.[54] Though he never self-consciously distinguishes these two strands, and indeed they often intersect or overlap in his middle works, for the sake of clarity we can distinguish his usage of these two "exercises."[55] As we shall see, these two variations of the ancient trope of the view from above, the Olympian and Stoic are woven into the fabric of Nietzsche's philosophical "naturalism."

In *Daybreak*, Nietzsche revises the ground of his commitment to naturalism or science. In *Human All Too Human*, as we have seen, he suggests that through their scientific drive free spirits *unintentionally* cause those wedded to metaphysical illusions to suffer nihilistic despair. By contrast, in *Daybreak*, he identifies the free spirit's enjoyment of the suffering they create for others as one important motive fuelling their pursuit of science. Nietzsche suggests that science not only purifies free spirits of fear and desire, but also that it is motivated or inspired by a certain type of passion. Science, Nietzsche claims, "sublimates" the ancient gods' delight in the spectacle of suffering.

In *Daybreak* 45, he suggests exaltation in human sacrifice has been humanity's highest and most powerful ideal. Nietzsche posits this divine cruelty as a potential motive force of science. Nietzsche speculates that the ancient moral exaltation in sacrifice, which he traces to early *Sittichlichkeit* communities and their religious "imaginary," might be harnessed to a new end: the pursuit of knowledge.[56] He believes that free spirits might now sublimate or transfigure the exaltation the gods derived from the spectacle of human sacrifice; it might become the motive driving their commitment to knowledge at any price.[57] Nietzsche countenances the view that it might be "worth" sacrificing humanity to satisfy this passion for knowledge:

> If ever the constellation of [a *self-sacrificing mankind*] appears above the horizon, the knowledge of truth would remain as the *one* tremendous goal commensurate with such sacrifice, because for this goal no sacrifice is too great.[58]

From the free spirit's god-like perspective, knowledge of truth trumps all other values, including life itself. Science, he acknowledges, may have a "tragic ending"—the species' extinction—but this is of no matter, or more precisely this is the best outcome for those who like Olympian gods are exalted by this spectacle. Free spirits tie the knot between knowledge and sacrifice. We might identify their motto as "*Fiat veritas, et pereat mundus.*"[59] They sacrifice humanity to satisfy their passion for knowledge:

> Perhaps mankind will even perish of this passion for knowledge! – even this thought has no power over us! But did Christianity ever shun such a thought? . . . (If) mankind does not perish of a *passion* it will perish of a *weakness*: which do you prefer? This is the main question. Do we desire for mankind an end in fire and light or one in the sand?[60]

Nietzsche's free spirits are intoxicated by knowledge as a fatal passion:

> Indeed we are perishing from this passion for knowledge! But that is no argument against it. Otherwise death would be an argument against the life of the individual. We *must* perish as individuals and as humanity![61]

Nietzsche constructs an apparently tragic dilemma for humanity: whether it chooses the path of passion or weakness, it risks annihilation; it is simply a question of whether we want it to go out with a "bang" or a "whimper."[62] We might compare Nietzsche's account of the free spirit's sacrificial passion for knowledge in *Daybreak* to Kierkegaard's famous "teleological suspension of the ethical."[63] Nietzsche logic of cruelty inverts Kierkegaard's logic of sacrifice. Kierkegaard's Abraham suspends the ethical in obedience to a higher, divine commandment; he sacrifices his son for the sake of a higher moral duty: unconditional piety or fidelity. Nietzsche, by contrast, imagines his free spirits in the position of gods who demand that mortals sacrifice themselves for their pleasure. Kierkegaard depicts mortal creatures sacrificing themselves (or their own) for the sake of fidelity to God. Nietzsche pictures free spirits as gods sacrificing mortals for the sake of their own elevation or exaltation. Nietzsche's free spirits are analogous to Olympian gods enjoying the spectacle of suffering, not to Christian moralists sacrificing themselves for God. In this sense, Nietzsche conceives sacrifice as a mechanism through which free spirits can participate in the joys of immortal, god-like creatures. He conceives knowledge and the intellect as motivated by "evil" drives, that is, drives that find satisfaction in witnessing or causing harm.[64] Science, he implies, is a "sublimation" of the ancient gods' delight in the spectacle of mortal suffering. In short, science is a sublimation of archaic cruelty. [65]

Nietzsche believes we are mistaken to think that "the evil drives of humanity" play no part in science.[66] The evil drives, he claims, play an important role in motivating the pursuit of knowledge. "To think otherwise than is customary" he observes "is . . . the effect of . . . strong, evil inclinations: detaching, isolating, defiant, gloating (*schadenfroher*), and malicious (*hämischer*) inclinations."[67] Their pursuit of knowledge is an effort to satisfy this *Schadenfreude*. However, we need to carefully distinguish between Nietzsche's diagnosis and his evaluation of science's motives and effects. He identifies evil inclinations like *Schadenfreude* and malice as among the causes of science; anyone who breaks with custom and opinion, in the manner of heretics and free spirits, is motivated by such drives. When Nietzsche evaluates this circumstance he is acutely aware of the potential damage free spirits cause others in satisfying their "evil" drives. Yet, ultimately, he judges that this malice and the damage it causes is a tragic necessity of greatness.

In *Daybreak* 562, for example, Nietzsche suggests that free spirits *produce* tragedies—they break the hearts of those who love them best by breaking with their opinions. He suggests that free spirits must assuage the grief they cause their loved ones by deserting or rejecting shared opinions (*Meinungen*). Here, in one of his most tender meditations, he stresses that free spirits need to make reparations to their loved ones for inflicting on them this unwanted, undeserved suffering. Nietzsche uses Odysseus' trip to Hades or his down-going ("*untergehen*") to illustrate this reparative impulse.[68] By using this *Odyssey* allusion, Nietzsche also implies that he thinks it is impossible for free spirits to undo or heal the sorrow they cause through the pursuit of knowledge. In the relevant passage, Odyssey meets the shade of his mother who tells him that she died of grief and longing for him while he was away at war. Three times Odysseus attempts to embrace her, but he discovers that like all shades she is incorporeal and his arms simply pass through her body. Tragically, Nietzsche implies, the free spirit's pursuit of knowledge irreparably damages those nearest to him or her.

Nietzsche claims that the harm free spirits cause others is a tragic necessity. It is a necessity not in the sense that the harm is unforseeable or unavoidable, but in the sense that it is a condition of their existence. For Nietzsche, inflicting harm is a necessary condition of greatness. In GS 28, Nietzsche identifies greatness with hard-heartedness, or more literally an absence of charity (*Unbarmherzigkeit*).[69] Great individuals pay no heed to cries for compassion. "At times," he writes, "our strengths propel us so far ahead that we can no longer stand our weaknesses and perish from them. We may even foresee this outcome and still have it no other way. Thus we become hard against that within us that wants to be spared; and our greatness is also our mercilessness [or heartlessness]."[70] Greatness entails acting without regard for one's own preservation. Great individuals spare themselves nothing. Compassion, mercy, charity—all, so he claims, stands in the way of their greatness.

Nietzsche characterizes GS 28 as "a parable for the whole effect of great human beings on others and on their age: precisely with what is best in them, with what only they can do, they destroy many who are weak, insecure, in the process of becoming, of willing, and thus they are harmful." In GS 325, Nietzsche makes it clear that he thinks individuals can only attain greatness by *inflicting* great pain on others and resisting the temptations of compassion:

> What belongs to greatness – Who will attain something great if he does not feel in himself the power to *inflict* great pain? Being able to suffer is the least; weak women and even slaves often achieve mastery at that. But not to perish of inner distress and uncertainty when one inflicts great suffering and hears the cry of this suffering that is great; that belongs to greatness.[71]

How do great individuals and free spirits overcome their compassionate distress for those they harm? Nietzsche identifies the Olympian gods enjoyment of human tragedy as the alternative to compassion, the primary moral prejudice he aims to eliminate as the species' guiding morality. Nietzsche sees Olympian spectatorship as one way great individuals overcome their distress over the general purposelessness of existence, especially the purposelessness of suffering, and their distress over inflicting suffering on others. In *Daybreak* 144, he contrasts two responses to others' misfortune and suffering: suffering with them (*Mitleid*), and the "art of the Olympians." We can only aid or comfort these sufferers, he suggests, if we have learned this art and henceforth "*edified*" (*erbauten*) ourselves by their misfortunes instead of being made unhappy by them. What does Nietzsche mean by "edified" in this context? What would it mean in his terms to be edified by the spectacle of others' suffering? We might assume that Nietzsche identifies edification with acquiring knowledge that might be useful in helping to respond to or treat this suffering.

However, in D 144, Nietzsche does not connect being edified by others' misfortune with therapeutic knowledge. Consider the sentence that immediately follows on and elaborates his suggestion that we learn to edify ourselves by others' misfortune: "But that is somewhat too Olympian even for us: even though we have, with our enjoyment of tragedy, already taken a step in the direction of this ideal divine cannibalism." [72]Here Nietzsche spells out the nature of this "edification" as enjoyment or pleasure in the tragic hero's misfortune, through which, he suggests, "we" have moved toward a form of "ideal divine cannibalism." In this closing sentence of D 144, Nietzsche is decidedly not suggesting that we should learn more about others' suffering for the sake of curing it or helping them overcome it. Rather, he suggests that we learn how to feed off it for our own pleasure or enjoyment. Nietzsche's analogy makes this clear: spectators should be to those they see suffering as cannibals are to their human sacrifices. They feast on others' suffering. That Nietzsche thinks that this may be beyond "us" now, or be too Olympian for "us," in no way implies he eschews this as a positive response. On the contrary, he identifies his "spectatorial" cannibalism as both "ideal" and "divine."

Of course, this Olympian perspective is not the only response to suffering Nietzsche canvasses in D (or elsewhere). However, as we shall see, he clearly takes this as the philosophical free spirit's best or ideal direction. Elsewhere in D and even more clearly in unpublished drafts, Nietzsche identifies a very different alternative to the morality of compassion: not god-like gloating over human suffering, but practical effective care. In these notes, Nietzsche objects to compassion/*Mitleid* not in the name of this higher Olympian delight, but in the name of a more effective treatment of suffering. Glossing Kant's "Doctrine of Virtue" *in* section 34 of the *Metaphysics of Morals*, Nietzsche claims that "real pity [*Mitleid*] actually only doubles the suffering [*Leid*]."[73] To this utilitarian criticism of pity, understood as a contagious sharing of suffering, he adds the following observation: "[pity/*Mitleid*] is perhaps itself the source of the inability to help."[74]

Nietzsche's point is acute. Contemporary empirical psychologists claim that in sharing in others' suffering, we are unable to effectively help them because we need to attend to our own suffering.[75] Indeed, Nietzsche observes that not only do we inhibit our capacity for helping others by sharing their suffering, we may also reinforce their suffering by mirroring it back to them: "If we let ourselves be made gloomy by the lamentation and suffering of other mortals, and cover our own sky with clouds, who is it who will have to bear the consequences of this gloom? These other mortals, of course . . . ."[76] Nietzsche recognizes that emotional contagion can engender a negative mimetic feedback loop. In the unpublished notes, he offers an alternative to emotional contagion: "only when one knows about [suffering], but does not suffer, can one act for the sake of the other, as a doctor."[77] Nietzsche's unpublished reflections therefore offer a promising theory of practical compassion, which hinges on *knowing* that and how others suffer, rather than on *sharing* their suffering.

However, Nietzsche himself values the Olympian view from above as the highest or "ideal" response to mortal suffering. Compared with this Olympian view, he suggests, compassion can only make matters worse for both the sympathizer and the sufferer.[78] We can aid and comfort sufferers, he suggests, not by echoing their lamentations, but only by learning the Olympian art of delighting in human misfortune. Nietzsche thinks we somehow help our fellows by ascending to these Olympian heights. Presumably he means that, since taking the Olympian view is the only worthwhile response to human suffering, we can aid others by exemplifying this god-like enjoyment of human misfortune. We show them how they too might ascend above humanity. Nietzsche unequivocally values the Olympian view from above as the highest or "ideal" response to mortal suffering. The Nietzschean physician counsels us to ascend to Olympus in order to extirpate ordinary, mortal emotional responses to misfortune: fear, distress, pity, and so on.

Nietzsche's later explicit evaluation of Olympian spectatorship as the "highest" philosophical perspective underscores this point. In BGE, Nietzsche identifies the highest ranked philosophers as those who can assume the Olympian view of humanity as an object of amusement or *Schadenfreude*.[79] Like the Olympians, they enjoy mockery and they cannot contain their laughter even during the holy rites of mortals. They laugh at the "expense of all serious things."[80] Nietzsche underlines the fact that the "golden laughter" of those he dubs the highest-ranked philosophers derives from their mockery of others. He does so by identifying their laughter with the type of laughter Hobbes proscribed. Hobbes conceived laughter as a type of pusillanimous vainglory. Laughter, he claimed, is the expression of the feeling of superiority we derive from comparing ourselves against others' imperfections and deformities.[81] Nietzsche rehabilitates the Olympians' mocking, vain, and superior laughter at the defects of mortals as the model of philosophical wisdom:

> *The Olympian vice*. – In despite of that philosopher who, being a real Englishman, tried to bring laughter into ill-repute among all thinking men – 'laughing is a bad infirmity of human nature, which every thinking mind will strive to overcome'

> (Hobbes) – I should actually risk an order of rank among philosophers depending on the rank of their laughter – all the way up to those capable of *golden* laughter. And supposing that gods, too, philosophize, which has been suggested to me by many an inference – I should not doubt that they also know how to laugh the while in a superhuman and new way – and at the expense of all serious things. Gods enjoy mockery: it seems they cannot suppress laughter even during holy rites.[82]

Nietzsche's highest-ranked philosophers (or joyful scientists) derive their superiority from their god-like philosophical perspective and its mocking laughter. [83]Ultimately, then, Nietzsche privileges the Olympian view from above as the ideal response to mortal suffering. It enables free spirits to enjoy the spectacle of human tragedy, and it prevents them from succumbing to the great distress they feel when they inflict suffering on others. Nietzsche's free spirits cannot afford to sympathize with human suffering; they must rise above it and enjoy it. That Nietzsche advocates this Olympian vice is a measure of just how strongly he felt the temptation of compassion. Though he suggests that free spirits must inflict suffering on others for the sake of their own greatness, he also recognizes that they risk perishing by resisting their own "inner distress" at causing others "great suffering." According to Nietzsche, greatness requires inflicting suffering *and* overcoming compassion for the victims.

In *Daybreak*, however, Nietzsche oscillates between this Olympian "view from above" and its *Schadenfreude* and the Stoic/sage-like "view from above" and its *euthumiē*. In some passages, Nietzsche explicitly draws attention to his dependence on the classical and Stoic conception of the relationship between knowledge, the self and its evaluative and affective orientation toward existence. In *Daybreak* 450, Nietzsche suggests that the allure of knowledge for passionate spirits is precisely as a Stoic exercise in freeing oneself from a partial or "egocentric" perspective on nature:

> Does it not thrill through all your senses – this sound of sweet allurement with which science has proclaimed its glad tidings, in a hundred phrases and in the hundred and first and fairest: 'Let delusion vanish! Then "woe is me!" will vanish too; and with "woe is me!" woe itself will be gone'. (Marcus Aurelius)[84]

Here Nietzsche first connects the scientific elimination of delusion (*den Wahn*) with the purging of individuals' unhappiness about their *own* condition (woe is me!). From this, Stoic perspective individuals lament their own fate ("woe is me!") only because they suffer from delusions about nature or their place within the cosmos. These delusions must be such that they justify and inflame grievances regarding their own individual fate. Science, Nietzsche maintains, seduces passionate individuals with the promise that it will eliminate the grounds not simply of their own personal discontent, but all sources of distress and lamentation. To this extent, it seems to promise a new happiness or joy. The Stoic sage, we might recall, has his own kind of good emotions (*eupatheia*), which includes joy (*chara*). In antiquity, materialist philosophies and cosmologies were tightly connected with good emotions. The Stoic sage, for example, had his own kind of good pathos including "well reasoned elevation" or joy, and cheerful spirit (*euthumia*), which derives from the joy the sage takes in the universe's self-sufficiency.[85] Physics or science redeems its promise by eliminating the egocentric view of nature that fails to see how every event is a necessary part of the whole. That it is to say, science rejects the egocentric view that evaluates nature in terms of its satisfaction of individuals' prudential concerns.

Nietzsche's identification of this perspective with Marcus Aurelius makes it clear that he thinks Stoicism exemplifies how science informs or shapes one's ethical and affective comportment. Nietzsche sees Stoic philosophy as an example of how individuals can accede to the truth about nature in a way that extirpates painful, disturbing "passions," or more specifically, eliminates the need to lament their individual fate. For the Stoics, science or physics is a spiritual exercise, which consists in looking down at things from above, including oneself, or from the point of view of nature as a whole. Referring to Seneca's *Natural Questions*, Hadot notes that the "soul of the philosopher, looking down from the heights of the heavens, becomes aware of the puniness of the earth, and the ridiculousness of the wars fought by human armies . . . over miniscule stretches of territory."[86] In Stoic philosophy, physics is an exercise that enables philosophers to see human matters in their true dimensions; the view from above, for example, makes it possible for them to "see" the insignificance of individual cares and in doing so it eliminates the passions that disturb their serenity. "The goal of physics as a spiritual exercise" Hadot writes "was to relocate human existence within the infinity of time and space, and the perspective of the great laws of nature."[87] Marcus Aurelius exemplifies this philosophical exercise: "When you are reasoning about mankind, *look upon earthly things below as if from some vantage point above them.*"[88]

Once we see things independently of this ego-standpoint, as Marcus Aurelius exhorts, it becomes possible to make different esthetic and moral evaluations of nature and the cosmos. From the point of view of nature, a view the Stoic philosophers identify as seeing things from above, egoistic cares are correctly identified as matters of indifference. Physics is an exercise that corrects mistaken evaluations. In Stoic philosophy, therefore, the importance of physics lies in its effect on the soul's emotional order. It frees the Stoic from pathological disorders. Hadot suggests that the ancient philosophers, particularly the Roman Stoics, practiced "physics" as a spiritual exercise that transformed their value-judgment of the world. Marcus Aurelius, he observes, claimed that all the phenomena we judge to be repugnant or ugly are in fact intimately linked to the processes, course, and development of the world, which in turn can be traced back to universal Reason.[89] "If one possesses experience and a thorough knowledge of the workings of the universe," Aurelius writes, "there will be scarcely a single one of those phenomena which accompany natural processes as a consequence which will not appear to him, under some aspect at least, as pleasant. Such a person will derive no less pleasure from contemplating the actual gaping jaws of wild beasts than he does from all the imitations, which painters and sculptors provide thereof . . . it is not just anyone who can derive pleasure from [such phenomena]. Rather, only that person who has become truly familiar with Nature and her works will do so."[90]

In *Daybreak* 551, Nietzsche explicitly turns to ancient philosophers to identify what he calls "future virtues." Ancient philosophy, he suggests, establishes the exemplary model for these virtues. To cultivate these virtues, he implies, free spirits must reclaim the ancient philosophers' practice of natural knowledge or physics as a spiritual exercise.

Nietzsche rehabilitates the sage's view from above as the key to a certain "generous" or "magnanimous" ethical disposition towards nature:

> Perhaps there will come a time when . . . courage in thinking will have grown so great that, as the supreme form of arrogance it will feel itself *above* man and things - when the sage will as the most courageous man, also be the man who sees himself and existence farthest beneath him – This species of courage, which is not far from being an extravagant generosity, has hitherto been *lacking* in mankind.[91]

Nietzsche associates this courage in thinking with seeing things from a great height, one of the standard tropes of ancient philosophy. It is the ancient sage who takes this god-like, empyrean view of temporal, worldly affairs. Nietzsche speculates that our future virtues may in some sense reprise the ancient sage's virtues. Nietzsche obviously and self-consciously borrows the "view from above" from the ancient philosophical tradition. He highlights the fact that he is recycling the classical philosophical tradition and its spiritual exercises by explicitly associating the view from above with the classical/Hellenistic figure of the sage (*der Weise*). In ancient philosophy, of course, the sage represents the fulfillment of the philosophical way of life. Nietzsche claims that the effects of modern science may prove to be similar to those that classical and Hellenistic philosophers sought to realize through ancient "physics": *viz.*, the greatness of soul that remains unmoved or untroubled by existence. Just as classical philosophers understood "physics" as a spiritual exercise intended to bring about greatness of soul that assents to the world, so too Nietzsche believes science might have a similar outcome: an extravagant generosity.

In *Daybreak* 551, Nietzsche highlights the view from above as fundamental to his joyful science; it is the "view from above" that he hopes might engender an extravagant generosity toward the world. Nietzsche had earlier suggested that "miserliness" is one of the primary dangers of the postmetaphysical condition. We have discovered, he maintains, that our evaluative and esthetic predicates (good, beautiful sublime, evil) are projections of our soul, not intrinsic features of the world. For this reason, he suggests, we are tempted to retract all these predicates on the grounds that they do not properly belong to objects. Nothing is good, beautiful, sublime or evil in itself. "Let us take care" he warns "that this insight does not deprive us of the capacity to lend, and that we have not become at the same time *richer* and *greedier*."[92] How is it possible to recover this capacity to give away these predicates; and on what basis might we distribute them once we no longer conceive them as intrinsic attributes of objects but as projections of states of our soul? Or, as he frames it in *Daybreak* 551, how is it possible for abject, fearful dependents to become gift-bestowing sovereigns? It is precisely this issue of learning how to apply the predicate "beautiful" to that which is necessary that Nietzsche places at the heart of the doctrine of *amor fati*.[93] *Nietzsche identifies the sage's "view from above" as the lynchpin of this conversion.* It is by seeing nature as a whole that free spirits establish grounds for a positive or "generous" evaluation of natural phenomena.

Nietzsche's use of this figure of the sage's view from above is central to his concept of a joyful science and its doctrine of *amor fati*. Hadot notes how Nietzsche anchors his doctrine of *amor fati* in a version of the classical view from above: "that is the soul's flight above all things, in the immensity of the universe."[94] In order to grasp the meaning of Nietzsche's Latin motto, therefore, we need to understand how he transposes this ancient model of philosophy into the late-nineteenth-century philosophical context and its naturalistic doctrines. Hadot identifies a remarkable similarity between the Stoicism's love of fate and Nietzsche's doctrine of *amor fati*. [95]As Hadot conceives it, the aim of Stoicism's spiritual exercises or discipline of desire is to make it possible for individuals to lovingly consent to the will of the Whole. In many ways, he argues, Nietzsche's Latin phrase "*amor fati*" coincides with the aim of Stoic philosophy. Epictetus encapsulated the objective of the Stoic discipline of desire in his famous apothegm: "Do not seek for things to happen the way you want them to; rather, wish that what happens happen the way it happens: then you will be happy."[96] Hadot claims that the Stoic consent to fate required individuals to identify with the Whole or universal reason, and to that extent it entailed that they transcend their own individuality. "If then the self's awareness is accompanied by a consent to events" he writes "it is opened up to the whole of cosmic becoming, to the extent that the self elevates itself from its limited situation and partial, restricted individual viewpoint, toward a universal perspective."[97] It is because the Stoic love of fate hinges on this "cosmic consciousness," as he calls it, that the discipline of desire corresponds to the physical part of philosophy. Stoic physics is a spiritual exercise through which individuals elevate themselves to the view of the Whole and the self *qua* will or liberty coincides with the will of universal reason, or *logos*, which extends throughout all things. Through physics as a spiritual exercise "the self as guiding principle coincides with the guiding principle of the universe."[98]

Now, as we have seen, Hadot notes that the "view from above" is also an integral feature of Nietzsche's doctrine of *amor fati*. According to Hadot, Nietzsche shares with Stoicism the conception of philosophy as an art of living, the aim of which is to consent to all events, and he deploys the very same type of spiritual exercise, *viz.*, the so-called view from above. It is a sage-like view from above that Nietzsche later conceives as the basis of his doctrine of *amor fati*. The view from above is the enthymeme in Nietzsche's first statement of this doctrine.[99] Nietzsche makes this premise explicit in *Nietzsche contra Wagner*:

> Everything which is necessary *when seen from above and from the point of view of the vast economy of the whole*, is in itself equally useful. We must not only put up with it, but *love* it. *Amor fati*: that is my innermost nature.[100]

Conclusion

This chapter has shown how Nietzsche's positivist commitments in the middle period challenge his classical commitment to philosophy as a way of life. Truth and flourishing, he concedes, are not necessarily compatible. It demonstrates that in *Human, All Too Human*, Nietzsche attempts to resolve this dilemma by conceiving positivism's evaluative neutrality as itself directly contributing to human flourishing insofar as it liberates free spirits from painful moral passions. Positivism might disenchant the world, but it also liberates free spirits to enjoy the spectacle of nature free from the tumult of the passions. Without metaphysical morality darkening the skies above nature, free spirits can enjoy the innocence of nature. However, in *The Wanderer and his Shadow*, Nietzsche acknowledges that free spirits can only delight in contemplating nature, if they can take pleasure in the purposeless suffering it inflicts on humanity. Nietzsche deploys the ancient trope of the Olympian view from above as a means of cognitively reframing nature. Taking the view from above, he implies, might make it possible for free spirits to emulate the Olympians and take delight in nature's tragic spectacle.

In *Daybreak*, Nietzsche oscillates between a quasi-Stoic and Olympian view from above. In his Olympian moment, he identifies the god's enjoyment of tragedy as one way great individuals can overcome their distress over the general purposelessness of existence, especially the purposelessness of suffering, and their distress over inflicting suffering on others. In the later parts of *Daybreak*, Nietzsche draws explicitly on the Hellenistic model of philosophy, the image of the sage, and the spiritual exercise of the view from above. He draws on this Hellenistic exercise to explore how free spirits might incorporate the insights of the new nonteleological, evolutionary conception of nature. Nietzsche identifies the Olympian "view from above" as a framing device enabling free spirits to delight in the spectacle of nature and the Stoic "view from above" as a device that makes it possible to affirm nature as a whole.

Notes

1 I would like to thank Keith Ansell-Pearson, Eli Friedland, Bill MacDonald, Matthew Sharpe, Gudrun von Tevenar, and especially Michael Janover for their generosity in providing critical comments on drafts of this chapter.

2 See, for example, Gregory Moore, *Nietzsche, Biology and Metaphor* (Cambridge: Cambridge University Press, 2002) and Robin Small, *Nietzsche and Rée: A Star Friendship* (Oxford: Oxford University Press, 2005).

3 See Martin Heidegger, *Nietzsche Volume III,* trans. J. Stambaugh, D. F. Krell, F. A. Capuzzi (New York: Harper, 1991), pp. 3947. See Claire Richter, *Nietzsche et les théorie biologiques contemperaines* (Paris: Mercure de France, 1911).

4 See John Richardson, *Nietzsche's New Darwinism* (Oxford: Oxford University Press, 2004); and Dirk Johnson, *Nietzsche's Anti-Darwinism* (Cambridge: Cambridge University Press, 2010). Cf. Robert B. Pippin, *Nietzsche, Psychology and First Philosophy* (Chicago: University of Chicago Press, 2010).

5 See, for example, Pierre Hadot, *Philosophy as a Way of Life: Spiritual Exercises from Socrates to Foucault,* trans. Michael Chase (Malden: Blackwell, 1995), p. 272; Horst Hutter, *Nietzsche's New Regime of the Soul and Its Ascetic Practices* (Lanham: Lexington Books, 2006); Michael Ure, *Nietzsche's Therapy: Self Cultivation in the Middle Works* (Lanham: Lexington Press, 2008); and Julian Young *Nietzsche: A Philosophical Biography* (Cambridge: Cambridge University Press, 2010), pp. 277–85.

6 KSA 1881 15[159].

7 Julian Young, *Nietzsche*, p. 278.

8 Halliwell shows that the idea of surveying life from above became embedded in Greek cultural consciousness as a result of the picture of the Olympian gods who view human existence from a certain distance as a kind of spectacle for their

own interest and consumption. The Olympian view was then taken up by Greek philosophy and incorporated into its notion of the human mind's own capacity for comprehensive contemplation or "*theoria*" (literally viewing). Greek philosophy converted the Olympian's external spectatorship into the spectatorship that takes place inside the philosopher's soul and places it cognitively "above the world." See Stephen Halliwell, *Greek Laughter: A Study of Cultural Psychology from Homer to Christianity* (Cambridge: Cambridge University Press, 2008), p. 337.

9 Pierre Hadot, *What is Ancient Philosophy?* (Cambridge: Harvard University Press, 2002), pp. 118–22, 128–31.

10 Hadot, *What is Ancient Philosophy*?, p. 209.

11 Christopher Janaway, *Beyond Selflessness: Reading Nietzsche's Genealogy* (Oxford: Oxford University Press, 2007), p. 39.

12 See Martha Nussbaum, *Therapy of Desire* (New Jersey: Princeton University Press, 1994), pp. 37–40.

13 HH 517.

14 HH 34.

15 Ibid.

16 E.g. D 52.

17 HH 7; see also HH 30. Nietzsche reiterates this point in later notes, see, for example, WP 442; KSA 1888 14[141]. Nietzsche shared his contemporaries' concerns about the epistemic dangers of the ancient model of philosophy. See Friedrich Albert Lange, *History of Materialism and Criticisms of its Present Importance* (London: Kegan Paul, Trench, Trübner and Co., 1892), p. 103; and pp. 95–6.

18 HH 34.

19 Jürgen Habermas, *Knowledge and Human Interests,* trans. J. Shapiro (London: Heinemann, 1972), p. 292.

20 D 10.

21 HH 34.

22 Habermas, *Knowledge and Human Interests*, p. 293.

23 Ibid.

24 GS 1.

25 Habermas, *Knowledge and Human Interests*, p. 292.

26 D 424.

27 See also the following unpublished 1880 note: "The passion for knowledge sees *itself* as the *purpose* of existence - if it denies purposes, it sees itself as the most *valuable result* of all accidents. Will it *deny* the value?" KSA 9, 11 [69].

28 D 424.

29 HH 33.

30 HH 34.

31 Ibid.

32 See Arthur Schopenhauer, *The World as Will and Representation, vol. 2,* trans. E. F. J. Payne (New York: Dover Publications, 1958), pp. 638–9.

33 On Nietzsche's "error theory" of morality in the middle period, see Maudemarie Clark & David Dudrick, 'Nietzsche and Moral Objectivity: the Development of Nietzsche's Metaethics,' in B. Leiter & N. Sinhababu (eds), *Nietzsche and Morality* (Oxford: Clarendon Press, 2007), pp. 192–226, pp. 198–201.

34 GM III.24.

35 Adam Smith draws a similar distinction within Stoicism, see, *The Theory of Moral Sentiments* (Cambridge: Cambridge University Press, 2002), VII. ii, 36–7.

36 HH 34.
37 Ibid.
38 Ibid.
39 Ibid.
40 Ibid.
41 WS 14.
42 WS 12.
43 See GM 2.7.
44 WS 12.
45 WS 14.
46 See also D 37.
47 WS 14
48 Ibid.
49 I use scare quotes around the word "Olympian" here to indicate that Nietzsche significantly modifies the Homeric concept of divine laughter. According to Halliwell, the Olympian gods never laugh at the absurdity or vanity of human existence as such nor does human suffering cause divine laughter. "Nietzsche" as he explains "uses Homeric laughter to echo the ultimate insignificance of reality [HH 16], but such existential laughter is never actually sounded, by gods or men, in Homer." See Halliwell, *Greek Laughter*, p. 59, fn 20, and p. 367. Hereafter, I use the term Olympian in this Nietzschean sense.
50 Bernard Williams, *The Sense of the Past* (Princeton: Princeton University Press, 2006), pp. 331–7, p. 333.
51 See also *D* 562.
52 HH 34.
53 I borrow this distinction from Halliwell, *Greek Laughter*, pp. 353–71.
54 Halliwell, *Greek Laughter*, p. 59.
55 Halliwell notes that Nietzsche is sometimes an advocate of a laughter of "existential absurdity," but also of "euthumic" cheerfulness. Haliwell, *Greek Laughter*, p. 367. See also Jessica Berry, 'Nietzsche and Democritus: The Origin of Ethical Eudaimonism,' in Paul Bishop (ed.), *Nietzsche and Antiquity* (Rochester: Camden House 2004), pp. 98–113.
56 D 18.
57 In conceiving of scientific inquiry as potentially motivated by god-like joy, Nietzsche deliberately recalls his earlier discussion at *Daybreak* 18 of the *Sittlichkeit* gods who "are amused and put into good humour by our suffering." In this religious "imaginary," he observes, human suffering "steams up (to the gods) like a perpetual propitiatory offering on the altar." In *Daybreak* 45, Nietzsche conceives free-spirited scientists' relationship to humanity as analogous to these evil gods' relationship to humanity. What motivates their pursuit of science is their desire to exalt in sacrificing humanity.
58 D 45.
59 KSA 1873 8[29].
60 D 429.
61 See KSA 1881 9: 7[171].
62 See also KSA 1881 9: 7[302]. "The passion for knowledge can come to a *tragic* end: are you scared? As much as with any passion! – Usually, however, you scholars are without passion, instead, you have *got use to your boredom*!."
63 See Søren Kierkegaard, *Fear & Trembling*. trans. Sylvia Walsh (Cambridge: Cambridge University Press, 2006).

64 See also GS 35.
65 See also BGE 229: "(T)he seeker after knowledge . . . acts as an artist and transfigurer of cruelty."
66 GS 37.
67 GS 35.
68 Homer, *Odyssey*, Book XI.
69 GS 28.
70 Ibid.
71 GS 325. Nietzsche's emphasis.
72 D 144. Thomas Bartscherer plausibly suggests that Nietzsche derives this idea of ideal divine cannibalism *(Götter-Kanibalenthum)* from Herbert Spencer's *Data of Ethics* (1879), a German translation of which he read and annotated while composing *Daybreak*. See Thomas Bartscherer, 'The Spectacle of Suffering: On Tragedy in Nietzsche's *Daybreak*', *Phænex* 1(2), 2006: pp. 71–93. This is the relevant passage: ". . . supposing that from the savage who immolates victims to a cannibal god [*cannibalischen Gotte*], there are descendants among the civilized who hold that mankind was made for suffering, and that it is their duty to continue to live in misery for the delight of their maker, we can only recognize the fact that devil-worshippers are not yet extinct."
73 *KSW* 9, 2[35].
74 Ibid.
75 See C. Daniel Batson, "These things called empathy: eight related but distinct phenomena," J. Decety and W. Ickes (eds), *The Social Neuroscience of Empathy* (Cambridge, MA: The MIT Press, 2009), pp. 3–15.
76 D 144.
77 *KSW* 9, 2[35].
78 See, respectively, D 134, 144.
79 Nietzsche also identifies Zarathustra/Dionysus with this malicious laughter; see Z III 16: The Seven Seals (Or: Yes and Amen Song) and Z IV, 1: The Honey Sacrifice. I thank Gudrun von Tevenar for drawing my attention to Zarathustra's malicious laughter. See Gudrun von Tevenar, 'The Malicious Dionysian,' in K. Gemes and J. Richardson (eds), *Oxford Handbook on Nietzsche* (Oxford: Oxford University Press, forthcoming).
80 In considering Nietzsche's point, we do well to remember that the Greek tragedians identified the following as serious disasters potentially worthy of pity: *viz*., death, bodily assault or ill-treatment, old age, illness, lack of food, lack of friends, separation from friends, physical weakness, immobility, reversals of expectations, absence of good prospects. See Aristotle, *Rhetoric*, 1386a6-13.
81 Thomas Hobbes, *Leviathan* (Harmondsworth: Penguin, 1985), I.6 'Sudden Glory Laughter.'
82 BGE 294.
83 Elsewhere I have argued that in his middle period, Nietzsche often diagnoses this kind of Olympian or heroic laughter of total affirmation as a psychological malady and identifies healthy self-cultivation with smiling, antiheroic acknowledgment of finitude and vulnerability. Here I am suggesting that in his later works, Nietzsche tends to identify with rather than diagnose this "Olympian" ethos and that it eclipses his earlier notion of self-cultivation. See Michael Ure. 'Stoic Comedians: Nietzsche and Freud on the Art of Arranging One's Humours.' *Nietzsche-Studien* 34(2005): 183–216; and *Nietzsche's Therapy; The Ethics of Self-Cultivation in the Middle Works* (Lanham: Lexington, 2008).

84 D 450.
85 See Margaret Graver, *Stoicism and Emotion* (Chicago: University of Chicago Press, 2007), pp. 58–9.
86 Pierre Hadot, *Philosophy as a Way of Life*, p. 245.
87 Hadot, *Philosophy as a Way of Life*, p. 244.
88 Marcus Aurelius, *Meditations* VII, pp. 47–8.
89 Pierre Hadot, *The Inner Citadel*, trans. Michael Chase (Cambridge: Harvard University Press, 1998), p. 168.
90 Marcus Aurelius, *Meditations* III, p. 2.
91 D 551.
92 D 210.
93 GS 276.
94 Hadot, *The Inner Citadel*, p. 172; p. 331, n. 6.
95 Hadot, *The Inner Citadel*, pp. 143–46. Nietzsche's enthusiasm for Hellenistic eudaimonism and the sage's joyful assent to the universe is evident throughout HH and D. In HH 2 334, for example, he affirms the Hellenistic ideal of the sage's self-sufficiency. See Michael Ure, 'Nietzsche's Free-Spirit Trilogy and Stoic Therapy,' *Journal of Nietzsche Studies* 38(2009): 60–84.
96 Epictetus, *Manual*, p. 8.
97 Pierre Hadot, *The Inner Citadel*, p. 146.
98 Hadot, *The Inner Citadel*, p. 146.
99 GS 276.
100 NCW, Epilogue, 1, italics added. This passage shows how Nietzsche brings together the Stoic view from above and evolutionary biology ("the economy of the whole"). Here Nietzsche is much closer to the Stoics in his metaphysical assumption that from the point of view of the whole of nature, every event is useful or functional. Elsewhere, by contrast, Nietzsche assumes that nature blindly produces countless random, useless, or dysfunctional variations, see, for example, HH 224.

11

Zarathustra's Stillness: Dreaming and the Art of Incubation

Rainer J. Hanshe

In an immediate understanding of the dream there is joy, all of its forms speak to us, there is nothing indifferent and unnecessary. Nevertheless, while this dream-reality is at its peak, the feeling creeps in that it is an appearance: [. . .but] reality too is appearance.

– Nietzsche[1]

In the *Birth of Tragedy*, Nietzsche claims that it is not the waking but the dreaming half of life that is "the more privileged, important, dignified, and worthy of being lived, indeed the only half that is truly lived."[2] Similarly, in *Beyond Good and Evil*, he proclaims that what "we experience in dreams, if we experience it often, is in the end just as much a part of the total economy of our soul as is anything we 'really' experience."[3] If Nietzsche accords an exceptional degree of significance to the oneiric dimension of life, suggesting that in and of itself it warrants as much if not more value than our waking life, he also maintains that our dreams' habits guide us during our waking hours and lead us "even in our most cheerful moments."[4] Thus, our predominant monarchs are dreams, navigating forces that direct not only our night journeys but, perhaps more significantly, our day journeys as well. While the structure and overall *Stimmung* of *Thus Spoke Zarathustra* are oneiric,[5] dreams function precisely as such helpful guides for Zarathustra. They have other functions also, including that of prophecy—as Zarathustra avows: "whoever had to create, he always also had prophetic dreams and astral signs—and believed in belief!"[6] While there are four crucial instances when he dreams during his *Untergang*, Zarathustra engages in one other unique kind of "dreaming" and it always occurs during his "stillest hours." Since to Zarathustra our "stillest hours" are our greatest events,[7] it is imperative to analyze Zarathustra's own stillest hours, in order to gain insight into precisely what they are constituted of and what Nietzsche reveals through them.

Of the numerous "still hours" in *Zarathustra*, each has a different function. Zarathustra engages in them to communicate with the earth, to enter into self-reflective states, to raise questions about his teaching during moments of crisis, and as a meditative but intense mode of wide-awake "sleeping," during which he receives visions, premonitions, wisdom, "still words," etc., all of which aid him during his *Untergang*. Of paramount importance is the state of concentrated stillness that Zarathustra enters into, a mode of incubation or temple-sleep practiced by, for instance, Amphiaraos, Parmenides, and Empedocles. Nietzsche would have been intimately familiar with incubation through reading of the devotees of Asclepius and numerous ancient sources from Homer to Strabo and Macrobius as well as, possibly, through Rohde's research for *Psyche*.[8] Rohde explains that it is through the legend of Amphiaraos "that we have a proof that already in the days when the quasi-Homeric poetry was still popular, people believed in deathless dwellers below the earth and in their active potency in the mantic act."[9] Akin to "a dream but not a dream," Peter Kingsley describes incubation as actually a "third type of consciousness quite different from either waking or sleeping."[10] In that heightened state of consciousness, Parmenides and Empedocles received the wisdom on which they formulated their teaching as opposed to developing it abstractly. It is not a form of ratiocinative thinking, misinterpreted, Heidegger argues, as rational, but a form of thought that includes feeling or mood, is "more reasonable—that is, more intelligently perceptive—because more open to Being."[11] When one reaches rationality's limits, it is through the phantastic that in dreams the imagination enables us to comprehend or reach otherwise inaccessible knowledge, sources of knowledge which exceed conscious understanding. In the dream or incubation state, the rational and the irrational intertwine, forcing us to recognize the thresholds of self-knowledge, that everything cannot be discerned through rationality alone.

Often, as Nietzsche elaborates, there is a form of thought more powerful than calculative and logical thought, a faculty Nietzsche refers to as "an alien, illogical power—the power of creative imagination." Such thought is not ruled by measure, but "leaps from possibility to possibility, using each one as a temporary resting place. . . . But the special strength of imagination is its lightning-quick seizure and illumination of analogies." Concluding, Nietzsche proclaims that "non-provable philosophic thinking has its value" and in it "lies an impelling force which is the hope of future fruitfulness."[12] This is of course not to say that rationality is opposed *in toto* by Nietzsche, but he demonstrates the necessity of understanding its limits, especially when it rules out affective perspectives. "Your spirit has been persuaded to despise what is earthly, but not your entrails: and they are what is strongest in you!"[13] The opposition to such forms of knowledge has been so strong that Zarathustra must dare us to believe in ourselves, and more, in our "entrails" for in ignoring them we have ignored a fundamental epistemological source. And when Zarathustra proclaims that the will to truth in part means that everything must be "transformed into what is—humanly thinkable—humanly visible—perceptible!"[14] he does not anthropomorphize truth but demarcates its earthly boundary. This is to set truth in opposition to metaphysics and all metaphysical modes of knowledge, as well as to extol the senses, intuition, and the imagination as valid epistemological sources. And during the phantasmatic state of dreaming or incubation, Zarathustra received the vision of the eternal return, the very *Grundconception* of his teaching, as well as other crucial insights about "life" upon which his tragic philosophy is based. In "The Return Home," Zarathustra directly alludes to incubation when lamenting that few still want "to sit quietly on the nest and hatch the eggs."[15] In *Daybreak*, when speaking of the venerable art of philology, Nietzsche asserts that the art "demands of its votaries one thing above all: to go aside, to take time, to become still, to become slow."[16] In construing philology as an art of rumination, Nietzsche aligns it with the act of a cow sitting in a field patiently chewing its cud. Since to incubate is to lie down like an animal in a lair, there is a clear parallel between the acts. Analyzing several critical moments in the narrative when Zarathustra incubates will then enable us to illustrate the instrumental role incubation has as a mode of askesis for Zarathustra. Its importance as a philosophical praxis for Nietzsche, who, I believe, seeks to recuperate the pre-Platonic art of incubation, in order to reinstitute a holistic askesis that also embodies intuition and the imagination, can also be demonstrated.[17] As part of Nietzsche's transvaluation of all values, the restitution of incubation is moreover a radical displacement of the orthodox philosophical valuation of reason as the sole legitimate epistemological mode through which knowledge is acquired. For Nietzsche, it is no longer through reason alone that one obtains knowledge, but through a meditative praxis that engages the entire body, which "is a great reason" and "a manifold with one sense,"[18] something which gives birth to "alien, illogical powers." If, as Nietzsche believes, the images of dreams are useful for interpreting life, and the events of dreams are helpful for "practicing life,"[19] our literal and incubatory dreams are valid means for obtaining knowledge, integral elements of our total economy. Through such oneiric modes, we gain a type of knowledge that incorporates both thinking and feeling, both the rational and the "irrational" aspects of existence. In opposition to the prevailing abnegation of the body in post-Christian/post-Cartesian culture, this is to honor the body (*Leib*, not *Körper*), which contains more reason than our finest wisdom[20] and gives free play to the flight of the imagination and its discoveries.

As Kingsley explains, incubation was a "specific and established technique . . . for making the journey to the world of the dead; for dying before you died." It involves isolating oneself "in a dark place, lying down in complete stillness, [and] staying motionless for hours or days."[21] Henriëtte Boas notes that the importance given to incubatory dreams "arisen out of the earth" was "supported by the view, that, as the earth was full of the seeds of future life, it also contained the mysteries of the future in general, and dreams in particular."[22] Although the passage is vastly overdetermined, Nietzsche speaks of visiting the dead in the intriguing aphorism "Descent into Hades." In the current context, such a claim receives its perhaps most germane reading, especially since, as Mary Hamilton points out, one of the customary preludes to incubation involved the sacrifice of a ram:[23] "I too have been in the underworld, like Odysseus, and will often be there again; and I have not sacrificed only rams to be able to talk with the dead, but have not spared my own blood as well."[24] Zarathustra engages in comparable incubatory activities in his cave and elsewhere, such as under trees at various critical moments throughout Zarathustra, and Boas explains that trees in particular, as well as springs and caves, were some of the sacred spots where one would incubate. When speaking of the divinatory act of visiting the future, Zarathustra professes that he would rather "be a day-laborer in the underworld and among the shades of times past!"[25] While incubating, the body and the mind become silent and one gains access to another realm, which Kingsley refers to as "a world of utter paradox" where one possesses "a totally different state of awareness," such as in dreams during sleep.[26] The first time Zarathustra sleeps in the narrative occurs subsequent to his burial of the ropedancer, whose perilous fall and death prefigures Zarathustra's *Untergang*. Significantly, it is stressed that both the dawn and the forenoon—two singular temporal moments for Nietzsche—pass over Zarathustra's countenance as he sleeps. In stating that the new truth came to him between "dawn of morning and dawn of morning," Nietzsche implies that Zarathustra had been "sleeping" for an entire day, which, as Kingsley and others explain, is precisely the length of time often spent incubating. Boas explains that one of the main points of incubation "was the strengthening effect, and in which revelation came in a more or less direct manner," often accompanied with dreams.[27] After opening his eyes, Zarathustra glances into the forest and the stillness; amazed, he looks into himself and quickly rises "for he has seen a new truth." This is the first announcement in the narrative of an important new insight or discovery, but Zarathustra does not achieve this insight through the act of abstract thinking. It is something he "receives" while in an awakened state of sleep, and this recalls Nietzsche's figure of "the genius of the heart who silences all that is loud and self-satisfied, teaching it to listen; who smoothes rough souls and lets them taste a new desire—to lie still as a mirror, that the deep sky may mirror itself in them" (BGE §295; KSA V.237). Nietzsche's image of the philosopher is similarly characterized as one who "seeks to hear within himself the echoes of the world symphony and to re-project them in the form of concepts. While he is contemplative-perceptive like the artist, compassionate like the religious, a seeker of purposes and causalities like the scientist, even while he feels himself swelling into a macrocosm, he all the while retains a certain self-possession, a way of viewing himself coldly as a mirror of the world" (PTAG §3; KSA I.817). If the psyche's hidden depths—Nietzsche's "*tiefe Himmel*"—are unconcealed in the dream or incubatory state after silencing all that is noisy and disruptive, such wisdom or knowledge would in his terms be knowledge that is nonrational, knowledge free of herd mentality consciousness, knowledge in part discovered through intuition and flights of imagination.

As Nietzsche makes clear, Zarathustra's mode of sleeping is distinctly different from everyone else's and it is virtue in particular that shapes the character of one's sleep. Shapiro describes Zarathustra's sleep simply as "peculiar" and does not analyze or refer to any other passages on sleep in the book, nor in relation to what he says of sleep, does he refer to the chapter "On the Professorial Chairs of Virtue."[28] There, Zarathustra comes to the realization that what people seek when they seek teachers of virtue is sound and dreamless sleep. Virtue can either be an opiate or stimulant. "For all these much-lauded wise men with their professorial chairs, wisdom was sleep without dreams; they knew no better sense for life."[29] In "At Midday," which includes another telling incubatory moment, Zarathustra reveals that, in opposition to all others, sleep for him is like a delicate unseen breeze that is feather-light. It is not heavy but dances upon him. "My eyes he does not press closed; my soul he leaves awake. Light is he, verily! feather-light. He persuades me, I know not how? He touches me inwardly with flattering hand, he compels me. Yes, he compels me, that my soul might stretch herself out."[30] Significantly, this passage is said while Zarathustra is incubating: "no sooner was he lying on the ground, in the stillness and secrecy of the colorful grasses, than he forgot his slight thirst and fell asleep. . . . Only his eyes remained open: for they were not tired of seeing and admiring the tree and the love of the vine. But in falling asleep

Zarathustra spoke thus to his heart: 'Still! Still! Did the world not just become perfect?'" And Zarathustra values the dreams that come to him during his sleep, because sleep itself does something to him—it compels him to "stretch out" his soul. In "On the Great Yearning," Nietzsche clarifies that stretching out the soul is an extraordinary ecstatic event, the release of the past and the future within the body in the present, or the kinetic enactment of the eternal return, which is an instant of gaining power over time.[31] Thus, it should be clear that, even if a specific praxis such as "stretching out the soul" is not explicitly delineated in such moments, sleep is a deeply meditative activity—whenever Zarathustra is "sleeping," it is imperative to remember that part of him remains active and alert and that his soul is "stretching out."

To return to Zarathustra's new discovery, by informing us that he has seen a new truth, Nietzsche indicates that Zarathustra observed his new truth in a dream or that it was an inner vision—it is not something consciously thought. This is certainly crucial since, for Nietzsche, pictorial truth is considered of greater veracity than conceptual truth, due to its closer proximity to what it metaphorizes. And since thought that rises to consciousness, as Nietzsche argues, is only "the most superficial and worst part," presumably, what rises to oneiric consciousness is the most profound and "best" part, for it does not take the form of words, but images, visions generated by the imagination. What we acquire in incubatory states is not what belongs to the social or herd nature, but to individual existence, the psyche's hidden depths, the "*tiefe Himmel*." Thoughts in this state are not governed by the "genius of the species" or the perspective of the herd, but by what Nietzsche believes is "incomparably personal, unique, and infinitely individual."[32] When incubating, one then moves beyond the surface and sign world, beyond the merely utilitarian into "everything strange, unusual, and questionable,"[33] what disturbs us because we do not know or understand it, or what we cannot access in waking life, due to the measure that we must observe in it, or to the demand to provide proof. And what the herald of the *Übermensch* realizes is that he needs living companions who are fellow creators and who inscribe new values on new tablets as opposed to dead companions and corpses. Since the latter only think conceptually instead of with the entirety of their bodies to comprehend his teaching, they are but dead or insensate companions. Further, and this is in line with a thinking not ordered by the "genius of the species," Zarathustra decides that he will no longer share his teaching with everyone, but only with those he considers his companions; as he, they are to be harvesters and celebrants. When the narrative first commences, Zarathustra avers that in order to bestow and distribute his wisdom—which he gained through a lengthy 10-year retreat during which one can reasonably assume he incubated frequently if not every day—he must as the sun descend into the depths and the underworld. Before embarking on this *Untergang*, he asks the sun, or Apollo, the "divine protector of those who lie down in lairs,"[34] to bless him with his tranquil eye. Thus, it is not Dionysos, but the tutelary figure of those who incubate who Zarathustra first addresses in the *Vorrede*. If Zarathustra is a "Dionysiac monster,"[35] his polestar is Apollo, "the god of all image-making energies" and "of prophecy."[36] Lampert recognizes that there is a relationship between Zarathustra and Apollo, but after his initial comparison and reference to Zarathustra as a healer, he does not pursue the insight further. Soon after seeing his new truth, Zarathustra witnesses his animals searching for him, wondering whether he is still alive, then begins his *Untergang*, which comprises almost the entirety of the first three books of Zarathustra. The *Untergang* comes to an end at the close of "On the Convalescent" after Zarathustra experiences the eternal return while in a state of incubation. And the following three chapters that close the third book all occur in absolute silence and stillness, as Zarathustra is incubating and conversing with, respectively, his soul, Life, and Eternity. While Zarathustra's animals speak to him of his task of teaching the eternal recurrence, he does not hear them because "he lay still with his eyes closed, like one who sleeps, though he was not asleep: for he was just then conversing with his soul. But the serpent and the eagle, on finding him thus silent, honored the great stillness around him and discreetly stole away."[37] This image of Zarathustra in stillness, with eyes closed, sleeping but not sleeping, correlates exactly to the description various scholars give of incubation.

Another of Zarathustra's stillest hours occurs in "On the Bite of the Adder." It is the second incubatory moment in the book and transpires while Zarathustra is sleeping under a fig tree. When visited by a serpent, Zarathustra is not tempted nor provoked into an act of transgression but aided, for through the serpent's bite he is forced awake "at the right time: my way," he says, "is still long."[38] However, the serpent informs Zarathustra that his way will be short for the poison (*Gift*) that he injected into his body is deadly. Smiling, Zarathustra informs the snake that, as a "dragon," he will never die from such poison. As Shapiro first noted in *Alcyone*, "the German *Gift* once had the sense of present as well as poison" while "*Gabe* is either a present or a dose, that is something possibly unpleasant and possibly administered against one's will."[39] After thanking the snake, Zarathustra commands it to retract its poison, since it is not rich enough to bestow such a gift. The snake obeys him and, in an almost erotic gesture, sucks the poison from out his neck. Zarathustra is not only able to communicate with animals but to command them, too. Instead of being largely commanded by a serpent, as were Adam and Eve, he is the commanding one, an Orpheus able to charm and control even animals.[40] Out of this event, Zarathustra creates a story that serves as a poetic pedagogical device for his disciples. It is not through concepts that Zarathustra educates and teaches, but through allegorical tales or images, what is developed largely by the imagination (and encourages further imaginative development by his listeners). "For the genuine poet metaphor is no rhetorical figure, but an image which takes the place of something else, something he can really see before him as a substitute for a concept."[41] To Nietzsche, it is only if one is a bad poet that one resorts to the use of abstractions, for it is through allegory that one rides to every truth.[42] Such events, then, illustrate not only that Zarathustra gains valuable wisdom from incubating, but also that each experience he undergoes is a moment wherein his wisdom or his virtue is tested. Further, and more pertinently, these events are transformed into potent images and serve as crystallizations of his teaching, which can be embodied by those to whom it is transmitted. Like Homer, Zarathustra is able to depict things so much more vividly than all other poets because his perception of things is more acute.[43]

If our stillest hours comprise the greatest events of our lives, one of the greatest events of Zarathustra's life must surely occur in the chapter of the same name. "The Stillest Hour" is the concluding section of the second book, the moment when Zarathustra leaves his disciples in order to return to his solitude. Specifically, he is returning to his cave, a place of incubation, though he returns to it unhappily. In the next book, he will depart the Isles of the Blest and soon after recount his vision of the eternal return, a riddle that he says he *saw*. "What happened to me? Who ordered this?—Ah," Zarathustra explains, "my angry mistress wills it thus, she has spoken to me: have I ever told you her name? Yesterday towards evening there spoke to me my Stillest Hour: that is the name of my terrible mistress."[44] It is not precisely clear what this entity is, if that can ever be clarified, but it may not need to be. Although Shapiro rightfully asserts that it is not the voice of the narrator or of other characters in the story, he proposes that it may be the voice of Zarathustra. Ultimately, he leaves the question open, as it seemingly must remain. Lampert refers to the same dialogue as "an enactment of the double will" but, oddly, does not address the very unique mode of silent communication and *why* Nietzsche employs it.[45] And what is more important than precisely who or what the Stillest Hour might be is *how* it communicates and is characterized—its silence is instrumental.

Stillness, or *hesychia*, is the state entered into when incubating. It is the term commonly translated as "the quiet life." As Kingsley opines though, to translate *hesychia* as "the quiet life" is misleading. It also elides what may in fact be one of the most central aspects of "the quiet life" that once was the philosopher's life.[46] "For the Greeks," Kingsley elaborates, "stillness had a whole side to it that they found intensely disquieting—and not just disquieting but also sinister, alien, profoundly inhuman."[47] The "quiet life" then is not a mode of ataraxia, some unperturbed state of pure contemplative ease, but something rife with exceptionally more tension.[48] To Nietzsche, philosophy is clearly not quiet in the sense of being peaceful, but disquieting, sinister, alien, and profoundly inhuman—such is living at the extremity of consciousness. In the *Untimely Meditations*, Nietzsche proclaims that one of the philosopher's tasks is to disturb[49] while in *Ecce Homo*, he refers to the philosopher as a terrible explosive.[50] In addition, to speak of another characteristic of *hesychia*, Nietzsche speaks of how his sickness compelled him to alter all of his habits; it bestowed on him "the necessity of lying still, of leisure, of waiting and being patient—But that means, of thinking!—" Precisely through this practice of stillness his nethermost self, which he said had "been buried and grown silent under the continual pressure of having to listen to other selves,"[51] finally spoke again as opposed to the chattering herd consciousness that generally speaks in us. Lastly, if there is a distinct parallel between the profoundly inhuman and the *Übermenschlich*, in referring to the Stillest Hour as both his "angry" and "terrible" "mistress," Nietzsche endows stillness with the disposition of intense disquiet. Relatedly, in reference to Rohde, Boas notes that the earth was "often conceived as a very strong and powerful numen," the "mistress of life and death," and it was precisely through "contact with the Earth" that one's "physical and psychical energies were strengthened" for "the Earth was possessed of oracular power."[52] The episode with the Stillest Hour also betrays something sinister, alien, and profoundly inhuman, and it is imperative to sustain these aspects of stillness whenever thinking of the still and incubatory moments that occur in *Zarathustra*. Let us further consider the "Stillest Hour."

"Do you know," Zarathustra asks his friends, "the terror of him who falls asleep?—He is terrified down to his toes, because the ground gives way and the dream begins."[53] As one whose sleep is not comfortable, as one whose virtue forces him in part to remain awake during sleep, Zarathustra's stillest hours are direct incubatory encounters with the psyche's hidden depths, the nethermost self in which the "*tiefe Himmel*" or "world symphony" is reflected. As Assoun notes, for Nietzsche, "dreams express the essence, the core of truth around which human reality gravitates, whose manifestations are only appearances. In the last analysis, dreams hold this privilege by constituting the appearance of appearance. Reality being appearance, dreams are such only to a second degree; for this reason, they are valued as 'yet higher satisfactions of the universal aspiration to appearance.'"[54] And in the encounter with the Stillest Hour, the intensely disquieting aspect of "the quiet life" is further evident. The stillness that Zarathustra hears around him—evidence that his mode of perception is synesthetic[55]—is so sinister that "the clock of his life draws breath" and he undergoes terror, which is to say, *time ceases*—we enter Zarathustra's time of dying. As noted earlier, incubation is a technique for dying before you die and to Nietzsche, being immortal requires dying "numerous times over the course of your life."[56] In dying multiple deaths, we learn to see anew, to be dead but with "open eyes," for it is then that we see "much that . . . has never been seen before, and for as far as [one] can see everything is spun into a net of light and as it were buried in it."[57] This continual "dying" is necessary because, as Nietzsche says in the same aphorism, "life" perpetually draws us to itself and occludes our vision. In his continual perishing then, Zarathustra seeks clarity, but this pursuit is not without its dangers. Throughout the encounter with the Stillest Hour, the entity speaks to Zarathustra without voice and her inaudible whispering is so profoundly unsettling that it makes even the courageous hermit of the mountains scream in terror and grow frighteningly pallid in complexion.[58] Zarathustra's angry mistress reveals that he knows some great truth or secret, but will not utter it. Presumably, it is the riddle of the eternal return, which we discover in the following book. When Zarathustra confesses that he does not possess the strength to announce the secret, the Stillest Hour continues to confront him, challenging him to an *agon* that he must overcome. "Do you not know who is most needed by all? The one who commands great things? To accomplish great things is difficult: but more difficult is to command great things. That is what is most unpardonable in you: you have the power, and you do not want to rule."[59] When Zarathustra replies that he lacks the lion's voice for commanding,[60] the Stillest Hour speaks to him again in her mute whisper, uttering one of the central passages of the book: "It is the stillest words that bring on the storm. Thoughts that come on doves' feet direct the world. O Zarathustra, you shall go as a shadow of that which must come: thus will you command, and commanding lead the way."[61] The fact that Zarathustra does not hear the voice of the Stillest Hour with his ear, but via some other means, is made emphatically clear by Nietzsche through his repeating ten times that the Stillest Hour speaks to Zarathustra without voice.[62] This is the only line in the book that is repeated with such frequency within one chapter but, strangely, to cite just two prominent scholars, neither Lampert nor Shapiro observed this very dramatic and informative repetition.[63] Through such calculated and instructive repetitions, Nietzsche not only compels us to apprehend this particular aspect of his thought, but also dramatically asserts its import. As Nietzsche indicates throughout his work and frequently in *Zarathustra*, things are sensed synesthetically.

After Zarathustra confesses to being ashamed, the Stillest Hour instructs him to become a child free of shame, for that is what he must achieve in order to convey the next stage of his teaching. When he refuses, laughter erupts around him, tears at his entrails, slashes open his heart, betraying bodily repercussions, that he has not been mentally but *physically* wounded by this ephemeral encounter. Although that may be meant figuratively, Nietzsche may be indicating that oneiric events can have effects as palpable as "real" ones. If dreams are as integral an aspect of the total economy of our lives and even direct our waking hours, that then they can have as palpable an effect as "real" events, is not difficult to accept. "Speaking" to Zarathustra one last time, the Stillest Hour informs him that, while his fruits are ripe, he is not yet ripe enough for them. "'So you must go back to your solitude: for you are yet to become mellow' [*mürbe*]."[64] Laughter erupts once more and flees, implying that the Stillest Hour has vanished, just as instantaneously as does the lion in "The Sign."[65] Once the Stillest Hour vanishes, it becomes still around Zarathustra "as if with a twofold stillness. But I lay on the ground, and the sweat poured from my limbs."[66] Aside from this indicating that the entire event occurred while Zarathustra was lying on the ground in an incubatory state, the Stillest Hour also instructs him to return to his cave in order to learn to become a child again. As Krell points out, "On the Vision and the Riddle" was originally to begin "with the sentence (crossed out at the proof-stage), 'But what is it I dreamt not long ago as I lay on my sickbed?' The suggestion is that the vision . . . and the riddle . . . are intrinsic to convalescence itself; they are not illnesses that one might leave behind, maladies from which one might totally convalesce."[67] If convalescence is construed as a mode of incubation, and it is viable to do so, what the original beginning of the chapter also reveals is an explicit reference to incubation, of the instructive visions that Zarathustra receives while in altered states of consciousness outside the confines of rational thinking.

Intriguingly, Zarathustra is not yet *mürbe* (mellow) enough to affirm the eternal return and this in part is what he must learn, a quality that seems out of odds with the brutal cast often given by many commentators to Zarathustra or the *Übermensch*. It is not through becoming more courageous or warlike as many might expect, or presume, that will enable Zarathustra to affirm the eternal return, but precisely through becoming *mürbe*.[68] What is toughest is what is humble, as the Stillest Hour says to Zarathustra: "'What do you matter? You are not yet humble enough for me. Humility has the toughest hide.'"[69] Yet, this is not perhaps that odd. In *Human, All Too Human*, Nietzsche observes that, while the most savage forces build pathways and are predominantly destructive, "their work was none the less necessary, in order that later a gentler civilization might raise its house. The frightful energies—those which are called evil—are the cyclopean architects and road-makers of humanity."[70] Similarly, aside from being made out of what is hard and fragrant, the other quality of those who have "turned out well" is that they are delicate.[71] And when speaking of the necessity of not expending energy to guard oneself against danger, Nietzsche notes that "to have spikes is an extravagance, a double luxury even if one is free to have no spikes but open hands . . . ."[72] It seems justifiable to claim that it is through the praxis of stillness that Zarathustra will accomplish the task of becoming *mürbe*, for such a mode of meditation would lead to a state of mellowness, the proper physiological frequency necessary for affirming the eternal return. In this episode of the narrative then, one of the functions of stillness or incubation is to aid Zarathustra during a time of crisis. He receives firm counsel at this moment, not pitying comfort, and is driven to fulfill the task he is destined to. As the Stillest Hour declares, he is "most needed by all," and this reveals the exigency of the situation and the significance of the teaching as well as its import for humanity, or for the creators and companions who will lead humanity toward the creation of the *Übermenschen*, the creation we might say of a Periclean polis where each individual is a self-governing being who moves between freedom and order and who links both through passion.

To conclude, through the praxis of incubation, Nietzsche enacts and obeys his own injunction to remain loyal to the earth; this enactment is not only figured imaginatively in Nietzsche's philosophical fiction, but in his own life. In June of 1883, while at work on the second book of *Zarathustra*, Nietzsche wrote to Carl von Gersdorff that he was "up in the Engadine again, for the third time, and again I feel that here and nowhere else is my proper home and place of incubation. Ah, how much everything lies hidden in me still, and wants to become word and form! Only here is it quiet and high and lonely enough for me to be able to perceive my innermost voices!"[73] Through this attentive praxis, quotidian consciousness is surpassed, language is abandoned, and in turning inward, one listens to what Nietzsche calls the "spirits [*geisterhaft*] that are all around us, every moment of our life" he observes "wants to say something to us, but we refuse to listen to these spirit-voices [*Geisterstimme*]. We are afraid that, when we are alone and quiet, something will be whispered into our ear, and so we hate quietness and deafen ourselves with sociability."[74] To use a term of Heidegger's, which may in fact be a transfiguration of Nietzsche's concept, with invoking the practice of incubation, Nietzsche is calling us to *hearken* to the earth. As the dweller of the Black Forest notes, to hearken is to be called and to be called is to obey, to dutifully listen "from below." Not to listen *to* something below, but to listen *from* below, from the depths of our being, the psyche's hidden depths or "*tiefe Himmel*," from the deepest strata of the earth,[75] from the source which may yield to us something to which we can attune ourselves. This is not to be enraptured, or to refuse to perceive with one's senses as Nietzsche warns in the *Nachlaß*, for to be overcome by such fantasies "is an illness of the intellect, not a path to knowledge."[76] Instead, it is to simultaneously perceive with the senses, to permit rationality its proper circumference, *and* to let the *tiefe Himmel* or "world symphony" mirror itself in one. If, as Heidegger avows, "to think is before all else to listen, to let ourselves be told something and not to ask questions,"[77] there is no thinking without listening—incubating, then, is a mode of thinking; to incubate is to listen, to learn to become *mürbe* enough to hear the music of *Dasein*. In *On the Essence of Language*, Heidegger directly connects hearkening with obedience, thus there is a conceptual parallel with Nietzsche's notion of staying loyal to the earth, for to sustain such loyalty is to move beyond the egoistic subject and, in Nietzsche's terms, to think or feel cosmically, to overcome one's worldly anthropomorphism and submit oneself to the earth—to obey it! It is to move into inorganic realms, to turn into a stone: "Slowly, slowly to become hard like a precious stone—and at last to lie there, silent and a joy to eternity."[78] To do this is to die, to let the human, all too human perish, and to encounter the "*tiefe Himmel*" or ground of being. This is perhaps to truly think, for as Deleuze and Guattari claim, "thought is sometimes closer to an animal that dies than to a living, even democratic, human being."[79] "Let us not think of the return to the inanimate as a regression!" Nietzsche pronounces. "We become quite true, we perfect ourselves. Death has to be reinterpreted! We thereby reconcile ourselves with what is actual, with the dead world."[80] If to incubate is to lie down like an animal in a cave or open field and meditate, not to think conceptually, as Kofman instructs, it is to allow the foreign and "illogical" forces, such as intuition and imagination, to flash and offer elucidations, allowing "meaning" and clarity to occur on their own and to transfigure us. It is thus that the free spirit, "without turning Jesuit, nonetheless penetrates," as Nietzsche exults, "the irrational constitution of existence."[81]

Notes

1 BT §1; KSA I.26.
2 BT §4; KSA I.38.
3 BGE §193; KSA V.114.
4 Ibid.
5 The sense of temporality in Z is rather ambiguous, with often no precise sense of time's passage in the narrative. For the most provocative and challenging reading of time in *Zarathustra*, see Paul S. Loeb, *The Death of Nietzsche's Zarathustra* (Cambridge University Press, 2010).
6 Z: II.14; KSA IV.154.
7 Z: II.18; KSA IV.169.
8 Pausanias, the record of the Epidaurian inscriptions, Iamblichus, and Cicero are just a few of the sources through which Nietzsche would have known of incubation. Aristophanes even lampoons it in *The Rich Man*, pp. 620–49. For transcriptions of the Asclepian testimonies, see Emma and Ludwig Edelstein, *Asclepius* (Maryland: Johns Hopkins University Press, 1945), I.338–442. For further material on incubation, including later accounts, see Ludovicus Deubner, *De Incubatione* (Leipzig: Teubneri, 1900), Mary Hamilton, *Incubation* (London: W. C. Henderson & Son, 1906), E. R. Dodds, *The Greeks and the Irrational* (California: University of California Press, 1951; 2004), 110–6, Karl Kerenyi, *Asklepios* (New York: Pantheon Books, 1959), and Patricia Miller, *Dreams in Late Antiquity* (New Jersey: Princeton University Press, 1997).
9 Erwin Rohde, *Psyche* (London: Routledge, 2000), p. 93. For the passages on incubation, see iii, 8, 28 (sleep and death), 46, 92–3, 104, 106, 107, 133 (heroic oracles of), 140, 150, 151, 260, 289 (prophecy by), 292, 311.
10 Peter Kingsley, *Reality* (California: Golden Sufi Center, 2003), p. 31.
11 Martin Heidegger, *Poetry, Language, Thought* (New York: Harper & Row, 1994), p. 24.
12 PTAG §3; KSA I.814. See also PTAG §§ 5, 7, 9, 11, and 12 (KSA I.822–6, 830–3, 835–9, 844–7, 847–50) for other passages on the imagination as well as intuition, both of which Nietzsche sets in opposition to rationality and logic, but without disavowing either of the latter. Although Nietzsche does not use the word *intuitiv* frequently, *Vorstellung* occurs nearly 200 times despite Parkes' contra claim. See Graham Parkes, "Nietzsche and East Asian Thought," in Bernd Magnus, and Kathleen Marie Higgins eds, *The Cambridge Companion to Nietzsche* (Cambridge University Press, 1996), p. 365. It seems doubtful too that Nietzsche does not exalt intuition

as Parkes also argues in the same text. It would be illuminating to consider the numerous passages where the term *Phantasie* occurs in Nietzsche's *oeuvre* and the relation of each faculty to art; in addition, whenever Nietzsche criticizes rationality, there is an implicit valorization or exalting of intuition or the imagination. For passages on intuition, see TL §2 (KSA I.886–90), D §544 (KSA III.314), TI: SUM §5 (KSA VI.113–4), and the *Nachlaß*. The passages on *Vorstellung* are too numerous to list.

13 Z: II.15: KSA IV.157.

14 Z: II.2; KSA IV.109–10.

15 Z: III.9; KSA IV.233.

16 D: P §5; KSA III.17.

17 In his poetic-historical work on the Paleolithic imagination, *Juniper Fuse*, Clayton Eshleman also points out that various sacred spaces which were once powerful places of incubation have become spaces of but mere docile reception, implying that recuperating such praxes is of fundamental import, what can transform them once again into active sources of power: "The cathedrals and churches in which humankind passively sits today, listening to watered-down statements based on utterances of visionaries and ecstatics, were, before being in effect turned inside out, active underground 'sanctuaries' or 'incubational pits.'"—Clayton Eshleman, *Juniper Fuse* (Connecticut: Wesleyan University Press, 2003), xxv.

18 Z: I.4: KSA IV.39.

19 BT §1; KSA I.27.

20 Z: I.4; KSA IV.40.

21 Kingsley 2003, p. 31.

22 Henriëtte Boas, *Aeneas' Arrival in Latium* (Amsterdam: Hoord-Hollandsche Uitgevers-Mij, 1938), p. 189.

23 Hamilton 1906, 84. See also Pausanias (i.34), *Aeneid* (vii.8) and Ovid, *Fasti* (vi.649).

24 AOM §408; KSA II.533–4.

25 The opening lines of "On the Land of Culture" are pertinent (KSA IV.153).

26 For a philosophical investigation of sleep, see Jean-Luc Nancy, *Fall of Sleep* (New York: Fordham University Press, 2009). Oddly, Nancy does not address Nietzsche or Z in his book. For a few representative passages by Nietzsche on sleep: D §376 (KSA III.246), GS §§ 59, 164 (KSA III.422–4, 498).

27 Boas 1938, p. 191.

28 Z: II.14; KSA IV.154. See Gary Shapiro, *Archaeologies of Vision* (Chicago: University of Chicago Press, 2003), pp. 188–9. Joan Stambaugh refers to it more particularly as a "mystical event," but that remains obscure. T. K. Seung refers to it as mysterious, which does not move beyond ambiguity. For Stambaugh, see *The Other Nietzsche* (Albany, NY: SUNY Press, 1994), 141–6; for Seung, see *Nietzsche's Epic of the Soul* (Kentucky: Lexington Books, 2005), 276–8, *passim.*

29 Z: I.2; KSA IV.34.

30 Z: IV.10; KSA IV.343.

31 For a further elaboration of this concept, see Rainer J. Hanshe, "Invisibly Revolving— —Inaudibly Revolving: The Riddle of the Double *Gedankenstrich*," *The Agonist* III (1), (spring 2010): 7–26.

32 GS §354; KSA III.590–3.

33 GS §355; KSA III.593–4.

34 Kingsley 2003, p. 42.

35 BT: ASC §7; KSA I.22.

36 BT §1; KSA I.27. On Zarathustra and Asklepius, see Lampert 1986, 74 and 82, and on Zarathustra, Apollo, and rhythm, 216 and 239. See also D.F. Krell, *Postponements* (Indiana University Press, 1986), and more recently, Babette Babich, *Words in Blood, Like Flowers* (Albany, NY: SUNY Press, 2006).
37 Z: III.13 §2; KSA IV.277.
38 Z: I.19; KSA IV.87.
39 Gary Shapiro, *Alcyone* (Albany, NY: SUNY Press, 1991), p. 32.
40 There is a parallel between Z and the Orphic tradition of *catabasis*. See Yulia Ustinova, *Caves and the Ancient Greek Mind* (Oxford: Oxford Universty Press, 2009), 239. See also W. K. C. Guthrie, *Orpheus and Greek Religion* (Princeton, NJ: Princeton University Press, 1993).
41 BT §8; KSA I.60.
42 Z: III.9; KSA IV.231.
43 BT §8; KSA I.60. This is but one way in which Nietzsche/Zarathustra is different from the poets he critiques. He is a dreaming poet who knows the limits that Apollo draws (see BT §1; KSA I.26–8).
44 Z: II.22; KSA IV.187.
45 Shapiro 1991, 110–1, as well as 58 and 122. Lampert 1986, p. 153.
46 Consider, in relation to this, the role and function of silence and the meaning silence had for the ancient Greeks. For one exploration: Silvia Montiglio, *Silence in the Land of Logos* (Princeton, NJ: Princeton University Press, 2000).
47 Peter Kingsley, *In the Dark Places of Wisdom* (California: Golden Sufi Center, 2001), p. 185.
48 For those who mistrust or doubt Kingsley's view, in Christian accounts, this aspect of incubation exists too. In *hesychia*, Christians believe that they are identifying "with the ineffable witness of our unfolding psycho-physical experiences." It is an understanding that "acts like a 'two-edged sword' which 'cuts so deeply it divides Consciousness from psyche.'" Even from this Christian perspective, *hesychia* has a disquieting and sinister aspect. See Timothy Freke and Peter Gandy, *Jesus and the Lost Goddess* (New York: Random House, 2002), p. 176, 288.
49 SE §8; KSA I.426.
50 EH: "Untimelies" §3; KSA VI.320.
51 EH: "Human" §4; KSA VI.326.
52 Boas 1931, pp. 188–9.
53 Z II.22; KSA IV.187.
54 Paul-Laurent Assoun, *Freud and Nietzsche* (London: Continuum, 2006), p. 121.
55 For a thorough exploration of synesthesia in Nietzsche, see Rainer J. Hanshe, "Nietzsche's Synaesthetic Epistemology & the Restitution of the Holistic Human," in Vanessa Lemm (ed.), *Nietzsche and the Becoming of Life* (New York: Fordham University Press, 2013), *forthcoming*. A different version of this paper is available here (last accessed on Monday 2 July 2012): http://www.nietzsche.cl/docs/Sesiones%20Paralelas_Parallel%20Sessions/10.1%20RAINER%20J.%20HANSHE.pdf.
56 EH: "Zarathustra" §5; KSA VI.342.
57 WS §308; KSA II.690.
58 There is a possible relation here with the voice of Faunus. See Boas, p. 193.
59 Z: II.22; KSA IV.189.
60 The enormous difficulty of the task is made clear in the following section—over Zarathustra's way of greatness "is written: Impossibility" (Z: III.1; KSA IV.194).
61 Ibid.

62 The Stillest Hour actually speaks a total of 11 times, but her last line is not described as silent or voiceless. At that point, it is clear that her mode of communication is unique; therefore, there are 11 repetitions of this phenomenon. Is there not then a connection here with the 11 bell strokes?

63 See Laurence Lampert, *Nietzsche's Teaching* (Connecticut: Yale University Press, 1989), 152–4; and Shapiro 1991, 110–1. Robert Gooding-Williams also does not observe the repetition. See his *Zarathustra's Dionysian Modernism* (California: Stanford University Press, 2001), pp. 294–5, *passim*. Although Seung acknowledges that the Stillest Hour is silent, he never asks *why* it is so. See his *Nietzsche's Epic of the Soul* (Kentucky: Lexington Books, 2005), pp. 106–50.

64 Z: II.22; KSA IV.189.

65 The instantaneous disappearance of the lion is but one of many events that forces us to question whether or not such encounters are "real" or whether they all occur within Zarathustra's consciousness during moments of incubation. This would offer one logical explanation for the vanishing lion and other peculiar events. The connection to the Orphic tradition of the *catabasis* is again quite palpable. One other possible explanation for such events is that Z is Nietzsche's Bardo Thodol, a book of the dead, and Z is a representation of Zarathustra's death journey, his passage from life to life, thus *he is actually dead throughout most of the book*, until the moment he reenters the cosmic life cycle.

66 Z: II.22; KSA IV.189.

67 Krell 1986, pp. 54–5.

68 Lampert does not observe this explicit instruction or task that the Stillest Hour sets for Zarathustra but simply says that he lacks the "resolve" to fulfill the task; while that may not be inaccurate, it is quite specifically through becoming "*mürbe*" that Zarathustra will be able to achieve the task. See Lampert 1989, pp. 153–4. Both Seung and Gooding-Williams also neglect to observe the specificity of this instruction.

69 Relatedly, consider Nietzsche's figuration of Zarathustra's body as extremely vulnerable and unprotected—he makes him into a reverse Achilles, invulnerable *only* in his heel. Another passage relates to this physical state: "I must be without caution: thus my lot wills it" (Z: IV.V §2; KSA IV.318).

70 HH §246; KSA II.205. For similarly oriented thoughts, see GS §§19, 313 (KSA III.390, 548), BGE §229 (KSA V.165–7), and TI "Anti-Nature" 3 (KSA VI.84) on the spiritualization of sensuality, which Nietzsche calls love, "a great triumph over Christianity." Strikingly, it is revealing that no exercise of violence is *ever* made against anyone by Zarathustra in the book, even against his enemies, whom he passes by with a "sleeping sword."

71 EH: "Wise" §2; KSA VI.267. Another way in which Nietzsche recognizes that someone has "turned out well" is that they are "good for our senses" (EH: "Books" §2; KSA VI.301–2), once again stressing the sensorial faculty as an orienting episteme. As Large points out in a footnote to his translation of EH, "turned out well" "is a paraphrase of the term '*Wohlgerathenheit*' (cf. III 1), which is most often applied to children but is also a close translation of the ancient Greek concept of virtue as *arête*." There is a clear relation here to the third type (the child) espoused in Z.

72 EH: Clever §8; KSA VI.292.

73 KSB VI.386.

74 SE §5; KSA I.379.

75 For an illuminating analysis of the geological aspect of Nietzsche's thought, see Graham Parkes, *Composing the Soul* (Chicago: University of Chicago Press, 1996).
76 KGW V, 4[321], p. 510; 4[152], p. 470.
77 Martin Heidegger, *On the Way to Language* (New York: Harper One, 1982), p. 76.
78 D §541; KSA III.309.
79 Gilles Deleuze, Felix Guattari, *What is Philosophy?* (London and New York: Verso Books, 1994), p. 108.
80 KSA 9:11[70].
81 KGW VII, 16[14], p. 529.

12

Nietzsche's Zarathustra, Nietzsche's Empedocles: The Time of Kings

Babette Babich

Politics and Nietzsche's sketches for the *Death of Empedocles*

Beyond the identification with Hölderlin often (and rightly) imputed to him,[1] Nietzsche drafted several attempts at a drama titled after Hölderlin's *Death of Empedocles*.[2] A classical philologist specializing in the works of Diogenes Laertius—the author of *The Lives and Doctrines of Famous Philosophers*—Nietzsche duly composed his drafts of the *Death of Empedocles* in a classical mode. Empedocles himself "imitates" his philosophical predecessors with "jealous" ambition[3], and we recall Nietzsche's characterization of "the ennobling of jealousy"[4]—the *agon* in Greek antiquity—as one of the stumbling blocks for contemporary scholars, as this also remains true to this day.

Empedocles is also represented as the philosopher who dies a free death: self-elected,[5] a death which also corresponds to his accession to divinity. Empedocles' refusal of kingship is part of this and Empedocles claims from the start when he speaks to shining Akragas "But unto ye I walk as god immortal now, no more as a man. On all sides honored fittingly and well, crowned both with fillets and with flowering wreaths."[6] By contrast with mortal life understood not merely as Nietzsche understands Anaximander's "ethical" reflection upon encroachment, one upon another, Empedocles' *Purifications* highlights the cycle of love yielding to strife, telling his own role as advocate precisely as outcast: "Of these I too am now one, an exile from the gods and a wanderer, having put my trust in raving strife."[7]

Lucian, the contemporary of Diogenes Laertius who also wrote of Empedocles in his *Icaromennipus*, wrote a number of parodic dialogues, or Menippean satires, dealing with death (and life) including his Κατάπλους ἤ Τύραννος[8] or *Downward Journey* also translated as *Journey to Hell*. And just to the extent that Nietzsche derives his Zarathustran *Übermensch* from Lucian's: 'υπεράνθρωπος in this same dialogue, an attention to Lucian's *Downward Journey* may aid our understanding and make this still more significant in the current context, the dialogue itself includes the very impolitic, that is, very political subtitle: *or the Tyrant*.

It is hard to resist an almost automatic comparison with Straussian readings of both Plato's *Republic* and Nietzsche's *Zarathustra* with Lucian's *Downward Journey* that examines the fate of the souls of the multifarious many, as contrasted with the fate of the exalted or the great, i.e., the tyrant, describing the "translation" of souls from life to the underworld and as contrasted with the world of the living up above and including a meditation on *vanitas*: human glory and its inevitable reversals.[9] A comparison of Nietzsche and Lucian illuminates the eternal (i.e., the ultimate) context of the "ought" in Zarathustra's teaching that the human being is something that "ought to be overcome" and, as cited above, "shall be."

If the vocations of shoemakers and rulers clearly allude to Plato's *Republic*, Christian readings are also important.[10] The same array of allusions also permits us to read Zarathustra as an explicitly Empedoclean figure. In this way, one can read the beginning of Empedocles' *Katharmoi* as detailing the "lives" or listing the roles one must appropriate: prophet, poet, healer, in order to be, as a figure of free death—as one who goes to ground—a mortal no more.

Thus it is the tale of Zarathustra's downgoing, told as the tale of one who dies, very paradoxically but also very philosophically, as we have already noted that the task of philosophy is always the task of learning to die. Just as Empedocles speaks to his Agrigentians, and leaves his own teaching of the eternal return of the same, just as he springs into his volcano and is thereby raised up (a claim reported, and controverted, in Diogenes Laertius as indeed, parodically, in Lucian who sets his Empedocles wafted up by the vapors of Etna as the man in the moon, living, a vegetarian to the end, on dew). Similarly, Zarathustra is the teacher of the eternal return and of the transmogrified (qua divine) Overhuman, liberated from or escaping the cycle of birth and rebirth, to a translation beyond death.

For more than a century, it has been noted that Nietzsche's plans for his *Zarathustra* included Zarathustra's death. Carl Jung and Theodor Ziegler contended that this death is also figuratively indicated toward the end of the text (although the locus in question depends upon whether one takes the text to end with the third part or, and the point is then still more explicit, with the fourth).[11]

Yet as I have argued, Zarathustra's death is announced already in the first book, if not with the conclusion of the *Prologue*: "— *Also begann Zarathustras Untergang*" allegorically qua down-going, going under or to ground, but very literally in *The Bite of the Adder*, where Zarathustra succumbs to a snake bite under a fig tree. Zarathustra chides the snake for biting him. Like Eve's talking serpent, shades of Harry Potter, Zarathustra speaks with snakes and understands them: "your way is short the adder said sadly, 'my poison kills.'"[12] The bitten Zarathustra bids the adder "take back" his poison (a dissonant request for the teacher of *amor fati*). And we read that the snake falls upon Zarathustra's neck a second time.

If the wish for such a second bite is real enough, the phantasm of such a second bite, efficacious in this way, suggests that the entirety of *Thus Spoke Zarathustra* is a dream before dying: just another philosopher's dream.

Nor does the text contradict this, and *On Free Death* details "the death that consummates," where Zarathustra describes death as a "festival." Here, with an explicit echo of Lucian's Ἀληθῆ διηγήματα or *True History*, Nietzsche titles the section *On the Blessed Isles* as does Lucian following Homer and Hesiod and Pindar, as well as Plato and so on. Nietzsche himself invokes the afterlife in utterly classical Greek terms. Rather than salvation or redemption or eternal life, it is "of time and becoming that the best parables should speak: let them be a praise and a justification of all impermanence."[13]

Apart from Zarathustra's own death, death is the point of the eternal recurrence, and in a direct parallel with Empedocles' Καθαρμοί or *Purifications*,[14] Zarathustra reflects: "Verily, through a hundred souls I have already passed on my way, and through a hundred cradles and birth pangs. Many a farewell have I taken; I know the heart rending last hours."[15] But "thus my creative will, my destiny, wills it. Or, to say it more honestly: this very destiny: my will wills."[16] In addition, Empedocles' teaching of rebirth echoes in the language of the "nuptial ring of rings, the ring of recurrence."[17]

Zarathustra's *Übermensch* is introduced in the context of the transition from the human to the eternal recurrence of the same. Nietzsche's Zarathustra thus gives a sermon in the marketplace, speaking of the human being as "a rope over an abyss," all against the backdrop of the dynamic tableau of the tightrope dancer of which Zarathustra seemingly notices nothing until it literally crashes down upon him. But Zarathustra's words are thus *visually* illuminated for his auditors who *see* what transpires above and behind him, as the speaking Zarathustra does not.

Those to whom Zarathustra speaks did not come to hear him. Much rather, those gathered in the marketplace are there for market reasons, for the sights to be seen, especially the unfolding spectacle of life and death, above and below.

The parallel with Empedocles as rhetorician is thus with Zarathustra as rhetorician. As Nietzsche observes, Aristotle in his lost *Sophist* describes Empedocles as "the inventor of rhetoric."[18] Nietzsche's *Thus Spoke Za*rathustra begins with Zarathustra's *Prologue*, his prespeech, followed by "Zarathustra's Speeches." Like Zarathustra's (non) listeners, the Agrigentians do not attend to what Empedocles teaches, as Hölderlin dramatizes this very political quandary. And yet this is the crux of rhetoric, and it is how esoteric and exoteric teachings work. As Jacob Boehme emphasizes the esoteric, those who have ears to hear may be addressed in a public discourse, because the many, as Heraclitus complains, are like those who hear a teaching and who are the same *both* before hearing it and after (and this is the kicker) hearing it.[19] By their fruits you shall know them.

Zarathustra's supper or "Evening Meal" contrasts in good Empedoclean (and better Cynic) fashion, a vegetarian's meal of ground corn and water, with lamb aromatically cooked with sage and served with wine and recommended in the context of gladness or delight[20]—we recall here that the historico-mythical figure of Zarathustra was said to have been born laughing[21]—as opposed to moral superiority or advantage.[22] The parodic fourth book of *Thus Spoke Zarathustra* sets the stage for the section entitled "The Higher Men" with a detailed allusion to the Lucianic or Mennippean equation of cooks and kings ("with Zarathustra even a king may be a cook,"[23] the same democratizing conversion reflected by Lucian's discussion of the kitchen smells and a dramatization of the reversal of circumstances for shoemakers (like Micyllus) and tyrants (like Megapenthes).

In the parodic section on the *Übermensch* following the supper of cooks and kings (or kings as cooks), Zarathustra highlights just this constellation and setting along with its motley cast of characters: "when I spoke unto all, I spoke unto none. In the evening, however, tightrope-dancers were my companions, and corpses; and I myself nearly a corpse."[24]

The time of kings

Politically speaking, philosophers—and Nietzsche was no exception—can seem to have been preoccupied with kingship. And if philosophers themselves are rarely rulers themselves, apart from the exceptional case of Pythagoras or the Stoic philosopher, Marcus Aurelius, they have, as this inspires both Jesuits and Straussians, kept company with kings, beginning with Thales and Plato to Descartes, as well as Heidegger and Žižek.

Perhaps most important to note in this lineage of philosophers and kingship, Aristotle was the son of the physician of Philip of Macedon and grew up at court, before he came to Athens to study with the Plato who argues that the best rule by the best suited to rule would be the rule of the philosopher. Similarly following Socrates, Diogenes the Cynic, rousted from his barrel and sold into slavery, when asked his particular skill as he was put up for auction, replied that his was the talent to rule human beings. Into this context, we should place the noble-born Empedocles as it was precisely in spite of his high provenance and wealth, that he "constantly refused sovereign power when it was offered him."[25]

This is the heart of Nietzsche's account of Empedocles as "reformer." And in a politicized rendering, keyed to his own time (and there is no other kind of political rendering but a timely one), Hölderlin dramatizes this same refusal. Here we note that following Plato, most classicists have contented themselves with thinking that Empedocles refused to be elevated to kingship owing to his distrust of the mob, i.e., the people. Alternately, Cornford gives the best articulation of this interpretation which is also the most prevalent and the most ancient. Empedocles refused kingship, because he did not want to be bothered (rhetorically this serves as the paradigm for Plato's argument for the need to compel the philosopher to rule in the *Republic*). In any case, as Diogenes Laertius explains, Empedocles opted for the simple life.[26] At the same time, Nietzsche emphasizes the care he took with his appearance, and Nietzsche's discussion of the friend and the way that one should present oneself before the friend, is indebted to this point. In the same fashion, Empedocles' so-called "simplicity" is not contradictory to the account of Empedocles' anger, expecting that he would be served wine at a feast without having to wait for his host before wine would be offered. Then as now, crassness ignores what is owed the guest: hospitality is always a matter of form, of what *should* be done,[27] and thus it is the basis of ethics.

Both Hölderlin and Nietzsche highlight the political in their engagement with Empedocles.[28] On Empedocles' own account, he refuses "kingship" because his "kingdom" can no longer be of this world. Logically: he is, as he tells us from the start, mortal no more. In addition, and this is the same thing, he is about to elect to die. This means that Empedocles' refusal of kingship is not merely complicated by Empedocles' "greatness of soul", but also his numerously attributed associations with familial nobility, as well as popular political influence.

For just this reason, the offer of kingship cannot but fall short for Empedocles, and in the case of Zarathustra, the same reasons recur, as Zarathustra speaks to his heart, as he also speaks to his shade:

> "Whither hath my lonesomeness gone?" spake he.
>
> "It is verily becoming too much for me; these mountains swarm; my kingdom is no longer of THIS world; I require new mountains.
>
> My shadow calleth me? What matter about my shadow! Let it run after me! I — run away from it."[29]

We return to the question of death and the realm of the shades below. Here it is essential to note that the language of Hölderlin's Empedocles explores the reformer's claim: "This is the age of kings no longer" [*Diß ist die Zeit der Könige nicht mehr*][30] together with the conflicted source of this resistance from one who felt himself a god in exile, derelict, and in deficiency: "You offer /me a crown, you men/seizing from me/ my holiness thereby." [*Ihr botet/Mir eine Kron', ihr Männer! nimmt von mir/Dafür mein Heiligtum*].[31]

To the extent that Nietzsche follows Hölderlin's own schemas as he does, one must add the further political complexities of Hölderlin's account of the same, given the influence of the terror in Germany. As Nietzsche outlines this in his own Empedocles draft: "The Agrigentians want to make him king, an unheard of honor. He recognizes the madness of religion, after a long battle."[32]

One may hear Empedocles' refusal of kingship and resistance to religion as a sign of his enlightenment *avant la lettre*, as scholars are inclined to do, or we may hear it in terms of his excessive ego, impetuosity, foolishness, or just and still more idealistically, as a vote for a new democratic mode (and Empedocles was both fond of and popular with the people). In either case, we read in Hölderlin's Empedocles as in Nietzsche's Zarathustra, *the time of kings is past*.

Nietzsche's account of Empedocles on kingship, reform, as on democracy and rhetoric must be understood in terms of Nietzsche's understanding of nobility and sovereignty, an understanding all too easily conflated with the common understanding of such terms as the noble and the sovereign. For like Lucian, Nietzsche always targets popular conflations. And thus we should ask, especially when it comes to the philosopher who brings us the distinction between master, i.e., noble and slave morality: *What do we mean by the noble?* Thus and where the second part of *On the Genealogy of Morals* also reprises the structure of the first part on the terms of debt and contract or law, so too the question of the sovereign and we need to ask: *What do we mean by the sovereign?*

Both questions must be posed afresh; yet most readings of *On the Genealogy of Morals* have yet to engage the challenge of Nietzsche's "sovereign individual" conceived as Nietzsche himself presents this to us. In the context of bonds that one makes and breaks, the context of the bond that one sets upon oneself as one gives one's word, precisely as only one who *can* hold himself to his own word is a human being with the *right* to make a promise, as only such a human being is *able* to keep the promises he makes. Here it is important to note the Kantian allusion in Nietzsche's discussion of the promise only the sovereign individual has the right to make, because only sovereign individuals can hold themselves to their word, despite external or empirical contingency: "they know themselves strong enough to maintain it in the face of accidents, even 'in the face of fate' —."[33] Nietzsche argues that one must have the "right to make promises"[34] by contrast with "the feeble windbags who promise without the right to do so . . . [or] the liar who breaks his word even at the moment that he utters it."[35] Nietzsche's engagement with Kant is typically expressed in terms of legitimacy—indicting the very idea of synthetic *a priori* judgments *an sich*, that is: in terms of their possibility for us, that is to say: *speaking epistemologically*:

> Kant asked himself: How are synthetic judgments *a priori* possible?—And what really did he answer? By means of a faculty: but unfortunately not in a few words, but so circumspectly, venerably, and with such an expenditure of German profundity and flourishes that the comical *niaiserie allemande* involved in such an answer was overlooked. . . . Or, to speak more plainly and coarsely— synthetic judgments *a priori* should not "be possible" at all: we have no right to them; in our mouths they are nothing but false judgments."[36]

Like the preconditions for the possibility of synthetic *a priori* judgments, the point here has everything to do with what is needed to claim sovereignty. Effectively, so Nietzsche claims, the sovereign individual defies fate and should therefore by some accounts "not 'be possible' at all,"[37] nevertheless, in terms of what is needful in order to have the right to make a promise, that is, the right to give one's word in the first place, the sovereign individual must be, in order to be sovereign, possessed of the power needed to keep one's own word.

Here, like the centurion who once trusted a particular Syrian's promise, a word alone would suffice, because of the power of the one who gave his word. Thus Nietzsche argues that in order to have the "right" to make promises, one must to be able to keep the promise one makes without, this is his point about the feeble windbags, having it "break in one's mouth as one utters it." And that means, and now the comparison with that same Syrian is apt, that one has to be able to keep one's word in the face of fate, beyond death itself.

Nietzsche's reflections on nobility are intimations of mortality and immortality. Thus in *On Old and New Tablets*, in a seeming anticipation of his later epigraph to *Ecce Homo*, we read Zarathustra's musing: "when will my hour come? The hour of my going down and going under . . . the laughing lion with the flock of doves. Meanwhile I talk to myself as one who has time. Nobody tells me anything new: so I tell myself—myself."[38] I argue that there is here little of the putatively Emersonian tone so often read into these words in its later appearance in Nietzsche's *Ecce Homo—pace* George Stack, Stanley Cavell, and others.

Beyond New World transcendentalism, or what we like today to speak of as perfectionism, beyond pragmatism, we read a sustained reflection on nobility as Nietzsche's Zarathustra goes on to trace the values of this world, of worldliness, characterized in terms of its smallness or triviality. In this way, Nietzsche calls for a "new" kind of nobility

> to be the adversary of all rabble and all that is despotic. . . . For many who are noble are needed, and noble men are of many kinds, that there may be a nobility. Or as I said once in a parable: 'Precisely this is godlike, that there are gods, but no God.[39]

The focus on plurality is key, thus Nietzsche repeatedly emphasizes that Empedocles is rare among the ancients to the extent that his attention is on the people. Today in an age that is proud to call itself democratic no matter how the political dynamics of the real world of regulations and finances and wars works itself out in actual practice, we continue to suppose that class is a matter of money, nobility a matter of popular esteem and recognition: hence to be well-born is to be famous and vice versa, fame proves it. But Nietzsche's Zarathustra urges:

> O my brothers, I dedicate and direct you to a new nobility: you shall become procreators and cultivators and sowers of the future—verily, not to a nobility that you might buy like shopkeepers with shopkeepers' gold; for whatever has its price has little value.[40]

Thus Nietzsche, like Kant, speaks of the esteem for what is beyond estimation, beyond price.[41]

If we set aside the relevance of Nietzsche's own anxieties as some have detailed these,[42] nobility, for Nietzsche, has little to do with keeping company with the middle-class or esteeming the noble-born and here we read, and again we note the resonance with Hölderlin's Empedocles: "— what do princes matter now?—."[43] Later in the same section, Nietzsche's Zarathustra urges: "Go your *own* ways! And let the people and peoples go theirs—dark ways, verily, on which not a single hope flashes anymore. Let the shopkeeper rule where all that still glitters is—shopkeepers' gold."[44] Nietzsche, we recall from *Beyond Good and Evil* and *On the Genealogy of Morals* as well as *Human, All-too-Human*, is more inclined to tell us what nobility is than to take instruction. In his Zarathustra text, the echo is again to the same Syrian who reminded us that Caesar must be rendered what is his. Recollecting Hölderlin's Empedoclean reflection, Nietzsche writes: "The time of kings is past; what calls itself a people today deserves no kings. Look how these peoples are now like shopkeepers: they pick up the smallest advantage from every kind of rubbish . . ."[45]

In Nietzsche's *Nachlaß* sketch for the second act of his *Death of Empedocles*, he describes the pestilence often noted in association with Empedocles as physician. It is as purifier that Nietzsche's own notion of the philosopher as the physician of culture is related and this purification is also the point of the overman. The reference to plague recurs in Diogenes Laertius and Hölderlin (not to mention Sophocles' *Oedipus* trilogy, both at the start and the end); Nietzsche outlines that "Empedocles prepares great theatrical festivals, Dionysian bacchanales, art reveals itself as the prophet of human agony."[46] And, shades of Goethe and Wagner and the emphasis on the lie, we also read (this is of course a play on Pantheia's name): "Woman as Nature."[47]

In the third act of Nietzsche's first draft, we find a parallel to Zarathustra's initial or first revelation, which, like Lucian's *Dialogues of the Dead* or like his *Downward Journey*, includes a dialogue with a corpse and spending time with or keeping company with the same. Yet Zarathustra does not claim the power, as does Empedocles to "bring back from Hades a dead man's strength."[48] This point is complicated, given the claims made for Empedocles both in popular accounts of the mystical variety as well as scholarly accounts.[49]

Where Empedocles claims, and the parallel with Jesus and Lazarus is no accident, to have the power to "bring back from Hades a dead man's strength" (ibid.) insight into the tragic nature of life becomes both a paradox and a potential object of mockery. It is the last that we find in marvelous evidence in Lucian's presentation of Empedocles in his *Icaromenippus*. Thus with dark humor, Zarathustra gives straightforward comfort to the living corpse that is the dying, and thus literally overcome, tightrope walker, rope dancer, or overman: "You have made danger your calling, and there is nothing contemptible in that. Now you perish of your vocation: for that I will bury you with my own hands."[50]

If we turn from Nietzsche's Zarathustra to Nietzsche's Empedocles, the scene cuts to Empedocles at a wake, the resolution as we are informed is "to destroy the people so that they might be freed from devastation." This is euthanasia, as Nietzsche also writes "One has been a poor observer of life, if one has not also seen the hand that out of solicitude — kills."[51] Empedocles, as a physician, has seen this and more, and the point also made real sense to the Nietzsche who worked in his military service as an orderly. By contrast with the mercy of death, for Empedocles, we read that those "who survive the pestilence seem still more pitiable to him." Then, and the movement of the drama follows Hölderlin, we cut to a scene at the Temple of Pan where we hear the lament, "The Great Pan is dead," a cry which should be set in the context of Nietzsche's reference to the sculptural tableau of the tragic artwork which he also compares to "the world of statues," invoking the "drunken 'science' (in place of 'wisdom')."[52] Here the context Nietzsche describes corresponds to the "decline of the gods,"[53] conveying the spirit of Nietzsche's most memorable, and most Lucian indebted regret as he writes in *The Antichrist*, "Almost two thousand years and not a single new god!"[54]

"A woman in the audience sees her beloved fall, wants to go to him."[55] This point exceeds the space allotted here, but we may note that the allusion to Nietzsche's later discussion of the complex question of interfering with the tragedy is complicated in the case of this woman who is herself a poet, Corinna, and her situation[56] and further with respect to the various theories of the chorus, as Nietzsche notes these in *The Birth of Tragedy*. Here, Empedocles restrains her and discovers his own love for her, not unlike Achilles and the queen of the Amazons, Penthesilea. And like Achilles and Penthesilea, this is a death scene, almost operatic. "She surrenders; the dying one speaks. Empedocles is horrified before the aspect of nature thereby unveiled before him."[57]

In this tragic constellation, Nietzsche writes "Empedocles is driven through all levels, religion, art, science, directing the final dissolution against himself."[58] Nietzsche's 1870 sketch anticipates Zarathustra's own hermit-existence and above all, Zarathustra's down-going more Lucianic than Platonic, if only because the beginning of this down-going is almost literally articulated in connection with death, first off as downgoing, and then as Nietzsche invokes the death of god, the light of dead stars, along with the fall of the tightrope walker and the image of Zarathustra carrying a corpse, which is at the same time a traditional way of referring to the body and its always already consummate destiny, as distinct from the soul. Add to this many other references, including dreams with coffins, howling dogs, the old hermit himself and his proximity to death. If all this (and more) were not enough, we may consider the dreadful bathos of the death of the tightrope dancer. A dwarf or a demon "springing over" one's head also bespeaks death, as does, and as Jung reminds us, the later image of the flying Zarathustra, who also obligingly descends into hell.[59]

That Nietzsche reflects on death in this way is clear as we recall he will speak of himself as dead as father—and so too this is overdetermined, his brother as well, if indeed still living, as his mother (and sister). The reference to death is also, we noted, evident in Zarathustra's allusion to the archaic thought of eternal recurrence, which is after all an event that transpires in the fullness of the time of one's life, that is, it is what becomes of one after one's death (instead of the nothing that Socrates, long before science, already mentions as a then-current supposition, and instead of heaven, or what Zarathustra refers to, as Erwin Rohde also refers to, as the ancient Greek conventionality of the *Blessed Isles*. In a longer discussion than is possible here, we might be able further to detail the relation between Nietzsche's *Zarathustra* and Hölderlin's *Hyperion*. Here we note the reflections in Nietzsche's *Death of Empedocles*:

> . . . Now as an anatomist, he contemplates the suffering of the world, becomes a tyrant, uses religion and art, more and more hardening himself. He has decided upon the destruction of the people inasmuch as he recognizes their incurability. The people gather around the crater: he goes mad and proclaims the truth of rebirth before his disappearance. A friend perishes with him.[60]

Summarizing the trajectory of Empedocles' life and his death, Nietzsche understands Empedocles as a tragic political figure, in a democratic kingly, thus tragically kingly and indeed, following Sophocles, as Nietzsche does in his *The Birth of Tragedy*, sacrificial modality. And so Hölderlin depicts his Empedocles.

In this context of peoples and of kings, the political question Nietzsche poses asks, "How does the political artwork [*Staatskunstwerk*] go to ground?" (KSA 7, 148). As we have come to recognize from Nietzsche's analysis of both Socrates and Euripides in *The Birth of Tragedy*, explicitly diagnosing the devastation of the Greek polity, Nietzsche offers the today still dissonant reply, when he answers that the state is done to ground not by art, not by philosophy and certainly not by religion or myth, but precisely "By means of science [*Wissenschaft*]. Why so? Failure of art, refusal of wisdom." (Ibid.)

By contrast with this first of his sketches for the death of Empedocles, the focus of Nietzsche's aesthetic effort in *The Birth of Tragedy out of the Spirit of Music* explores the political transfiguration of suffering, not for a people who simply, oddly, or dissonantly found in tragedy a cult focus for their entire civilization, but, and much rather for a people exquisitely sensitive to suffering, a people who as Nietzsche writes in *Schopenhauer as Educator*, "evinced the most powerful and exuberant lust for life." (SE §3)

But how is one to explain the tragic aesthetic? Posing this question, Nietzsche counters the then and still popular notion of Greek cheerfulness [*Heiterkeit*], a debate that continues even today between the classic sculptural relief of Winkelmann[61] and Lessing's poetic account. For Nietzsche, the notion of Greek "cheerfulness" simply cannot be sustained, and he follows the positive rigor of his teacher Friedrich Ritschl as he makes this claim. In "Socrates and Greek Tragedy" Nietzsche despairs, citing the resilience of the notion of cheerfulness

> as if there had never been a 6th century with its birth of tragedy, its mysteries, its Empedocles and Heraclitus, indeed as if the works of art of the great age were not present, which however, one for one, can not be explained on the basis of such a doddering and slavely pleasure in existence and cheerfulness and refer instead as their existential foundation to an entirely different world perspective.[62]

Going to ground: Nietzsche's *Übermensch* and Lucian's ʽυπεράνθρωπος

I have noted that parody is essential for this political reading and the Canadian scholar Northrop Frye had already laid the ground rules of this kind of comparison for Anglophone readers, as Frye explained in a section of his *Anatomy of Criticism*:

> whenever the "other world" appears in satire, it appears as an ironic counterpart to our own, a reversal of accepted social standards. This form of satire is represented in Lucian's *Kataplous* and *Charon*, journeys to the other world in which the eminent in this one are shown doing appropriate but unaccustomed things, a form incorporated in Rabelais, and in the medieval *danse macabre*. In the last named the very plain or simple equality of death is set against the complex inequalities of life.[63]

In his monograph on the ancient Greek novel and its antecedents, Nietzsche's friend Rohde highlights the oddness and the importance of "travelling in the underworld, for the sake of philosophical knowledge."[64] This subterranean undertaking is featured in both Nietzsche's Zarathustra and Lucian's dialogues, and this same translation is the point of Empedocles' leap into the Volcano. Just as the jester leaps after the tightrope dancer (as the literal "over"-man at the start of *Thus Spoke Zarathustra*) and similarly threatens to drag Zarathustra himself down to hell, the story Lucian tells in his play on the tyrant's mortal downgoing, articulates the morality tale of those who appear in everyday life in the guise of apparent or supposed "Higher-Men."

Lucian's provocative contrast in his *Downward Journey, or the Tyrant* highlights the superficial vision of the overman as a man of the wealthy, or "higher" power class, a man who towers above others regarded as lower, or lesser, in this life, and the same man transposed into the afterlife: the "superman" ['υπεράνθρωπος] is a man of power "like a tyrant." These political attributes allowed Micyllus, the shoemaker, to report that in life, the tyrant Megapenthes

> appeared to [him] as a superman, thrice-blessed, better looking and a full royal cubit taller than the rest of mankind." [. . .'υπεράνθρωπος τις ἀνὴρ καὶ τρισόβιός μοι κατεφαίνετο καὶ μονονουχὶ πάντων καλλίων καὶ 'υψηλ ότερος 'όλω πήχει βασιλικῶ . . .].[65]

Thus in Lucian's little comic play, *Menippus or the Descent into Hades*, Croesus, the former tyrant complains to Pluto that Menippus is giving them a hard time in hell, and Menippus admits: "Pluto, it's all true, I hate them. They're spineless good-for-nothings. . . . I enjoy needling them." The lord of the underworld urges: ". . . you shouldn't. They left a great deal behind. That's why they take it so seriously." But Menippus will not be swayed and Croesus complains, "This is terrible!" to which Menippus retorts:

> It is not. Yet what you people used to do on the earth was: making other people grovel before you, lording it over free men, never giving the slightest thought to death. Well you can start whimpering because you've lost everything.[66]

For Menippus, the problem is that the tyrant lived a callous and a blind life, both cruel *and* stupid. What matters for Nietzsche is the same blindness or stupidity.

In *The Downward Journey*, when the shoemaker Mycillus contrasted his original impression of the tyrant in life, what strikes him is his own blindness and to this extent complicity in his own misapprehension of the actual qualities of the tyrant Megapenthes. "But",—and of course this Lucianic "but" is the point of the satire "When he was dead, not only did he cut an utterly ridiculous figure in my eyes on being stripped of his pomp, but I laughed at myself even more than at him because I had marveled at such a worthless creature, inferring his happiness from the savour of his kitchen and counting him lucky because of his purple derived from the blood of mussels in the Laconian sea."[67]

If we can consider Lucian's overhuman so unmasked, then Nietzsche's Zarathustra by teaching the crowd the overhuman (if we can hear this in Lucian's spirit) turns out to be teaching something other than a simple promise of being elevated to the status of the overhuman. The parallel promise today of transhumanized humanity,[68] "enhanced" by some technologically mediated state of grace, for those with the money to claim this state, corresponds to the life of the tyrant, Megapenthes. Where mortality is the heart of Lucian's parody—sic transit gloria—today's faith in technology promises the tyrant eternal life. Hence although it is a current enthusiasm to argue that Nietzsche would have been a proponent of transhumanism, the parallel with Lucian seems to suggest that the promised transhuman condition might be one more vanity, one more "value" to be revalued. Once again is Zarathustra's "overhuman" a truly higher human being—or does one simply mistake him for such, as outer trappings and the smells of fine foods took in Mycillus? What are higher values indeed? This question is always the question that Nietzsche teaches us to ask as he calls for a revaluation of values.

For Lucian, as he repeatedly reminds his readers, one is stripped of everything in the passage from life to death, not merely one's position or possessions but also of one's looks, one's athleticism, or one's lack of it, for the Greeks did not teach the resurrection of the body (this will take a Christian conviction) but only the barest shadow of the self, the underworld is a world of shades. It is not for nothing that Lucian hilariously reflects on the difficulty of recognizing anyone at all in the underworld, where all that remains are shadows, no flesh, no muscles, no skin, only skulls, only bones in the place of the beauty of a Helen or the warrior's prowess of an Achilles.

Philosophy as the art of attending to life means just as Lucian says in the mouth of Menippus, denouncing the vanity of an earthly king, giving one's attention to the thought of death. Thus in *The Gay Science* aphorism, Nietzsche asks *What is Life?* and answers very scientifically, precisely accurately in fact, not a touch of hyperbole: "Life—that is, continually shedding something that wants to die" (GS §26). Just so Nietzsche reflects in his *The Thought of Death* in the same locus, that the one thing we do not want to do is reflect on death. We do not think of it. Here I note that Nietzsche's metaphor is Lucian's metaphor, the same metaphor that works in Lucian's figure of Charon and Hermes as messenger, but also in Epictetus and Marcus Aurelius: we live as travelers embarked on a ship's journey, tarrying here and there, gathering this and that but who must be prepared to drop everything when the captain calls, as Epictetus puts it.

If we add Lucian's resonances, what then becomes of the traditional reading of Nietzsche's doctrine of the overman? In its Aryan configuration, set into what some claim to have been its original constellation in Nietzsche's *The Will to Power*, the idea of the *Übermensch* has been invoked as the causal factor in both world wars and indeed every war.[69] Toward the end of Sloterdijk's *Critique of Cynical Reason*, we read this enthusiasm for the mechanically improved human being as ideal soldier, not necessarily as a causative agent, but certainly as a concomitant and indeed, as Sloterdijk maintains, and Günther Anders is with him on this, as an accelerator.[70]

But no matter how one analyzes the titanic ideal of technology, as so many imagine that, if only we allow it (as if, in our times of all times), we were somehow holding science and technology back we would have the possibility of triumphing over death: delaying that ship's departure, perhaps for eternity. Nietzsche argues that such a desire is antilife. And it is hard to understand this, because we suppose that illness, age, death are signs not of life but of something gone terribly wrong.

In this way, Nietzsche's Zarathustra does not teach that humans should aspire to a higher status, think only of the man on the tightrope and the constant invocation, a chorus bordering on a mantra, that the human being is something that should be overcome. Hence rather and to the extent that we are all on the tightrope of our lives, the human must overcome that human, all too human desire for worldly supremacy, this-worldly and all too slavish power.

To what end?

Nietzsche tells us: for the sake of life.

Notes and references

1 See for further bibliographic references and discussion, Babich, "Between Hölderlin and Heidegger: Nietzsche's Transfiguration of Philosophy," *Nietzsche-Studien* 29 (2000): 267–301.

2 Discussions of Nietzsche and Empedocles date back to the beginning of Nietzsche scholarship, for example, Johann Piatek, *Fr. Nietzsches Empedokles-Fragmente* (Struj: Olbrich, 1910). More recent discussions include Raymond Furness, "Nietzsche and Empedocles," *Journal of the British Society for Phenomenolog*, 2/2 (1971): 91–4 as well as Anke Bennholdt-Thomsen's discussion of Nietzsche and Empedocles in her *Nietzsches Also Sprach Zarathustra als literarisches Phänomen. Eine Revision* (Frankfurt am Main: Athenäum, 1974), pp. 151–2. Recent conventional accounts such as Glenn Most's "The Stillbirth of a Tragedy: Nietzsche and Empedocles," in A. L. Pierris, (ed.), *The Empedoclean kosmos: Structure, Process and the Question of Cyclicity* (Patras: Institute for Philosophical Research, 2005), pp. 31–44 sidestep context and Walther Kranz's *Empedokles: Antike Gestalt und romantische Neuschöpfung* (Zürich: Artemis, 1949) includes Hölderlin as does Karl Reinhardt's reflections in *Vermächtnis der Antike*: *Gesammelte Essays zur Philosophie und Geschichtsschreibung* (Göttingen: Vandenhoeck & Ruprecht, 1966). See too David Farrell Krell, *Postponements: Woman, Sensuality and Death in Nietzsche* (Indianapolis: Indiana University Press, 1986) as well as Jürgen Söring, "Nietzsches Empedokles-Plan," *Nietzsche Studien* 19 (1990): 176–211. Although similarly opting to bracket the wide range of the scholarship on this theme, Krell addresses Nietzsche and Hölderlin in his translation of Hölderlin's *The Death of Empedocles: A Mourning-Play* (Albany: State University of New York Press, 2008). See too Véronique Foti's theoretically hermetic and insightful, *Epochal Discordance: Hölderlin's Philosophy of Tragedy* (Albany: State University of New York Press, 2007).

3 Nietzsche, "Die vorplatonische Philosophen," KGW, II/5, p. 3161. I offer further references in Babich, " Le Zarathoustra de Nietzsche et le style parodique. À propos de l'*hyperanthropos* de Lucien et du surhomme de Nietzsche, " *Diogène. Revue internationale des sciences humaines* 232 (October 2010 [2011]): 70–93.

4 Nietzsche, KGW IV/1, p. 126.

5 What is in dispute among most scholars who find this issue captivating is whether this death was real or actual or merely "staged." The discussion of Empedocles' manner of death in Diogenes Laertius and in Lucian who was also Laertius's more satirical contemporary, makes it plain that this was an issue in antiquity. I discuss this further in Babich, "The Philosopher and the Volcano," *Philosophy Today* 36 (Summer 2011): 213–31 as well as in more detail in Babich, "Le Zarathoustra de Nietzsche et le style parodique."

6 KRS 399; DK 112.

7 KRS 401; DK 115.Thus Nietzsche reminds us: "I believe in the old German saying, all gods must die." KSA 7, 124.

8 See the mid-nineteenth-century edition of Lucian available in the Loeb edition by A. M. Harmon, K. Kilburn and M. D. Macleod (Cambridge: Harvard University Press, 1913–67) or the Everyman edition, *Selected Satires of Lucian*, trans. Lionel Casson (New York: Norton, 1968), "Kataplous," pp. 175–93.

9 I note this in Babich, "Le Zarathoustra de Nietzsche et le style parodique. "

10 See, for example, of such a theological discussion of reversal, Ronald F. Hock, "Lazarus and Micyllus: Greco-Roman Backgrounds to Luke 16:19-31," *Journal of Biblical Literature* 106(3), (September 1987): 447–63.

11 Among others, like, most recently, Paul Loeb, David Allison invokes the structural necessity of Nietzsche's plans for Zarathustra's dying in his *Reading the New Nietzsche* (Lanham: Rowman and Littlefield, 2001) and as I show in the essays cited above, the notion is central to C. G. Jung's seminars. Contemporaneously with Jung's first account of this in his dissertation, Nietzsche's contemporary, Theobald Ziegler in his own account of Nietzsche in his lecture courses given in 1897/98 in Strasbourg (Berlin: Bondi, 1900), also makes this same point, using Nietzsche's rather obvious language to do so: " 'also begann Zarathustras Untergang'" Ziegler, *Friedrich Nietzsche*, p. 126. In his 1905 dissertation, the Russian Nicolaus Awxentieff argues that Zarathustra dies in the fourth, unpublished part of *Thus Spoke Zarathustra*. See Awxentieff, *Kultur-ethisches ideal Nietzsches. Darstellung und Kritik* (Halle a. S.: Hofbuchdruckerei von C. A. Kaemmerer & Co., 1905), p. 30.

12 Nietzsche, Z, Part I: *The Adder's Bite.*

13 Nietzsche, Z, Part II: On the Blessed Isles.

14 Cf. Empedocles, "For already I have once been a boy and a girl, a bush and a bird and a (dumb) fish from the sea." KRS 417; DK B117.

15 Nietzsche, Z, Part II: *On the Blessed Isles.*

16 Ibid.

17 Nietzsche, Z, Part III, *The Yes and Amen Song.*

18 Nietzsche, "Geschichte der Griechischen Literatur <I und II>," KGW, II/5 (Berlin: de Gruyter, 1995), p. 191 and cf. p. 192.

19 Heraclitus, DK 1, KRS 197.

20 Derrida is an invaluable inspiration for many reflections on this topic, where Derrida draws on Nietzsche's Zarathustra (with Brillat-Savarin happily haunting the background) in his "'Eating Well,' or the Calculation of the Subject." In *Points . . . Interviews, 1974–1994*, trans. Peter Connor and Avital Ronell (Stanford: Stanford University Press, 1995), pp. 255–87. See too Tobias Nikolaus Klass, "Veredelnde Inocculation. Nietzsche und das Essen," in I. Därmann and H. Lemke, (eds), *Die Tischgesellschaft. Philosophische und kulturwissenschaftliche Annäherungen* (Bielefeld: Transkript, 2007), pp. 11–156. Lucian's discussion of nobility and refinement bears upon Zarathustra in general. See here Nietzsche, KSA 9, p. 460; cf. 11, pp. 105, 106.

21 Anke Bennholdt-Thomsen draws upon both Charles Andler and Karl Schlechta for the legend detailed by Pliny, that Zoroaster laughs on the day of his birth. See again Bennholdt-Thomsen, *Nietzsches Also Sprach Zarathustra als literarisches Phänomen*, p. 88.

22 Nietzsche does not argue for the moral 'virtues' of such pleasures and eating meat remains morally invidious.

23 Nietzsche, Z, Part IV, *Evening Meal.*

24 Nietzsche, Z, Part IV, *The Higher Man.*

25 Diogenes Laertius, *The Lives and Opinions of Eminent Philosophers* (Cambridge, MA: Harvard University Press, 1901), esp. p. 363 and p. 367.

26 It should also be said that his manner of dress, insistence on gracious manners when it comes to serving wine, and other details are consistent with the claim of simplicity.

27 Empedocles is so offended by the contradiction of good form, that he punishes the offenders, NB: without sullying his hands, as it were, arranging for their death by indirect, that is, political means. See Diogenes Laertius, *Life of Empedocles*, IX.

28 I discuss the political overtones of both Hölderlin and Nietzsche in Babich, "Between Hölderlin and Heidegger," in Babich (ed.), *Words in Blood, Like Flowers: Philosophy and Poetry, Music and Eros in Hölderlin, Nietzsche, Heidegger* (Albany: State University of New York Press, 2006). See Pierre Bertaux, *Hölderlin, ou, Le temps d'un poète* (Paris: Gallimard, 1983) as well as, in conjunction with Hegel (and Dieter Henrich), Frank Völkel, "Im Zeichen der französischen Revolution. Philosophie und Poesie im Ausgang vom Tübinger Stift," in Andreas Grossmann und Christoph Jamme, (eds), *Metaphysik der praktischen Welt* (Amsterdam: Rodopi, 2000), pp. 96–120. See too Loralea Michaelis, "The Deadly Goddess: Friedrich Hölderlin on Politics and Fate," *History of Political Thought* 20(2), (1999): 225–49. On the contemporary reception of Hölderlin's politics, see Barton Byg's *Landscapes of Resistance: The German Films of Danièle Huillet and Jean-Marie Straub* (Berkeley: University of California Press, 1995), pp. 178–98, particularly pp. 184ff.

29 Nietzsche, Z, Part IV: *The Shadow*.

30 Hölderlin, StA II, iv, 1449.

31 Ibid., pp. 1498–500. A full discussion of this issue would take us beyond the limits of the current study, but it must be noted with regard to the political significance of both Zarathustra and Empedocles, including Hölderlin's, Empedocles, Nietzsche emphasizes Empedocles' failure in his bid for political reform and as pointing to nothing but his attention, unique among most ancient philosophers, to the people. In consequence of this failure "only Socrates is left." Nietzsche, KSA 8, 104.

32 Nietzsche, KSA 7, 527.

33 Nietzsche, GM II:2.

34 Ibid.

35 Ibid. This is a complex topic. I offer a preliminary discussion of some of these complexities in Babich, "The Genealogy of Morals and Right Reading: On the Nietzschean Aphorism and the Art of the Polemic," in Christa Davis Acampora (ed.), *Nietzsche's On the Genealogy of Morals* (Lanham: Rowman & Littlefield, 2006), pp. 171–90.

36 Nietzsche, BGE § 11.

37 Ibid.

38 Nietzsche, Z, Part Three: *Old and New Tablets*, §1.

39 Ibid., §11.

40 Ibid., §12.

41 See Kant, *The Foundations of the Metaphysics of Morals*, from Lewis White Beck, (ed.), *Kant Selections* (New York: Macmillan, 1988), pp. 277ff.

42 See for example, David F. Krell, *The Good European* (Chicago: University of Chicago Press, 1997), p. 16.

43 Nietzsche, Z, Part Three: *Old and New Tablets*, §12.

44 Ibid., §21.

45 Ibid.

46 Nietzsche, KSA 7, 126.

47 Ibid.

48 Diogenes Laertius, VIII.59.

49 I refer to Peter Kingsley et al. elsewhere.

50 Nietzsche, Z, *Zarathustra's Prologue* §7.

51 Nietzsche, *Jenseits von Gut und Böse*, §69.

52 I discuss this in Babich, "Zu Nietzsches Statuen: Skulptur und das Erhabene," in Beatrix Vogel and Nikolaus Gerdes, (eds.), *Grenzen der Rationalität: Teilband 2* (München: Allitera, 2011), pp. 391–421.

53 Nietzsche, KSA 7, 139; cf. KSA 7, 236.
54 Nietzsche, AC §19.
55 Nietzsche, KSA 7, 139.
56 Compare this wanting intention with Aristotle's description of intention and responsibility in the *Nicomachean Ethics* of *pretending* to spar with a *pretended* blunted weapon.
57 Nietzsche, KSA 7, 139.
58 Ibid., 126.
59 See for references and further discussion, my essays cited above.
60 Nietzsche, KSA, 7 126.
61 I discuss the erotic durability of Winckelmann's vision with a number of further references in Babich, "Die Naturkunde der Griechischen Bronze im Spiegel des Lebens: Betrachtungen über Heideggers ästhetische Phänomenologie und Nietzsches agonale Politik," *Internationales Jahrbuch für Hermeneutik* (Tübingen: Mohr, 2008), pp. 127–89 and still more recently in Babich, "The Aesthetics of the Between: Space and Beauty," in Vinzenz Brinkmann, Matthias Ulrich, and Joachim Pissarro, (eds), *Jeff Koons. The Painter & The Sculptor* (Frankfurt: Schirn Kunsthalle, 2012).
62 Nietzsche, KSA 1, 603.
63 Frye, *Anatomy of Criticism: Four Essays* (Princeton: Princeton University Press, 1957), p. 232.
64 Erwin Rohde, *Der griechische Roman und seine Vorläufer* (Leipzig: Breitkopf und Härtel, 1900), p. 261.
65 Lucian, *Dialogues*, Loeb edition, Vol. II, p. 35 [Greek: p. 34]. Modified.
66 Ibid.
67 Ibid.
68 See further, Babich, "On the "All-too-Human" Dream of Transhumanism," *The Agonist*, 4/II (2012): http://www.nietzschecircle.com/AGONIST/2011_08/Dream_of_Transhumanism.html as well as "Geworfenheit und Prometheischen Scham im Zeitalter der Transhumanen Kybernetik: Technik und Machenschaft bei Martin Heidegger und Günther Anders". In Christian Steckhardt, (ed.), *Die Neugier des Glücklichen* (Weimar: Bauhaus Universitätsverlag, 2012), pp. 7–35.
69 See William Macintire Salter, "Nietzsche and War," in Tracy Strong, (ed.), *Friedrich Nietzsche* (Aldershot: Ashgate, 2009), pp. 3–26. See here on the question of war and the political Strong's "Introduction," Ibid. pp. xi–xxxiii and my own discussion in Babich, "Nietzsche's Will to Power: Politics and Destiny," Ibid., pp. 281–96.
70 I discuss this with further references in Babich, "Sloterdijk's Cynicism: Diogenes in the Marketplace," in Stuart Elden, (ed.), *Sloterdijk Now* (Oxford: Polity, 2011), pp. 17–36; 186–9 and see for a discussion of Anders and the politics of the contemporary digital realm, Babich, "Geworfenheit und Prometheischen Scham im Zeitalter der Transhumanen Kybernetik." Paul Virilio reprises, again, this same notion in his *The Great Accelerator* (London: Polity 2012).

Literature

Allison, David B. *Reading the New Nietzsche*. Lanham: Rowman and Littlefield, 2001.
Awxentieff, Nicolaus. *Kultur-ethisches ideal Nietzsches. Darstellung und Kritik*. Diss, Halle, 1905.
Babich, Babette. "Between Hölderlin and Heidegger: Nietzsche's Transfiguration of Philosophy." *Nietzsche-Studien* 29 (2000): 267–301.

—"Die Naturkunde der Griechischen Bronze im Spiegel des Lebens: Betrachtungen über Heideggers ästhetische Phänomenologie und Nietzsches agonale Politik." In Günther Figal, (ed.), *Internationales Jahrbuch für Hermeneutik* (Tübingen: Mohr, 2008), pp. 127–89.

—"Geworfenheit und Prometheischen Scham im Zeitalter der Transhumanen Kybernetik: Technik und Machenschaft bei Martin Heidegger und Günther Anders." In Christian Steckhardt, (ed.), *Die Neugier des Glücklichen* (Weimar: Bauhaus Universitätsverlag, 2012), pp. 7–35.

— "Le Zarathoustra de Nietzsche et le style parodique. A propos de l'*hyperanthropos* de Lucien et du surhomme de Nietzsche." *Diogène. Revue internationale des sciences humaines* 232 (October 2011): 70–93.

—"Nietzsche's Will to Power: Politics and Destiny." In Tracy B. Strong, (ed.), *Friedrich Nietzsche* (Aldershot: Ashgate, 2009), pp. 281–96.

—"On the "All-too-Human" Dream of Transhumanism." *The Agonist*, 4/II (2012) http://www.nietzschecircle.com/AGONIST/2011_08/Dream_of_Transhumanism.html.

— "Sloterdijk's Cynicism: Diogenes in the Marketplace. " In: Stuart Elden, (ed.), *Sloterdijk Now* (Oxford: Polity, 2011), pp. 17–36; 186–9.

— "The Philosopher and the Volcano." *Philosophy Today* 36 (Summer 2011): 213–31.

— "The Aesthetics of the Between: Space and Beauty." In Vinzenz Brinkmann, Matthias Ulrich, and Joachim Pissarro, (eds), *Jeff Koons. The Painter & The Sculptor* (Frankfurt: Schirn Kunsthalle, 2012).

— "The Genealogy of Morals and Right Reading: On the Nietzschean Aphorism and the Art of the Polemic." In Christa Davis Acampora, (ed.), *Nietzsche's On the Genealogy of Morals*. (Lanham: Rowman & Littlefield, 2006), pp. 171–90.

—*Words in Blood, Like Flowers: Philosophy and Poetry, Music and Eros in Hölderlin, Nietzsche, Heidegger.* Albany, NY: SUNY Press, 2006.

— "Zu Nietzsches Statuen: Skulptur und das Erhabene." In Beatrix Vogel and Nikolaus Gerdes, (eds), *Grenzen der Rationalität: Teilband 2* (München: Allitera, 2011), pp. 391–421.

Bennholdt-Thomsen, Anke. *Nietzsches Also Sprach Zarathustra als literarisches Phänomen. Eine Revision*. Frankfurt am Main: Athenäum, 1974.

Bertaux, Pierre. *Hölderlin, ou, Le temps d'un poète*. Paris: Gallimard, 1983.

Byg, Barton. *Landscapes of Resistance: The German Films of Danièle Huillet and Jean-Marie Straub*. Berkeley: University of California Press, 1995.

Derrida, Jacques. "'Eating Well', or the Calculation of the Subject." In Elisabeth Weber, (ed.), *Points . . . Interviews, 1974–1994*, trans. Peggy Kamuf et al. (Stanford: Stanford University Press, 1995), pp. 255–87.

Diels, Herman and Walther Kranz. *Die Fragmente der Vorsokratiker*. 5th edition. Berlin: Wiedmannsche Buchhandlung, 1934; 1922. [DK].

Diogenes Laertius. *The Lives and Opinions of Eminent Philosophers*, trans. C. D. Yonge. Cambridge, MA: Harvard University Press, 1901. [1853].

Foti, Véronique. *Epochal Discordance: Hölderlin's Philosophy of Tragedy*. Albany, NY: State University of New York Press, 2007.

Furness, Raymond. "Nietzsche and Empedocles." *Journal of the British Society for Phenomenology* 2/2 (1971): 91–4.

Frye, Northrop. *Anatomy of Criticism: Four Essays*. Princeton, NJ: Princeton University Press, 1957.

Hock, Ronald F. "Lazarus and Micyllus: Greco-Roman Backgrounds to Luke 16:19-31." *Journal of Biblical Literature* 106(3), (September 1987): 447–63.

Hölderlin, Friedrich. *The Death of Empedocles: A Mourning-Play*, trans. D. F. Krell. Albany, NY: State University of New York Press, 2008.

—*Sämtliche Werke*. Ed. Adolf Beck, Friedrich Beißner, Große Stuttgarter Ausgabe. Eight volumes. Stuttgart: Kohlhammer, 1943–85. [StA].

Kant, Immanuel. *The Foundations of the Metaphysics of Morals*. Ed. Lewis White Beck, *Kant Selections*. New York: Macmillan, 1988.

Kirk, G. S., J. E. Raven, and M. Schofield, *The Presocratic Philosophers: A Critical History with a Selection of Texts*. Cambridge: Cambridge University Press, 1984; 1957. [KRS].

Klass, Tobias Nikolaus "Veredelnde Inocculation. Nietzsche und das Essen." In I. Därmann and H. Lemke, (eds), *Die Tischgesellschaft. Philosophische und kulturwissenschaftliche Annäherungen*. (Bielefeld: Transkript, 2007), pp. 11–156.

Kranz, Walther. *Empedokles: Antike Gestalt und romantische Neuschöpfung*. Zürich: Artemis, 1949.

Krell, David Farrell. *Postponements: Woman, Sensuality and Death in Nietzsche*. Indianapolis: Indiana University Press, 1986.

—*The Good European*. Chicago: University of Chicago Press, 1997.

Lucian, Dialogues. Ed. and trans. A. M. Harmon, K. Kilburn and M. D. Macleod. Cambridge: Harvard University Press, 1913–67.

—*Selected Satires of Lucian*, trans. Lionel Casson. New York: Norton, 1968.

Michaelis, Loralea. "The Deadly Goddess: Friedrich Hölderlin on Politics and Fate." *History of Political Thought* 20(2), (1999): 225–49.

Most, Glenn. "The Stillbirth of a Tragedy: Nietzsche and Empedocles." In A. L. Pierris, (ed.), *The Empedoclean kosmos: Structure, Process and the Question of Cyclicity*. (Patras: Institute for Philosophical Research, 2005), pp. 31–44.

Nietzsche, Friedrich. *Kritische Gesammtausgabe*. Berlin: de Gruyter, 1995. KGW.

—*Kritische Studienausgabe*. Berlin: de Gruyter, 1980. KSA.

—*Also Sprach Zarathustra*, KSA Volume 4.

—*Der Antichrist*, KSA Volume 6.

—"Die vorplatonische Philosophen." *Kritische Gesammtausgabe* [KGW] II/5.

—"Geschichte der Griechischen Literatur <I und II>." KGW, II/5.

—*Jenseits von Gut und Böse*, KSA Volume 5.

—*Zur Genealogie der Moral*. KSA Volume 5.

Piatek, Johann. *Nietzsches Empedokles-Fragmente*. Progr. Gymn. Stryj, 1910.

Reinhardt, Karl. *Vermächtnis der Antike: Gesammelte Essays zur Philosophie und Geschichtsschreibung*. Göttingen: Vandenhoeck & Ruprecht, 1966.

Rohde, Erwin. *Der griechische Roman und seine Vorläufer*. Leipzig: Breitkopf und Härtel, 1900.

Salter, William Macintire. "Nietzsche and War." In Tracy B. Strong, (ed.), *Friedrich Nietzsche* (Aldershot: Ashgate, 2009), pp. 3–26.

Söring, Jürgen. "Nietzsches Empedokles-Plan." *Nietzsche Studien* 19 (1990): 176–211.

Strong, Tracy B. "Introduction." In Strong, (ed.), *Friedrich Nietzsche*. (Aldershot: Ashgate, 2009), pp. xi–xxxiii.

Robinson, Christopher. *Lucian and his Influence in Europe*. Chapel Hill: The University of North Carolina Press, 1979.

Virilio, Paul. *The Great Accelerator*. London: Polity 2012.

Völkel, Frank. "Im Zeichen der französischen Revolution. Philosophie und Poesie im Ausgang vom Tübinger Stift." In Andreas Grossmann and Christoph Jamme, (eds), *Metaphysik der praktischen Welt* (Amsterdam: Rodopi, 2000), pp. 96–120.

Ziegler, Theobald. *Nietzsche*. Berlin: Bondi, 1900.

13

Nietzsche's Care for Stone: The Dead, Dance, and Flying [1]

Graham Parkes

From his childhood through to the end of his career, Nietzsche greatly appreciated the therapeutic powers of the natural world, and he celebrated and advocated them in many passages in his writings.[2] The energies of animals and birds and beasts of prey and of burden, the forces of wind and storm, the rushing of streams and rivers, the massive heavings of the sea, the quiet majesty of forests, and the still power of mountains—since all of these belong, for Nietzsche, to what he calls the "great economy" of the soul, it is healing and whole-making to be aware of them and interact with them more fully. Since stone and rock hold a special place in this economy, a focus on these phenomena will render this vast topic manageable within the compass of a brief chapter.

A consideration of Nietzsche's views of rock and stone, and the role played by related imagery in his texts, reveals a generally unnoticed feature of his philosophy of nature as well as his philosophical therapeutics. He especially reveres unhewn rock, for what it can teach us about life, and for what its image tells us about what is unteachable in the depths of the soul. In this his ideas are unusual in western traditions of thought: although reverence for unworked stone is typical of most cultures in their beginnings (the Celts and the Polynesians, for example), among mature civilizations the East-Asian stand out in their zealous retention of it. In the West, Nietzsche's precursors in this respect are Goethe, Schopenhauer, and Ralph Waldo Emerson.[3]

For this task, we need to appreciate the relations between our *ideas* of stone, many of which come from our understanding of rock through natural science, and the archetypal *images* that flow from the same source, prefigured in myth and imaginally elaborated in poetry and literature, and in a way congruent with the ideas. Nietzsche's relations to rock, as the hardest, heaviest part of the earth, are most richly imagined in his "most personal" book, *Thus Spoke Zarathustra*, and especially in the protagonist's relations with his arch-enemy, the Spirit of Heaviness. Zarathustra's accomplishes his greatest therapeutic task, the overcoming of this powerful antagonist, through the medium of stone: the philosophers' stone and the stone of death, and the rock on which he sits and dances, and from which he ultimately takes off and flies.

Youth, death, and the stone of fate

In his youth, according to his early notebooks and letters, Nietzsche was something of a nature mystic. The first poem (and the second item) recorded in his juvenilia, dating from when he was 10 years old, begins with the (in German) rhyming couplet: "There on that outcrop of rock/There's my favourite place to sit."[4] At the age of 14 he wrote:

> From childhood on I would seek solitude and would feel best when I could abandon myself to myself undisturbed. This usually happened in the open temple of nature, where I would find the truest friends.[5]

Prominent among such friends is stone: following a list of what he calls "my enemies"—"mosquitoes, cloudy skies, and warm damp air"—the first in a list of "my friends" is: "rocks." Nietzsche records in his notebooks several childhood memories of digging up "calcite [a carbonate mineral] and other rocks" on a ridge near his home in Naumburg. Under the heading "Windlücke" (a spot not far away) he wrote: "Rocks as witnesses of prehistory. . . . What happy days!"[6] This childhood experience is at the basis of a later aphorism that imagines the human being—himself—seen "In the Mirror of Nature," and asks:

> Is a human being not well described when we hear that . . . from childhood on he experiences and reveres unhewn rocks as witnesses of prehistory which are eager to acquire language?[7]

Gravestones, stone bordering the underworld of the dead, weigh heavy in young Nietzsche's recollections of childhood. At the age of 14, he reminisces about his (now distant) home town: "How lively still the graveyard stands before me! How often I wondered, when I saw the ancient mortuary, about the biers and the black mourning crepes, the old grave inscriptions and monuments." And a few years later, he writes: "A little higher than the ponds stand the parsonage and the church, the former surrounded by gardens and groves of trees. And next to them the cemetery, full of sunken gravestones and crosses." At 19, Nietzsche writes yet another autobiographical sketch titled "My Life," in which he likens (his) life to a landscape where the "rock formations and kinds of stone" show the general structure of the life, while the vegetation provides the individuating physiognomy of "the small experiences and inner processes." "The following brief biographical notes," he goes on, "are smooth stones; in reality these stones are beautifully clad in moss and earth." And shortly after that he writes again of "the cemetery, full of sunken gravestones and crosses."[8]

During this period, Nietzsche developed a Hölderlin-influenced, hylozoist philosophy of life, according to which everything is alive and ordered in a hierarchy "beginning with stone . . . progressing to plants, animals, and human beings, and issuing in earth, air, heavenly bodies" and so forth, and which regards the entire world as being animated by *die Urseele*, the Primordial Soul.[9] At the age of 21, as a graduate student in Leipzig, Nietzsche came across a similar but highly elaborated philosophy of life and the lifeless when he first read Schopenhauer's masterpiece, *The World as Will and Representation*. Schopenhauer posits "will" as a cosmic force that drives all motion and transformation, including the human life that we live.

> The reader will recognize that same *will* not only in those phenomena that are quite similar to his own, in human beings and animals, as their innermost nature; but continued reflection will lead him to recognize the force that drives and vegetates in the plant, indeed the force by which the crystal is formed, the force that turns the magnet to the North Pole . . . and finally even gravitation, which acts so powerfully in all matter, pulling the stone to the earth and the earth to the sun; all these he will recognize as being different only in the phenomenon, but the same according to their inner nature . . . and as that which is immediately known to him as *will*.[10]

In the course of a series of lectures Nietzsche delivered in Basel "On the Future of Our Educational Institutions" (1872), he speaks through the persona of "an old philosopher":

> If you want to lead a young person onto the right path of education and culture, be careful not to disturb his naively trustful and personally immediate relationship with nature: forest and rock, storm and vulture, the single flower, the butterfly, the meadow and the mountainside must speak to him in their own tongues; at the same time he must recognize himself in them as in countless dispersed reflexes and reflections and in a multicolored whirl of changing appearances.[11]

Rock, among other natural phenomena, speaks to the open soul in the language of rock, such that the soul can then see itself in all of stone's aspects and facets. The old philosopher goes on to bemoan the fact that few youths are fortunate enough to enjoy such close personal relations with the natural world, since education teaches them early on how to subjugate nature toward one's own ends through "clever calculation and cunning."

Nietzsche's early experiences of stone in the graveyard, stone's connection with death, guide his subsequent reflections on the natural world beyond human life—and beyond all life, to the "lifeless." He had witnessed a move beyond biocentrism in his early readings of Emerson, who often reflects on rock and stone. In his mid-30s, Emerson recorded in his journal a kind of death experience that he had on stepping out of the house into a night illumined by the full moon.

> In the instant you leave behind all human relations . . . and live only with the savages—water, air, light, carbon, lime, & granite. . . . I become a moist, cold element. 'Nature grows over me.' . . . I have died out of the human world & come to feel a strange, cold, aqueous, terraqueous, aerial, ethereal sympathy and existence.[12]

Several of Nietzsche's unpublished notes similarly celebrate our intimacy with the so-called inanimate world: "To be redeemed from life and become dead nature again can be experienced as a festival—of one who wants to die. To love nature! To revere again what is dead!" For Nietzsche, what makes us from the start close relatives of this "dead" realm is our physical constitution as living organisms.

> How distant and superior is our attitude toward what is dead, the anorganic, and all the while we are three-quarters water, and have anorganic minerals in us that perhaps do more for our well- and ill-being than the whole of living society![13]

The idea of crossing over to the realm of the inanimate in the form of stone appears in the published works in the brief aphorism "How One Ought to Turn to Stone": "Slowly, slowly, to become hard like a precious stone—and finally to lie there, still and to the joy of eternity."[14] It is a long process: beginning with Nietzsche's experiences of dying away from the human world, burning his life into writing such notes and aphorisms, which are then subject to successive interpretations, until there emerges a gem of a thought that will consistently delight, when seen from different angles and in different lights.

By writing, Nietzsche is doing what all natural phenomena are already doing all the time. There's a magnificent characterization of nature as secular inscription at the beginning of Emerson's essay on Goethe:

> All things are engaged in writing their history. The planet, the pebble, goes attended by its shadow. The rolling rock leaves its scratches on the mountain; the river its channel in the soil; the animal its bones in the stratum; the fern and leaf their modest epitaph in the coal. The falling drop makes its sculpture in the sand or the stone. . . . The round is all memoranda and signatures, and every object covered over with hints which speak to the intelligent.[15]

And in his essay "Fate" (a favorite of Nietzsche's from his youth), Emerson emphasizes the interplay between fate, or "Nature as tyrannous circumstance," imagined as rock, and the dynamic powers of human life—the task being to integrate our own powers with the "negative power" of circumstance.

> The book of Nature is the book of Fate. She turns the gigantic pages—leaf after leaf—never re-turning one. One leaf she lays down, a floor of granite; then a thousand ages, and a bed of slate; a thousand ages, and a measure of coal; a thousand ages and a layer of marl and mud.[16]

Then come vegetation and animal life and, finally, human existence—where "when a race has lived its term, it comes no more again." Impermanence still reigns. But the rock remains, the leaf of granite slowly curls up, jutting out into the world of the human as adverse circumstance.

> Famine, typhus, frost, war, suicide, and effete races, must be reckoned calculable parts of the system of the world. They are pebbles from the mountains, hints of the terms by which our life is walled up. . . . We cannot trifle with this reality, this cropping-out in our planted gardens of the core of the world.[17]

We trifle with that core at our peril, and are doing so now, insofar as our persistence with ever deeper mining, hydraulic fracturing, and carbon sequestration evidence a stubborn refusal to face reality and accept limits to our powers to satisfy our insatiable desire to consume.

In one sense, we can turn to stone because we are already half way there.

The image of stone in self-fashioning

At the end of the first section of Nietzsche's first book, *The Birth of Tragedy*, after a glowing description of Apollo as the divine shaper of the dream-world and imagination, there is an account of the effects of *Rausch*, intoxication, as a manifestation of Dionysus as "loosener" or "dissolver."

> Under the magical spell of the Dionysian it is not only the bonds between humans that are restored: alienated, or hostile, or subjugated nature also celebrates again her festival of reconciliation with her lost son, the human being.

Nietzsche conjures here, and we should hear, Schiller's "Ode to Joy" as sung at the end of Beethoven's *Ninth*: "Be embraced, you millions! Take this kiss for the whole world!" A festival indeed, but important that Dionysus is the god of wine, and to have the "joy bubbling in the goblets, in the grape's golden blood," since he brings suffering as well as intoxication.[18] The rush of intoxication takes us out of ourselves, dissolving the bounds of the individual, both enacting and alleviating the suffering at the same time.

> This rending, the authentic Dionysian suffering, is like a transformation into air, water, earth and stone, plant and animal; where the condition of individuation is regarded as the source and primal ground of all suffering, as something inherently reprehensible.[19]

But Dionysus is the god not only of the vine but also of the dance. "In singing and dancing the human being expresses itself as a member of a higher communality," insofar as Dionysian intoxication undermines the principle of individuation that keeps us feeling ourselves separate from other human beings and the world of nature.

> The human being is no longer an artist but has become a work of art: the artistic power of the whole of nature, to the most blissful satisfaction of the Primal One, manifests itself here through the frissons of intoxication. The most noble clay, the most costly marble—the human being—is here kneaded and hewn, and to the chisel blows of the Dionysian worlds-artist there rings out the cry of the Eleusinian Mysteries: 'Do you prostrate yourselves, millions? Do you sense your creator, world?'[20]

The intoxicating power of the Dionysian, working through the whole of nature's artistic forces, makes human beings works of art by shaping and integrating them into the totality. But then "the Dionysian worlds-artist" is said to knead and hew and sculpt the human being through the distinctly Apolline art of sculpture, whereby the context of the stone is chiseled away to reveal the individual form.

In an unpublished note from 1880, Nietzsche abandons the idea that a divine artist fashions us, in favor of the notion of our forming the "authentic self" ourselves:

> *To make ourselves*, to *shape* a form from all the elements—that is the task! The task of a sculptor! Of a productive human being! It's *not* through knowledge but through practice and a model that we become *ourselves*![21]

This image is prefigured in Emerson, who writes that "Man is a stupendous antagonism, a dragging together of the poles of the Universe." As embodied in an evolved figure that retains all its previous forms, the human is also bedrock and core of nature, combined with elemental, solar power.

> The lightning which explodes and fashions planets, maker of planets and suns, is [also in the human being]. On one side, elemental order, sandstone and granite, rock-ledges, peat-bog, forest, sea and shore; and, on the other, thought, the spirit which composes and decomposes nature—here they are, side by side, god and devil, mind and matter, king and conspirator, belt and spasm, riding peacefully together in the eye and brain of every man.[22]

Nietzsche develops this idea, but with a heightened tension between the sides that would preclude the "peacefully," in a passage addressed to those who want to "*abolish suffering*."

> In the human being *creature* and *creator* are united: in the human there is material, fragment, abundance, clay, dirt, nonsense, chaos; but there is also in the human creator, sculptor, hammer-hardness, spectator divinity, and seventh day—do you understand this opposition? And that your pity is for the creature in the human, for that which has to be formed, broken, forged, torn, burned, annealed, and purified—for that which must necessarily *suffer* and *ought* to suffer?[23]

Now the Dionysian worlds-artist (shadowed by the Christian Creator), who molds the noble clay and sculpts the marble of the human, works through certain human beings so that they become artists of the human as well. This kind of work is performed by and on the body, through physical practice guided by a *Vorbild* (literally, preimage), a pattern or model. Yet, what subsequent generations appreciate in such work is often the substance of the corpus rather than its form.

> The philosopher believes that the value of his philosophy lies in the totality, in the building: posterity finds the value in the stone with which he built and with which others have since built often and better.[24]

The kind of artistic creation Nietzsche is talking about here takes place on an interpersonal level and a far grander scale. In the course of a diatribe against the shortsighted superficiality of the modern age in Europe, Nietzsche deplores the tendency for people to become mere actors (where all nature ceases and becomes art) and bemoans the lack of architects who would build a real society out of individuals. He calls for a regaining of the broad perspective that would see the present in the context of the vast sweep of history and the individual against the background of the development of the race.

> Who would still dare to undertake works that would take millennia to be completed? The basic faith is dying out . . . that the human being has value and meaning only insofar as it is a stone in a vast edifice: for which it would have to be first and foremost solid, a stone and above all not an actor![25]

And how does one attain such a condition? "Slowly, slowly, to become hard like a precious stone—and finally to lie there, still and to the joy of eternity."

This transformation is to take place in a world of perpetual becoming—all there really is in Nietzsche's Heraclitean world. In an allegory of "time and becoming," Zarathustra praises and justifies "all impermanence." The suffering that derives from a life of impermanence is redeemed by his creating will, through which "life becomes lighter." Having worked on himself, sculpted his life into shape, his formative will then turns outward.

> To the human being it drives me again and again, my fervent creating-will; thus is the hammer driven to the stone.
>
> Ah, you humans, in the stone there sleeps an image, the image of my images! Ah, that it must sleep in the hardest, ugliest stone!
>
> Now my hammer rages fiercely against the prison. Fragments fly from the stone: what is that to me?
>
> I want to perfect it: for a shadow came to me—of all things the stillest and lightest once came to me!
>
> The beauty of the Overhuman came to me as a shadow. (*Z* 2.2)

Zarathustra, the awakened one, having seen in the raw material of the human the *Vorbild* of the Overhuman, will awaken the image to life by demolishing the prison from the outside, liberating the figure crushed into the dense conformity of stone. There will be fragmentation, pulverizing, suffering in shards and fragments. But this is what thinking in action, philosophizing with a hammer, sometimes entails.

Rock and fate in *Zarathustra*

When Nietzsche writes about *Thus Spoke Zarathustra* in *Ecce Homo*, he says that the work's "basic conception" is "the *thought of eternal return*, the highest formula of affirmation that can ever be attained."

> [This thought] dates from August of 1881. . . . I was walking along the lake of Silvaplana through the woods; I stopped beside a powerfully towering pyramidal block of stone not far from Surlei. The thought came to me there.[26]

The thought that enables the greatest affirmation of life struck the thinker as he stood by a pyramid of rock that most people would see as inanimate and lifeless. But let us remember what Nietzsche wrote not long after about the living by contrast with the lifeless: "Let us be wary of saying that life is opposed to death. The living is only a species of the dead, and a very rare species at that."[27] The living is not opposed to the dead because they are equally manifestations of will to power. After Nietzsche first presents the idea of will to power in *Zarathustra*, where we learn that "all life is . . . will to power," he then suggests in *Beyond Good and Evil* that the whole world is "will to power and nothing besides."[28] It is thus no surprise that rock should play a major role in the process recounted in *Zarathustra* whereby will to power learns to will eternal return.

In "The Grave-Song," Zarathustra voyages across the sea to "the Isle of the Graves," bringing "an evergreen wreath of life . . . to the graves of [his] youth" (*Z* 2.11). He laments that the "visions and apparitions" of his youth—"godlike moments" he calls them—died away so quickly, and now lie here buried. He laments that they were "murdered" by his enemies (Nietzsche's sister in collusion with the Wagners, according to allusions to personal betrayals he had recently experienced) who had cut short moments he thought were eternal in their capacity to return. He was ready to affirm the Emersonian maxim, "Godlike shall all beings be to me," when they assailed him in a distinctly ungod-like manner. When he was ready "to dance as [he] had never danced before, away beyond all heavens," they cut him short again, by cutting him off from "the visions and consolations of [his] youth." How is he to redeem these moments, resurrect these memories? The significance of the answer is emphasized by its being sung rather than spoken.

> Yes, something invulnerable, unburiable is within me, something that explodes rock: that is *my will*. Silently it strides and unchanging through the years. . . .
>
> To this day you continue to break through all graves! . . .
>
> Yes, you are still for me the demolisher of every grave: hail to thee, my will! And only where there are graves are there resurrections. —[29]
>
> Thus sang Zarathustra. —

However, as we learn from his speech "On Redemption," Zarathustra's liberating will is still itself a prisoner and impotent with respect to the past: "That time does not run backwards, this arouses the will's fury; 'That which was'—that is the stone which it cannot roll away" (Z 2.20). This fury turns into "the spirit of revenge" against all impermanence, which condemns everything in its flux to pass away into an unalterable, petrified past. This spirit affirms that the stone *can* be rolled away, in a resurrection that rises above impermanence and death to a realm of immortality.[30]

But toward the end of this speech, Zarathustra realizes that the *creative* will can say to "that which was," to the past: "But thus I willed it . . . thus do I will it!." Once the will realizes itself as will to power, as a play of constantly self-renewing interpretive forces, it can achieve "something higher than any reconciliation [with the passing of time]" which Zarathustra calls *zurückwollen*. This means that one learns to *will backward*, and thereby to roll away with a different motion the stone that blocks redemption of the past and explode the rock that impedes resurrection of those god-like moments of one's life that appeared to be dead and gone. Then one will also *want the past back* and come to love fate and all the unalterable events that make up one's becoming in the present moment. This is ultimately to will the eternal recurrence of the moment.

Stone plays a central role in Zarathustra's first full presentation of the thought of eternal recurrence, in his account of the "Vision and Riddle." In the previous speech, he prepares himself:

> Before my highest mountain I stand and before my longest wandering: therefore I must first descend deeper than I have ever done before: . . .
>
> Where do the highest mountains come from? I once asked. Then I learned that they come from out of the sea.
>
> The evidence is inscribed in their stone and in the walls of their summits. It is from the deepest that the highest must come to its height. —(*Z* 3.1)

The strata of softer stone bespeak the sea's floor and bear the inscriptions of ancient marine life in the form of fossils, while the layers of granite evidence an igneous extrusion from nearer the earth's core. But then long ago the granite floor curled up like a light leaf from the depths into the highest height, the rock itself taking slow and gradual flight. Correspondingly, Zarathustra must turn to stone, sinking to the deepest layers of the soul before ascending to its peaks.

The passage evokes Goethe's gem of an essay "On Granite" (which Nietzsche surely knew), where the poet-scientist writes of "the ancient discovery that granite is both the highest and the deepest . . . the solid ground of our earth," and of "the serene tranquility afforded by that solitary, mute nearness of great, soft-voiced nature." In contrast to the fertile valleys, the granite peaks "have never generated anything nor devoured anything living: they exist prior to and superior to all life." [31]

In the context of discussing Nietzsche's idea of fate, the Japanese philosopher Keiji Nishitani makes the following comments on this essay of Goethe's:

> Sitting atop a mountain on an outcrop of granite, overlooking a vast vista stretching out from beneath him, Goethe immersed himself in the thought that the vista had undergone numerous changes in the long history of the earth; that the granite on which he was sitting extended down deep into the earth's strata to form the backbone of the earth's crust throughout all its changes and movements. The image illustrates the idea of the self as a fate deep down within our foundations: fate as self—"this is I."[32]

Nishitani connects Goethe's granite essay with a powerful passage on granite in *Beyond Good and Evil*. There Nietzsche takes on the strange and wonderful task of "translating the human being back into nature," in the hope of revealing "the terrifying [and] eternal ground-text of homo natura."[33] The next aphorism describes this natural ground of the human.

> Learning transforms us, it does what all nourishment does that does not merely "preserve"—as the physiologist knows. But in our ground, "deep down inside," there is something unteachable, *some granite of spiritual fate*, of predetermined decision and answer to predetermined selected questions. In every cardinal problem there speaks an unchangeable "this is I": about man and woman for example a thinker cannot relearn but only finish learning—only fully discover what on that topic "stands firm" in him. . . . Later one sees [any solutions] as mere

> steps toward self-knowledge, signposts to the problem that we *are*—or, better, to the colossal stupidity that we are, to our spiritual fate, to what is *unteachable* "deep down inside."

The immediate background to this idea of an immutable foundation to the human psyche is provided by Schopenhauer, who argued that the empirical character is unalterable on the grounds that it is the unfolding of an act of the will, which stands outside time altogether.[34] Nietzsche alludes to this idea in his untimely meditation on Schopenhauer when he writes:

> Your true educators and formative teachers [*Bildner*] reveal to you what the true primal sense and basic material of your being is, something absolutely ineducable and unformable [*unbildbar*], but in any case hard to reach, bonded, lamed: your educators can be nothing other than your liberators. . . . Education is liberation, a clearing away of all weeds, talus, vermin that would touch the tender sprouts of vegetation, outpouring of light and warmth, affectionate downrushing of nighttime rain.[35]

Granite is a fitting image for the very bottom of the soul, for that in us that we cannot change, a fate of which we are innocently unconscious and which we become aware of only slowly and with difficulty, if at all. As the core of our being, which reaches back down through the deepest strata of history, it is the most deeply embodied stratum of our, our innermost incorporation. It is therefore the layer that is the hardest to sculpt, just as granite is far harder to shape than sedimentary rock.

Stone in eternal return

The account of Zarathustra's initial vision of eternal return opens in the ominous atmosphere of "a corpse-coloured twilight."

> A path that climbed defiantly through boulders, malicious, desolate, not graced by weed or shrub: a mountain-path crunched beneath my foot's defiance.
>
> Mutely striding over the mocking clatter of pebbles, trampling the stone that made it slide: thus my foot forced its way upward. (*Z* 3.2, 1)

Zarathustra is working his way up through a field of boulders, with pebbles and stones underfoot. On top of it, he defies the force of gravity by trampling the stone to make his ascent, even though the sliding sometimes sets him back.

> Upward:—in defiance of the spirit that drew it downward, drew it abyssward, the Spirit of Heaviness, my Devil and arch-enemy.
>
> Upward:—although he sat on me, half dwarf, half mole; lame; laming; dripping lead into my ear, lead-drop thoughts into my brain.[36]

In climbing, Zarathustra's foot is defying gravity, the Spirit of Heaviness, imagined as a subhuman dwarf who drips "lead-drop thoughts into his brain." If the weight of this base metal, poisonous in high doses, is not to bring him down and take him under, Zarathustra will have to learn (as Nietzsche said to his friend Overbeck he himself would have to learn) the trick of the alchemist: of turning the base metal of experience into gold by willing its eternal return. But the dwarf mocks this ambitious project, saying to him:

> "O Zarathustra, you Philosophers' Stone, you slingshot-stone, you star-pulverizer! You threw yourself so high—but every upthrown stone—must fall.
>
> "Sentenced to yourself and to your own stoning: O Zarathustra, far indeed you threw the stone—but onto *you* will it come falling back!"

Just as the alchemists strove to transform base metals into gold, the depth-psychologist in Nietzsche has to transform the base dross of experience into something invaluably radiant. The Spirit of Heaviness derides this aspiration by pointing out that the end of all his striving is death: being mortal, his exertions condemn him to his own stoning. The dwarf mocks his titanic pride in his will's ability to explode the rock that blocks redemption of his past, by calling him a star-pulverizer. What is the point of being the slingshot-stone that slays giants if, no matter how often one picks oneself up and projects oneself into the future again, the Spirit of Heaviness always "draws one downward" back to earth, "abyssward" into the underworld of death?

But during the silence that follows, Zarathustra manages to summon the courage to challenge the Spirit of Heaviness to a fight to the death:

> For courage is the best of dead-strikers (*Todtschläger*), courage that attacks: it even strikes death dead, for it says: "Was that life? Well then! One more time!"

Through this idea, which the Spirit of Heaviness is incapable of thinking, the affirmation of the fleeting moment in the prospect of its eternal return, Zarathustra overcomes his arch-enemy. By intimating the thought of eternal return in front of the gateway of the "Moment," he reduces the dwarf to silence and disappearance.

After returning home to the solitude of his cave Zarathustra says, in a speech "On the Spirit of Heaviness," that enmity toward that spirit "makes me of the bird's kind" (Z 3.11, 1). Making the medium appropriate to the topic, he will "sing a song" about his avian enmity, and about how he will overcome the Spirit of Heaviness by learning to fly.

> Whoever one day teaches human beings to fly will have shifted all boundary stones; all boundary stones will themselves fly into the air before him, and the earth itself he will baptize anew as "the Light One."
>
> . . .[As for] the human who cannot yet fly:
>
> Heavy are both earth and life for him; and thus the Spirit of Heaviness *wills* it! But whoever wants to become light and like a bird, he must love himself:—thus *I* teach. (Z 3.11, 2)

This passage intimates the possibility of a self-reorientation with respect to the fundamental forces of the world, in which what gives things their weight is no longer a single force—gravity, or God, or the human intellect—setting all things uniformly in one direction, but rather a dynamic matrix of ever-changing energies. Under such conditions values are easily invertible and perspectives reversible, and the demarcations (boundary stones) between categories are no longer fixed and immutable. These boundaries do not, however, disappear, giving rise to anarchy and indeterminacy; but they fly into the air and become light enough to be easily moved and removed by one who understands the greater patterning of the interconnection of all things.

To combat the Spirit of Heaviness, which makes human life such a burden, one must learn to love oneself—and to do that one must know oneself.

> And verily, this is no commandment for today and tomorrow, to *learn* to love oneself. Rather, of all arts this is the most subtle, cunning, ultimate, and most patient.
>
> For all that is one's own is well hidden from its owner; and of all treasure hoards it is one's own that is excavated last—thus the Spirit of Heaviness brings it about.

Knowing oneself is hard—Zarathustra repeatedly calls the task *schwer*, which also means "heavy"—because the Spirit of Heaviness, working through and as the cultural traditions of (in our case) Platonism and Christianity, endows us with "heavy words and values" such as "good" and "evil," before which those who have the strength will kneel reverentially, "like the camel," in order to assume the weighty burden of tradition.

While such cultural values are necessary for our becoming what we are, they are not only heavy enough to crush creativity in all but the strongest, but also *alien* in relation to the deepest strata of the soul, which are necessities—compacted into the body over many millennia—by comparison with the contingencies of one's contemporary culture. This is why the phase of the camel lands us in the desert, a zone infertile as rock, where no creative growth takes place (*Z* 3.11, 2).

The ancient incorporation of cultural and historical forces has been deformed by too many wrongheaded flights of the spirit, undertaken during the ages when humans had forgotten how to be true to the earth, as Zarathustra explains in his speech "On the Bestowing Virtue."

> In a hundred ways up to now has spirit as well as virtue flown away and made mistakes. Ah, in our bodies all this delusion and mistaking still dwell: body and will it has become there.
>
> In a hundred ways up to now has spirit as well as virtue experimented and gone astray. Yes, the human has been an experiment. Ah, much ignorance and error has become body in us!
>
> Not only the reason of millennia—but also their madness breaks out in us. Dangerous it is to be an heir. (*Z* 1.22, 2)

The task of knowing oneself is made harder by all this ignorance and error and madness at the core of our somatic endowment. Being so deeply incorporated, they cannot be shaken loose by mere intellection but need physical movement to turn them to our advantage.

But the task of loving oneself is made harder still by the difficulty of engaging what is not alien or foreign but most deeply one's own.

> And verily! Much that is one's *own* is a heavy burden too! And much that is within the human being is like an oyster: namely, disgusting and slippery and hard to grasp —
>
> — such that a noble shell with noble decoration must intercede. But this art too must one learn: to *have* a shell and handsome sheen and clever blindness! (Z 3.11, 2)

So hard is it to love what is disgusting in ourselves that we shy away from acknowledging it by masking it from others and ourselves, cultivating a selective blindness to what we are "deep down."

> The human is hard [*schwer*] to discover and its own self hardest of all; often the spirit lies about the soul. Thus the Spirit of Heaviness brings it about.
>
> But he has discovered himself who can say: This is *my* good and evil; with that he has struck dumb the mole and dwarf who says: "Good for all, evil for all."

The Spirit of Heaviness can be overcome only gradually, in stages. First one must sink like a stone, "descend deeper than [one has] ever done before" in order to confront one's basic "colossal stupidity"; then, on that basis, one can learn to move over and rise above it.

> And above all I learned how to stand and walk and run and jump and climb and dance.
>
> But this is my teaching: whoever wants to learn to fly must first learn to stand and walk and run and climb and dance:—one cannot fly into flying!

Near the beginning of his next speech, "On Old and New Tablets" (the old modeled on Mosaic stone), Zarathustra tells of how his "great wing-beating yearning . . . often tore [him] up and out and in the midst of laughing" so that he "flew quivering, an arrow, through sun-drunken rapture":

> — out into far futures that no dream as yet had seen, into hotter souths than artists had ever dreamed of: to where Gods in their dances are ashamed of all clothes . . .
>
> Where I also found my old Devil and arch-enemy again, the Spirit of Heaviness and all that he created: —
>
> For must there not exist that *over* which one dances and dances away? Must there not exist, for the sake of the light and the lightest, moles and heavy dwarves? — (Z 3.12, 2)

The Spirit of Heaviness was right to say that Zarathustra, like the rest of us, is ever "sentenced to his own stoning," since even when he flies into those farther futures and hotter souths he still encounters his arch-enemy, who is always there.

While it is only on the basis of those deepest layers of the soul that one can properly dance—over the realm of the dead—the dance that may lead to flight, this dance is, like play, devoid of any purpose beyond itself. After all, as Zarathustra says: "We should consider any day lost, on which we have not danced once!" (Z 3.12, 23).

And indeed the Third Part of *Zarathustra*, which Nietzsche originally intended as the last of the book, ends with "The Seven Seals (or The Yea- and Amen-Song)" and two sections on the dance and flying. The first celebrates the virtue of the dancer, Zarathustra's "Alpha and Omega," whereby "that all that is heavy becomes light, all body becomes dancer, all spirit becomes bird" (*Z* 3.16, 6).

> If ever I spread tranquil heavens over me and soared with my own wings into my own heavens:
>
> If I swam playfully in deep light-distances, and if to my freedom some bird-wisdom came: —
>
> — but thus bird-wisdom speaks: "See, there is no above, no below! Throw yourself around, and out, and back, you who are light! Sing! speak no more!" (*Z* 3.16, 7)

This is the human spirit liberated by the thought of eternal return, freed finally from the weight of all that is created by the Spirit of Heaviness: "compulsion, statute, need and consequence and purpose and will and good and evil." But this is no transcendent flight of the spirit into a realm beyond heaven and earth, but rather the flight of the bird, which always eventually comes down to earth in order to rest and nest.

The "Fourth and Last Part" of *Zarathustra* begins "as he sat on a rock in front of his cave and quietly looked out—out over the sea, and away over winding abysses" (*Z* 4.1). Then, with his eagle and serpent, Zarathustra climbs a high mountain in order to make the offering of honey, to bait his fishing line to catch the most wondrous human beings he can. For this he must take a firm stand:

> — with both feet I stand securely on this ground,
>
> — on an eternal ground, on hard primeval rock, on this highest hardest primeval mountain-range, to which all winds come as to a weather-divide, asking Where? and Whence? and Whither?

If this affirmation sounds strange, coming as it does from the great anti-foundationalist Zarathustra, we should recall that the rock of the peak is continuous with the "granite of fate" that supports the mountain and sustains the soul, and that Zarathustra can speak like this only because he has already learned to dance and to fly.

At the end of Part Four, Zarathustra returns to his cave. "And once more Zarathustra sank into himself and sat down on the large rock again and meditated." It is thanks to this meditation, seated on his rock, that he is able to speak his final speech and leave his cave, "glowing and strong, like a morning sun coming out of dark mountains" (*Z* 4.20).

* * *

In terms of contemporary therapies, Nietzsche is not advocating anything as literal as the putative healing powers of gemstones and crystals, nor is he counseling regular conversations with our rock collections, insofar as the language that unhewn rocks may speak is no human language. They speak rather "in their own tongues," in the primordial language of nature—which we nonetheless may, with practice, learn to understand at least in part. What he is advocating is that we attend to the images of stone that occur in our dreams and fantasies, and get in touch with "our inner rock." Just as Emerson's experience of living with "carbon, lime & granite" undergirds his talk about "how much firmness the sea-beaten rock has taught the fisherman," so Nietzsche's acknowledgment of the "anorganic minerals" in the human body is at the basis of his idea that we have within us, psychologically, the firmness of stone: indeed not only "some granite of spiritual fate" but also "something that explodes rock."[37] Stone is also emblematic of the "dead nature" that we need to participate in if we are to live a full and fulfilled existence.

Unlike Zarathustra, most of us will not manage to learn to fly, but at least we can dance. A man who knew a thing or two about dancing as well as flying once sang about the power of philosophy in these striking images:

> The power of philosophy—yeah
> floats through my head,
> Light like a feather,
> heavy as lead.[38]

Among the so-called "heavy metals," some (iron and zinc, for example) are necessary to life, whereas others (like lead and mercury) are of no benefit to the living—and in sufficient quantities are even deadly. Recall Zarathustra's characterization of the Spirit of Heaviness as "half dwarf, half mole; lame; laming; dripping lead into my ear, lead-drop thoughts into my brain" (Z 3.2, 1). It is fitting, then, that the dance should draw from that vitality in the body which is "light like a feather" to counteract that death-related element which is closest to the densest stone, "heavy as lead."

Notes

1 An earlier version of this chapter appeared under the title "Nietzsche on Rock and Stone: The Dead World, Dance and Flight," *International Journal of Philosophical Studies* 21/1 (2013): 20–40. Permission to reuse some of this essay here is gratefully acknowledged. Translations of passages from Nietzsche's works are my own, from the Colli & Montinari critical editions, since the extant English versions fail to capture some of the nuances necessary for the argument—with the exception of *Thus Spoke Zarathustra*, trans. Graham Parkes (Oxford: Oxford World's Classics, 2005).

2 See my essay "Staying Loyal to the Earth: Nietzsche as an Ecological Thinker," in John Lippitt, (ed.), *Nietzsche's Futures* (Basingstoke: Macmillan, 1998), pp. 167–88.

3 For an overview of the role of unhewn rock in the development of the classical Chinese garden, see my essay "Thinking Rocks, Living Stones: Reflections on Chinese Lithophilia," *Diogenes* 52/4 (2005): 75–87; and for the Japanese tradition, "The Role of Rock in the Japanese Dry Landscape Garden: A Philosophical Essay," in François Berthier (ed.), *Reading Zen in the Rocks: The Japanese Dry Landscape Garden* (Chicago: University of Chicago Press, 2000), pp. 85–155. The parallels with Nietzsche's understanding of stone are remarkable, though it is not possible to draw

them here. For a comparison of Nietzsche's ideas with Emerson's, see my "Floods of Life around Granite of Fate: Nietzsche and Emerson as Thinkers of Nature," *ESQ: A Journal of the American Renaissance* 43 (1997): 207–40.

4 Nietzsche, *KGW* I,1: p. 6.
5 Nietzsche, "From My Life," *KGW* I,1: p. 288.
6 Nietzsche, *KSA* 8: 41[21], 1879; 11[11], 28[6], 1878.
7 Nietzsche, *Assorted Opinions and Maxims*, aphorism 49.
8 Nietzsche, "From My Life," *KGW* I,1: p. 283; "The Course of My Life," *KGW* I,2: p. 259; "My Life," *KGW* 1,3: pp. 89–91.
9 Nietzsche, "The Course of My Life," *KGW* I,2: p. 256.
10 Schopenhauer, *The World as Will and Representation*, vol. 1, § 21; see also §§ 22 and 23.
11 Nietzsche, *KSA* 1:715–16.
12 Emerson, *The Journals of Ralph Waldo Emerson* (New York: Houghton Mifflin, 1914), 5:496–67.
13 Nietzsche, *KSA* 9: 11[125], 1881; 9: 11[207], 1881.
14 Nietzsche, *Dawn of Morning*, aph. 541.
15 Ralph Waldo Emerson, "Goethe," *Ralph Waldo Emerson: Essays & Lectures* (New York: The Library of America, 1983), p. 746.
16 Emerson, "Fate," in *Essays & Lectures*, p. 949.
17 Emerson, 'Fate', pp. 951–52.
18 Schiller, "Ode to Joy," lines 9–10, 73–4.
19 Nietzsche, *KSA* 7: 176.
20 Nietzsche, *The Birth of Tragedy*, § 1.
21 Nietzsche, *KSA* 9: 7 [213], 1880.
22 Emerson, "Fate," p. 953.
23 Nietzsche, *Beyond Good and Evil*, aph. 225.
24 Nietzsche, *The Wanderer and His Shadow*, aph. 201.
25 Nietzsche, *The Gay Science*, aph. 356.
26 Nietzsche, *Ecce Homo*, "Why I Write Such Good Books," *Thus Spoke Zarathustra*, §1.
27 Nietzsche, *The Gay Science*, aph. 109.
28 Nietzsche, *Thus Spoke Zarathustra*, 2.12; *Beyond Good and Evil*, aph. 36.
29 Compare *Matthew* 27:51-3: "And the earth did quake, and the rocks rent; and the graves were opened; and many bodies of the saints which slept arose, and came out of the graves after his resurrection."
30 See *Luke* 24:2, where after the Resurrection the women "found the stone rolled away from the sepulcher."
31 Goethe, "On Granite," in *Goethe: Collected Works*, vol. 12, (Princeton: Princeton University Press, 1988), pp. 131–34.
32 Nishitani, *The Self-Overcoming of Nihilism,* trans. Graham Parkes with Setsuko Aihara (Albany, NY: SUNY Press, 1990), pp. 91–2.
33 Nietzsche, *Beyond Good and Evil*, aph. 230.
34 Schopenhauer, *The World as Will and Representation*, especially vol. 1, § 55.
35 Nietzsche, "Schopenhauer as Educator," § 1. The word translated by "talus," *Schuttwerk*, carries a connotation of boulders, scree, or rock-fragments.
36 There is a parallel between Zarathustra's encounter with the dwarf and Siegfried's encounter with the dwarf Mime in Wagner's *Ring*.
37 Emerson, *Nature*, ch. 5, "Discipline."
38 Bob Marley and the Wailers, "Misty Morning," *Kaya* (1978), 1:00–1:24.

14

Nietzsche on Consciousness and Language[1]

Lawrence J. Hatab

What can be said about the kind of beings we are, about our "selves?" Nietzsche's thinking on human selfhood is enormously complicated. With his philosophy of radical becoming, any talk of a "self" has to confront the ambiguities of an ungrounded phenomenon, which cannot be grasped as a "kind." Selfhood, for Nietzsche, is always emergent within a dynamic of life forces that will disallow any impulse toward "identity." Nietzsche therefore rejects the modern model of an individual, unified, substantive, autonomous self. Selfhood cannot involve an enduring substance or a unified subject that grounds attributes, that stands "behind" activities as a causal source (*BGE* 19–21). There is no substantive self behind or even distinct from performance: "There is no 'being' behind doing, effecting, becoming; 'the doer' is merely a fiction added to the deed—the deed is everything" (*GM* I, 13; *KSA* 5, 279).

More than anything it is language that subsidizes these mistaken models of selfhood. Human experience and thinking are decentered processes, but the "grammatical habit" of using subjects and predicates, nouns, and verbs, tricks us into assigning an "I" as the source of thinking (*BGE* 17; *KSA* 5, 31). Human experience is much too fluid and complicated to be reducible to linguistic units (*BGE* 19), and the vaunted philosophical categories of "subject," "ego," and "consciousness" are nothing more than linguistic fictions that cover up the dynamics of experience and that in fact are created to protect us from the precariousness of an ungrounded process. Such a protection-project is the source of human "illness," for Nietzsche, namely, the incapacity to accept the finitude of natural life.

Selfhood, for Nietzsche, is also not a stable unity, but an arena for an irresolvable contest of differing drives, each seeking mastery (*BGE* 6, 36). There is no single subject, but rather a "multiplicity of subjects, whose interplay and struggle is the basis of our thought and our consciousness" (*WP* 490; *KSA* 11, 650). Nietzsche's agonistic psychology does not suggest that the self is an utter chaos. He does allow for a shaping of the self, but this requires a difficult and demanding procedure of counter-cropping the drives so that a certain mastery can be achieved. This is one reason why Nietzsche thinks that the modern promotion of universal freedom is careless and even dangerous (*TI* Skirmishes, 41). Contrary to modern optimism about the rational pursuit of happiness, Nietzsche sees the natural and social field of play as much more precarious and taxing. So according to Nietzsche (and this is missed in many interpretations) freedom and creative self-development are not for everyone: "Independence is for the very few; it is a privilege of the strong" (*BGE* 29; *KSA* 5, 47). Simply being unconstrained is not an appropriate mark of freedom; being free should only serve the pursuit of great achievement, a pursuit that most people cannot endure (*Z* I, Creator).

That the majority of human beings are bound by rules and are not free to cut their own path is not regretted by Nietzsche. The "exception" and the "rule" are *both* important for human culture, and neither one should be universalized. Although exceptional types further the species, we should not forget the importance of the rule in *preserving* the species (*GS* 55). The exception as such can never become the rule, can never be a model for all humanity (*GS* 76). Absent this provision, Nietzsche's promotion of "creative individuals" is easily misunderstood. The freedom from constraints is restricted to those who are strong enough for, and capable of, high cultural production. "My philosophy aims at an ordering of rank: not at an individualistic morality. The ideas of the herd should rule in the herd—but not reach out beyond it" (*WP* 287; *KSA* 12, 280).

Nietzsche (before Freud, and borrowing from Schopenhauer) also dismisses the centrality of consciousness and the longstanding assumption that the conscious mind defines our identity and represents our highest nature in its capacity to control instinctive drives. According to Nietzsche, consciousness is a very late development of the human organism and therefore it is not preeminently strong or effective (*GS* 11). In GS 354 (*KSA* 3, 590–93), Nietzsche says that if we consider ourselves as animals, we should be suspicious of the claim that consciousness is necessary for our operations.

> The problem of consciousness (more precisely, of becoming conscious of something) confronts us only when we begin to comprehend how we could dispense with it; and now physiology and the history of animals place us at the beginning of such comprehension. . . . we could think, feel, will, and remember, and we could also "act" in every sense of that word, and yet none of all this would have to "enter our consciousness" (as one says metaphorically). The whole of life would be possible without, as it were, seeing itself in a mirror. For even now, for that matter, by far the greatest portion of our life actually takes place without this mirror effect; and this is true even of our thinking, feeling, and willing life, however offensive this may sound to older philosophers. (*GS* 354)

I must note here that by "consciousness," Nietzsche could not mean simple "awareness" but rather self-consciousness, a reflective "mirror." Accordingly, nonconsciousness would not exclusively mean "unconsciousness" but also nonreflective activity, since he includes *thinking* in what can operate without (self-)consciousness. In addition, consciousness is not the opposite of instinct, but rather an epiphenomenal *expression* of instincts; even the reflective thinking of a philosopher "is secretly guided and forced into certain channels by his instincts" (*BGE* 3; *KSA* 5, 17).

Since consciousness seems to arise in *internal* self-reflection, the emphasis on consciousness has been coordinated with atomic individualism, the idea that human beings are discrete individuals and that social relations are secondary to the self-relationship of consciousness. For Nietzsche, however, the notion of an atomic individual is an error (*TI* Skirmishes, 33; *BGE* 12). "Individuality" is not an eternal property, but a historical, emergent development (*GS* 117). In this respect, *GS* 354 offers the surprising notion that consciousness itself is a social and linguistic construction. Nietzsche's argument is that consciousness is a function of language, and with language understood as *communicative* practice, a *common* apprehension of signs goes all the way down.

> Consciousness is really only a net of communication (*Verbindungsnetz*) between human beings; it is only as such that it had to develop; a solitary human being who lived like a beast of prey would not have needed it. That our actions, thoughts, feelings, and movements enter our own consciousness—at least a part of them—that is the result of a "must" that for a terribly long time lorded it over man. As the most endangered animal, he *needed* help and protection, he needed his peers, he had to learn to express his distress and to make himself understood; and for all of this he needed "consciousness" first of all, he needed "know" himself what distressed him, he needed to "know" how he felt, he needed to "know" what he thought. For, to say it once more: Man, like every living being, thinks continually without knowing it; the thinking that rises to *consciousness* is only the smallest part of all this—the most superficial and worst part—for only his conscious thinking *takes the form of words, which is to say signs of communication*, and this fact uncovers the origin of consciousness.
>
> In brief, the development of language and the development of consciousness . . . go hand in hand. . . . The emergence of our sense impressions into our consciousness, the ability to fix them and, as it were, exhibit them externally, increased proportionately with the need to communicate them to *others* by means of signs. The human being inventing signs is at the same time the human being who becomes ever more keenly conscious of himself. It was only as a social animal that man acquired self-consciousness. (*GS* 354)[2]

If Nietzsche is right, then even *self*-consciousness, perceived as a kind of internal representation or dialogue, is a function of social relations and the commerce of common signs. Accordingly, even "self-knowledge" (a crucial ingredient in traditional philosophical methods) is in fact only a function of the internalization of sociolinguistic signs that operate by fixing experience into stable and common forms. What is truly "individual," then, is *not* indicated even in self-reflection, because the *instruments* of reflection are constituted by the *omission* of what is unique in experience.

> . . . given the best will in the world to understand ourselves as individually as possible, "to know ourselves," each of us will always succeed in becoming conscious only of what is not individual but "average."
>
> . . . Fundamentally, all our actions are altogether incomparably personal, unique, and infinitely individual; there is no doubt of that. But as soon as we translate them into consciousness *they no longer seem to be*. (*GS* 354)

For Nietzsche, "individualism" is disrupted by the fact that most of what we recognize as human is a *social* phenomenon; at the same time, we cannot ultimately *reduce* human life to conscious linguistic and conceptual categories, even when such structures have been appropriated by individuals in their own self-regard, because there is an element of nonconscious experience that eludes these structures.

Before moving on with questions stemming from this analysis, I want to interject that something like Nietzsche's account of consciousness and language can be backed up by findings in developmental psychology. The notion of "inner speech" or "private speech"—meaning self-directed verbalization—can account for *how* language is implicated in self-consciousness. Research shows that inner speech is the most important factor in the development of self-awareness, the capacity to become the object of one's own attention, one's own thoughts and behaviors.[3] Such a process occurs originally in children but in adults as well (2). Fully immersed experience is not self-conscious. A kind of "distance" between the observer and the observed is required for the self-awareness *of* observation. Inner speech provides this kind of distance (7). It is important to stress that such a development is derived from the original *social* milieu of language, so that self-awareness arises from the *reproduction* of social mechanisms by way of self-directed language (5). The case of Helen Keller is instructive because she claimed that consciousness first existed for her only after she gained access to language (9). There is also neurophysiological evidence mapping the processes here described (8ff).

Private speech in young children (talking to oneself in task performance) has often been met with concern by parents; and Piaget had taken it to be a stage of egocentrism. But L. S. Vygotsky initiated the dismissal of this scheme by arguing that private speech is essential for the cognitive and behavioral development of the child, because here the child takes over the regulative role of the social world.[4] Language begins as collaborative tasking and conversation; private speech is a redirection of this milieu toward independent functioning. Cognitive and behavioral capacities begin in a social-linguistic network, and private speech begins a process that over time leads to the *internalization* of these capacities that now can operate "silently," as it were (61, 77).

In sum, mature development, individuation, and self-consciousness are the result of an internalization of the social-linguistic environment, mediated by inner or private speech. Such research lends credence to Nietzsche's analysis, although the language-consciousness conjunction in his account raises more radical philosophical interrogation about the very nature of human selfhood and the meaning of individuation.

It should also be noted that the word "conscious" had an early meaning of sharing knowledge with another person (see the *OED*), hence the phrase "conscious to . . ." The same sense could apply to inner awareness as witnessing one's own thoughts, as in the phrase "conscious to oneself" (thus borrowed from the social structure of consciousness). The word "conscious" is derived from the Latin *conscientia*, meaning "knowing together," which could refer either to shared knowledge or the joining together of different thoughts in the mind or to self-awareness. Such meanings of *conscientia* were deployed by Descartes.[5] The German *Bewusstsein* and *Gewissen* bear a relation with knowledge, and *Bewusstsein* was originally associated with *conscientia*.[6]

A number of questions arise in considering Nietzsche's thesis concerning language and consciousness. How far does Nietzsche take the conjunction of self-consciousness and socially based language? Is selfhood nothing more than a linguistic-communal phenomenon? Is language nothing more than a network of common signs that averages out experience? Given Nietzsche's endorsement of creative types, and thus creative language, would this have to be distinguishable from the language-consciousness conjunction to render creative departures from the norm genuinely possible?

The issue of consciousness, language, and selfhood is a focused version of a central theme in Nietzsche's philosophy: that knowledge and other modes of formation run up against the limit of radical becoming; also that knowledge stems from the "fixing" effects of language and grammar. For instance:

> Our usual imprecise mode of observation takes a group of phenomena as one and calls it a fact: between this fact and another fact it imagines in addition an empty space, it *isolates* every fact. In reality, however, all our doing and knowing is not a succession of facts and empty spaces but a continuous flux. . . . The word and the concept are the most manifest ground for our belief in this isolation of groups of actions. (*WS* 11; *KSA* 2, 546–47)

GS 354 adds the matter of selfhood and startles us by seeming to deny individual self-awareness a privileged status. What is truly "individual" is not any kind of accessible "self." Both knowledge and self-consciousness appear to be "errors"—instigated by language—when measured against life forces that exceed formation. In *GS* 355, right after the section on the communal function of language, Nietzsche claims that knowledge originates in reducing the unfamiliar to the familiar, a reduction based on *fear* of the strangeness of experience. Yet Nietzsche often insists that "errors" such as these are necessary for human functioning and survival. Indeed, identifying such errors is not on that account an objection (*BGE* 4). In *BGE* 268 (*KSA* 5, 222), Nietzsche calls the communal character of words "the most powerful of all powers" because of its life-serving value. Even further, in *WP* 522 (*KSA* 12, 193–94), after outlining the prejudices of language, Nietzsche adds: "we think *only* in the form of language. . . . we cease to think when we refuse to do so under the constraint of language." The linguistic order of thinking is "a scheme that we cannot throw off." A comparable claim is given in a published work: "we have at any moment only the thought for which we have the words at hand" (*D* 257; *KSA* 3, 208).

Remarks such as these make it hard to read the "errors" in question as fitting any familiar sense of falsehood, especially if one cannot even *think* outside of such errors, and if the fluid excess of becoming cannot really count as a "measure" for any kind of discernible truth. Of course this is an enduring question in Nietzsche studies, which I will not address here. I do take my bearings, however, from *Twilight of the Idols* (Reason, 5), where Nietzsche admits that once the traditional measure of "reality" is rejected, it does not make sense to talk of an "apparent world," of mere appearance, because there is nothing "real" in comparison. An 1881 *Nachlass* passage is relevant (*KSA* 9, 500ff.). There Nietzsche distinguishes between three degrees of "error" in relation to an eternal flux: "the crude error of the species, the subtler error of the individual, and the subtlest error of the creative moment (*Augenblick*)." Species-form is the crudest error because it corrals differences into a common universal. The assertion of the individual is a "more refined error" that comes later, rebelling against commonality in favor of unique forms.

But then the individual learns that it itself is constantly changing and that "in the smallest twinkling of the eye (*im kleinsten Augenblick*) it is something other than it is in the next [moment]." The creative moment, "the *infinitely small moment* is the higher reality and truth, a lightning image out of the eternal flow." The "higher reality and truth" of the creative moment is thus an "error" in a quite different sense compared to the species-error, which seems also to be the case with the error of the individual. Even the notorious fragment "On Truth and Lie in an Extra-Moral Sense"—the supposed source of Nietzsche's critique of truth as an erroneous superimposition of form onto flux—shows some leeway. The metaphorical transfer of fluid experience to fixed words and concepts is actually preceded by original "intuited metaphors" and "images" that are closer to the flux of experience by being singular, unique apprehensions; and such preconceptual apprehension is then associated with an artistic imagination that does not fall into the trap of fixed words and concepts (*KSA* 1, 875–90).

With respect to individual selfhood, in the light of *GS* 354, it is hard to fathom how "individuality" is thinkable. What I would want to say is that individuality here is not "graspable," but perhaps thinkable as a negative trace, as something *relative* to consciousness and language in terms of what is *not* discernible in words and self-awareness. I cannot fully develop this idea here, but its sense might emerge in considering the next question: How is creativity thinkable in the light of *GS* 354 and the communal function of language?

GS 354 contains the following aside: Nietzsche says that after a long duration of the communicative practices of language, "the ultimate result is an excess of this strength and art of communication—as it were, a capacity that has gradually been accumulated and now waits for an heir who might squander it." He then includes artists and writers as among such heirs and squanderers. This remark makes room for creative language, and the idea of squandering may fit claims Nietzsche sometimes makes about artistic creativity being a nonvoluntary compulsion arising from an overflowing surplus of energy (e.g., *BGE* 213, *Z* I, Gift). Yet the question remains: How can language be truly creative if it is seemingly bound by common forms and effects? The question turns on what Nietzsche means by creativity.

We have noted that for Nietzsche the existence of the norm is essential for the maintenance of human culture, but in another sense he insists that it is necessary for, and intrinsic to, creativity itself. The freedom of the creative type does not do away with structures and constraint. Creativity breaks the hold of existing structures in order to shape new ones (see *WS* 122). Creativity is a complicated relationship between openness and form. Certain "fetters" (*Fesseln*) are required (1) to prepare cultural overcomings of purely natural states (*HAH* I, 221), and (2) to provide a comprehensible shape to new cultural forms (*WS* 140; *KSA* 2, 612). Creative freedom, therefore, is not the opposite of normalization, discipline, or constraint; it is a disruption of structure that yet needs structure to both prepare and consummate departures from the norm (see *GS* 295 and *BGE* 188). For Nietzsche, creativity is a kind of "dancing in chains" (*WS* 140). For this reason, even a creative "self" does not have a strict identity contrasted with "normal" selves.

In *WP* 767 (*KSA* 10, 663), Nietzsche suggests that creativity is an individual *interpretation* of inherited schemes of language. Yet even more, and surprisingly, in *WS* 122 and 127, Nietzsche expresses admiration for Greek poetry's deployment of conventions, and he questions "the modern rage for originality." And in *WP* 809 (*KSA* 296–97), he talks of the aesthetic state as "the source of languages" and as a "superabundance of means of communication," and "the high point of communication and transmission between living creatures." Furthermore, "every mature art has a host of conventions as its basis—insofar as it is a language. Convention is the condition of great art, *not* an obstacle." I find this perfectly right, and it should temper certain overheated accounts of Nietzschean transgression. Finally, listen to *GS* 173 (*KSA* 3, 500): "Those who know they are profound strive for clarity. Those who would like to seem profound to the crowd strive for obscurity."

Creative language, therefore, is not the opposite of common meanings and communication, although it will disrupt and alter ordinary familiarity, and it will likely not have a universal audience, but an audience nonetheless. At the same time, since the original fuel for creativity is not the conscious self but a dynamic of subliminal, sublinguistic drives and instincts, then the idea of a "creative individual" can be understood only in a performative sense, in the contrasting effects of innovation compared to established patterns. This is why Nietzsche calls the free spirit a "relative concept," rather than some discrete identity (*HAH* 225; *KSA* 2, 189). Although *GS* 354 seems to render individuality *in cognito*, inaccessible to self-awareness and language, we need not polarize this rendition into an unspeakable uniqueness on the one hand and communal speech on the other. Cultural creativity must manifest itself in communicative language and its "uniqueness" is both drawn from subliminal drives and indicated in its effects relative to normalcy. Moreover, the performative and relative character of the creative individual would be consonant with Nietzsche's insistence that there is no "doer" behind the deed, that the deed is all there is (*GM* I, 13).[7]

The idea that creativity cannot be based in individual consciousness is something expressed often in Nietzsche's work, and I want to offer some remarks on how we can read him on this score. *WP* 289 (*KSA* 13, 310) offers the stark claim that "all perfect acts are unconscious." And in *BGE* 17 (*KSA* 5, 31), we are told that "a thought comes when 'it' wishes, and not when 'I' wish." Returning to a point made earlier in this chapter, the word "unconscious" cannot be coextensive with sheer unawareness. I think there are two senses of "unconscious" operating in Nietzsche's analysis, a *depth* sense and a *surface* sense. The depth sense refers to instinctive drives and life forces that are not available to awareness; the surface sense refers to spontaneous, nonreflective activity, behavior, and cultural functions. On spontaneous, nonreflective action, consider these passages from *The Wanderer and His Shadow*:

> *Closing the eyes of one's mind.* – Even if one is accustomed to and practiced in reflecting on one's actions, when one is actually acting (though the action be no more than writing a letter or eating and drinking) one must nonetheless close one's inward eye. (*WS* 236; *KSA* 2, 659)
>
> For as long as one is experiencing something one must give oneself up to the experience and close one's eyes: that is to say, not be an observer of it while still *in the midst* of it. For that would disturb the absorption of the experience. (*WS* 297; *KSA* 2, 687)

Recall that Nietzsche includes even thinking among activities that can operate spontaneously, without being "mirrored" in consciousness. If Nietzsche holds that thinking is grounded in language, then we can also talk of nonreflective language as well. This would help us understand various occasions in his texts where Nietzsche talks about an *immediacy* in artistic language or thought processes, in other words, a direct disclosure not only without reflection but without *any* intercession beyond its self-presentation.[8] I will mention a few instances without detailed discussion, simply to put this matter on the table for consideration.

In *The Birth of Tragedy*, Nietzsche describes the immediate disclosive effects of tragic poetry on the audience, which is so direct as to not even be "symbolic" or "fictional" (see *BT* 7, 8, 21). The problem with Euripides was that he aligned with Socrates in bringing the critical "spectator" on stage, especially by way of his Prologues (*BT* 11). Modern audiences have been corrupted by such critical distance from drama's capacity to "enrapture the genuine listener" (*BT* 22; *KSA* 1, 140–44). In certain later discussions, Nietzsche reiterates this sense of poetic immediacy. The discussion of poetic convention in *WS* 122 (*KSA* 2, 604) includes the motivation of poets to be "understood immediately," because of the competitive, public conditions of oral performance. In *WP* 811 (*KSA* 13, 356–57), artists are described as intoxicated with an overwhelming force of extreme sensuous acuity, which produces a "contagious" compulsion to discharge images that are "immediately enacted" in bodily energies: "An image, rising up within, immediately turns into a movement of the limbs." *GS* 84 likewise discusses the origin of poetry in discharges of rhythmic force that compel both body and soul toward disclosive effects. And in *EH*, Nietzsche tells of how *Zarathustra* and eternal recurrence "came to" him in August 1881, as a quasi-prophetic inspiration that "invaded" and "overtook" him, an involuntary necessity that made him feel like a mere "mouthpiece," and where image, parable, and reality seemed indistinguishable (*EH* Books, TSZ, 1; *KSA* 6, 335–37).

A certain immediacy of experience is something that Nietzsche frequently celebrates to counter the primacy of self-consciousness in modern philosophy, and self-consciousness is the domain of reflection, of "this entirely dismal thing called reflection" (*GM* II, 3; *KSA* 5, 297). Reflection is "dismal" because it displaces what Nietzsche thinks are the healthy, instinctive, and spontaneous energies in life. In GM I, 10, noble behavior is described as spontaneous, which is one reason why nobles are less "clever" than slaves. Yet we cannot say that Nietzsche utterly dismisses reflection. Philosophy is impossible without some degree of reflection, and Nietzsche considered himself to be a philosopher. We could say that among the motivations behind his nontraditional writing styles and the elusive character of his thinking, one key element stands out: Philosophy has typically aimed for reflective criteria to *govern* experience and thought. Nietzsche advances the essentially ambiguous task of reflecting upon that which precedes and always eludes reflection, and which is always already driving things, even reflection itself—in a word, *life*.[9] If this makes sense, we might hear more pointedly the perplexing opening line of the *Genealogy*: "We are unknown to ourselves, we knowers, even to ourselves, and with good reason" (*GM* P, 1; *KSA* 5, 247). Nietzsche's thought is sometimes described as fitting the classification "philosophy of life," which sounds right. Yet Nietzsche seems unique in recognizing and sustaining the fundamental enigma in thinking about life. A philosopher, as a living being, is something like a dog chasing its own tail. Nietzsche's communicative practices aim to talk us out of "selfhood," if that names a "what" behind our always already *becoming* what we are (paraphrasing *GS* 270). In this light, another puzzling remark in *EH* might make more sense: "To become what one is, presupposes that one not have the faintest notion *what* one is" (*EH* Clever, 9; *KSA* 6, 293). Nietzsche's diagnosis of human "illness" is based on our false ascriptions of fixed states, which only magnify our dissatisfactions with life when conditions of becoming alter our lives. The therapy for this illness involves a willingness to surrender fixations and affirm the fluidity of life.

* * *

I will close with some reflections on the matter of language in Nietzsche's thought and how it might apply to the question of rhetoric. I suspect that the notion of style can be connected with the limits of conscious language. In *EH* Books, 4 (*KSA* 6, 304), Nietzsche calls (good) style "the actual communication of an inner state," which effectively enacts signs, tempo, rhythm, and gesture (which was mentioned in *GS* 354 as part of language) to render an inner state accessible to an audience (even if a selective one). Can "inner state" here refer to that which escapes the "common signs" of language in *GS* 354? If language is not to be utterly separated from prelinguistic experience, style can refer to the "sub-verbal" elements of language that even point back to how language as such emerged out of embodied forces in human experience. Such subverbal elements can be located in Nietzsche's accounts of language in relation to gesture and music.

In *HAH* 216, Nietzsche claims that language originated in gestures and facial expressions, together with the automatic, immediate imitation of these phenomena in face to face experience, which is natural in adults as well as children (called "motor mimicry" in modern psychology). Such was a direct communication of shared meanings (such as pleasure and pain). From such common comprehension, Nietzsche says, a "symbolism" of gestures could arise, with verbal sounds first coupled with the gestures, and then after familiarity operable by way of the sound symbols alone. We can understand the sense of this in how much gestures and facial expressions play an important role in face to face speech.

Nietzsche occasionally discusses what can be called mimetic psychology, especially in his reflections on Greek art. An early essay, "Greek Music Drama," mentions the audience's sympathetic identification with the sufferings of tragic heroes (*KSA* 1, 528). And *The Birth of Tragedy* contains several relevant treatments. Apollonian and Dionysian forces are exhibited in nature herself, *before* the mediation of artistic works (*BT* 2). Forming and deforming powers are intrinsic to nature's very course, and dreams and intoxicated states (both of which exceed conscious control) are preconditions for the more cultivated manifestation of Apollonian and Dionysian powers, particularly those of language and music. Artists are said to "imitate" such primal natural energies, which could not mean representational simulation, but rather the more performative sense of "impersonating" these energies in artistic practices (impersonation being one of the meanings of *mimēsis* in Greek). Indeed, nature itself urges expression in bodily gestures and movements (*BT* 21). Singing and dancing then exhibit an enchanted, ecstatic elevation, a quasi-divine transformation where one is not really an artist because one "has become a work of art" (*BT* 1; *KSA* 1, 25–30).

In many respects, Nietzsche associates the Dionysian with music (*BT* 6, 17), especially its immediate emotional force that "overwhelms" conscious individuation. The Apollonian is associated with poetic language and theatrical technologies that shape a more individuated world. But since music and language are coordinated in tragic drama (*BT* 21), immediate disclosive force still operates in its performances. Poetic metaphors are not "symbolic," they possess a living power to disclose (*BT* 8). For Greek audiences, dramatic fiction was not a departure from reality, it produced on stage powerful scenes of "a world with the same reality and irreducibility that Olympus with its inhabitants possessed for the believing Hellene" (*BT* 7; *KSA* 1, 52–7). Tragic drama produced a Dionysian effect of mimetic identification, originally embodied in choral impersonation, where one acts "as if one had actually entered into another body, another character" (*BT* 8; *KSA* 1, 57–64).

In general terms, Nietzsche considers music to be equiprimordial with gesture as a foundation for language, particularly in terms of how a speaker's *tone* accompanies gesture symbolism. Rhythm and pitch intonations, according to Nietzsche, provide an additional common field of comprehension that renders the communicative power of language possible.[10] This is one reason why the Dionysian was essential for Greek tragedy in Nietzsche's eyes, because the "universal" element behind Apollonian language could be presented through the combination of music, gesture, and dancing that embodied the poetic performance.[11] We could say that Nietzsche's answer to the question of how language could express something beyond its arbitrary phonic forms (given the differences in words across different languages) would not be in terms of universal cognitive conditions, but universal corporeal conditions of gesture and musicality. And his reasons for restricting language to a certain fictional status would follow from our tendency to separate distinct words from (1) the flux of experience and (2) the embodied forces behind verbal speech. Yet it seems that the first tendency is the more apt target because the corporeality of language in gesture and tone is said by Nietzsche to make language possible and it is not hard to intimate its indigenous function in embodied speech.

In any case, it is well known that Nietzsche rejects any realist or representational model of language, since he takes language to be a creative forming of an unstable flux and an expression that cannot function independently of metaphorical, rhetorical, and imaginative forces. The fragment "On Truth and Lies in an Extramoral Sense" (*KSA* 1, 875–90) presents Nietzsche's classic account of such forces that preclude any pretense of objective truth. Human thought cannot provide straightforward representations of things in the world, because from the start thinking is infused with rhetorical elements of language (e.g., metaphor and metonymy) that are not objective matters, even though we assume as much out of psychological need. Nietzsche's early lecture courses on rhetoric provide an extensive and detailed analysis of ancient discourse that sets the background for his provocative critique of truth.[12] We recall that the passage from *WS* 11 counter-posed flux to our assumption of isolated facts surrounded by empty space, an assumption grounded in the presence of words. It should be clear, however, that *written* words best satisfy this condition as fixed in visual space, rather than the temporal flow of oral speech. Moreover, the embodied elements of language we have considered are also best indicated in face-to-face oral speech rather than the detached objects of graphic signs. Nietzsche advances this very distinction in his rhetoric course. Against the idea that ancient rhetoric appears unnatural and ornamental, Nietzsche claims that rhetoric was the natural condition for the oral context of ancient discourse.

> . . . the true prose of antiquity is an echo of public *speech* and is built on its laws, whereas our prose is always to be explained more from *writing*, and our style presents itself as something to be perceived through *reading*. One who reads and one who hears desire wholly different presentational forms. (21)

In *WS* 110 (*KSA* 2, 600), Nietzsche points to what is missing in written language, "the modes of expression available only to the speaker: that is to say, gestures, emphases, tones of voice, glances." In the rhetoric course, Nietzsche also discusses the agonistic element in ancient speech, the competitive forces that combined persuasive power with outdoing other speakers in style, beauty, and flourish (37). This raises a topic too big to engage here, but the transition from orality to literacy in the Greek world was one of the prime factors in the advent of philosophy; and the absorbing *power* of oral speech and poetry was one of the key targets in philosophical culture critique, most prominently in Plato.[13] Our discussion of language can at least provide an important angle on why Nietzsche's emphasis on embodied, oral speech goes hand in hand with his critique of traditional philosophy, and why a defense of rhetoric against traditional complaints can emerge out of Nietzsche's reflections.

For Nietzsche, philosophy never operates on purely cognitive grounds, as though separable from rhetorical elements of persuasion, emotional appeal, even seduction. Plato's critique of the Sophists and rhetoric concerned both philosophical and political spheres, and much of political theory has inherited a Platonic suspicion of rhetorical forces in political practice and discourse. Nietzsche insists that a strict distinction between reason and passion is untenable, that a crossing effect shows that cognition has its passion and passion its cognition (*WP* 387; *KSA* 13, 131)—in other words, that instinctive intimations and passionate responses can have disclosive power. How can we be sure that the infamous propensity for "image over substance" in politics generates only defective results? Might there be something important in so-called noncognitive dimensions of political engagement?

In Nietzschean terms, I think we can say that rhetorical force is a necessary condition for political discourse (with rhetoric understood as the psychological, rather than logical, force of language). Plato's attack on the Sophists went hand in hand with his critique of democracy—the undisciplined, open condition of all citizens having a say in political judgment. In democracy, political decisions have no ground other than audience persuasion, and in this respect, the Sophists can be seen as realistic educators in democratic practice. This is not the place to rehearse my work on trying to think democracy through a Nietzschean lens.[14] Yet a mark of this work has been the application of a Nietzschean suspicion against moralistic complaints about democratic practice, even among democratic theorists. Nietzsche considered the Sophists to be political realists, and he claimed that "it was their honor not to indulge in any swindle of big words and virtues" (*WP* 429; *KSA* 13, 331–32). The Sophists in his eyes were thoroughly Greek in their emphasis on the powers of speech in competitive formats, at the expense of secured measures of value independent of rhetorical effect (see *WP* 427–28; *KSA* 13, 167–69, 291–93). In this respect, Plato's opposition to the Sophists was anti-Hellenic in Nietzsche's estimation (see *TI* Ancients, 2).

Platonic "idealism" opposed the Sophists' relativism, skepticism, pragmatism, and their willingness to engage in expedient political machinations. Plato's model of perfect virtue and justice untarnished by practical interests and power became a lasting measure for assigning many political dispositions and methods to the category of vice (e.g., expediency, ambition, aggressiveness, power plays, and rhetorical techniques to win over an audience). My contention is that much of the charge of "immorality" against democratic political practices (issued by opponents and proponents alike) is susceptible to a Nietzschean diagnosis of political "asceticism," an aversion to the natural conditions of political life. The forces of rhetoric are a significant focus of this problem. Nietzsche's emphasis on agonistic, embodied, passion-laden speech permits a defense of rhetoric in politics, not as a necessary evil but as suited to the context of political discourse—among natural human beings for whom language involves a complex array of affective, narrative, even instinctive forces that can never be reduced to objective description or rational inference. Even Aristotle recognized that political speech must include attention to noncognitive elements such as emotion and the personality of speakers. This does not make political speech thoughtless, but a politics without rhetoric, emotion, and personality would be lifeless and devoid of certain powers that figure in our sense of the world. Style and personality may in fact run deep and tap into less mediated intimations. Such forces can be dangerous, of course, but also noble: for every Adolph Hitler there is a Martin Luther King. The "content" of King's speeches cannot be separated from his existential bearing and oratorical gifts. The same speech in a different voice would not be the same speech. The hope for political discourse solely on "the issues" and by way of rational persuasion—divorced from the effects of style, character, and emotion—would be naïve or suspicious from a Nietzschean standpoint.

This venture into rhetoric is meant to reinforce my concerns in discussing Nietzsche's thoughts on selfhood, consciousness, and language. I think that Nietzsche's apparent segregation of language from the flux of experience and unconscious instinct really suits only certain models of language based on descriptive realism, psychological faculties, and written graphics. I believe that the social, corporeal, and rhetorical features of language highlighted by Nietzsche can be located "in between" a reified picture of language on the one hand and something nonlinguistic on the other. Nietzsche's own language is rich in styles, forces, and effects that enact, I think, the "medial" picture of language I am suggesting. Otherwise, Nietzsche's texts themselves would be susceptible to the charge of "error." Nietzsche's writings are meant not only to disabuse us of philosophical fictions, but also—*by way of their linguistic effects*—to draw out intimations of natural life, which can be hidden by language, but not on that account entirely without a voice.

Notes and references

1 This chapter is a revised and expanded version of a paper delivered at the 2009 meeting of the Friedrich Nietzsche Society at Oxford University: "Talking Ourselves into Selfhood: Consciousness and Language in *Gay Science* 354," which is published in *Nietzsche on Consciousness and the Embodied Mind*, ed. Manuel Dries (Berlin: Walter de Gruyter, 2011). With quotations from Nietzsche's works, I have occasionally modified published translations.

2 A similar point is made in later works: *BGE* 268 and *TI* Skirmishes, 26.

3 Alain Morin, "Possible links between self-awareness and inner speech," *Journal of Consciousness Studies* 12.4-5 (2005), 115–34. Page references above refer to this article.

4 Adam Winsler, Raphael M. Diaz and Ignacio Montero, "The Role of Private Speech in the Transition From Collaborative to Independent Task Performance in Young Children," *Early Childhood Research Quarterly* 12 (1997): 57–79. This particular point is on p. 60. Page references above refer to this article.

5 See Boris Henning, "Cartesian *Conscientia*," *British Journal for the History of Philosophy* 15/3 (August 2007): 455–85.

6 See Richard E. Aquila, "The Cartesian and a Certain 'Poetic' Notion of Consciousness," *Journal of the History of Ideas* 49/4 (Winter 1988): 561.

7 While culture-creation disrupts established forms of life, it is meant to settle into *new* forms of culture (rather than unhinged or indiscriminate anomalies). In this respect, we should consider Nietzsche's recognition of "second nature," which he calls a "new habit, a new instinct" that coalesces after a "first nature" of cultural inheritance has been altered or replaced—keeping in mind that the first nature in question was once a second nature replacing a first nature, and that this new second nature will become a first nature that will face disruption in the future after its own settlement (*UM*: UAH 3; *KSA* 1, 265–70).

8 As an aside, I wonder if the sense of linguistic immediacy can be related to Nietzsche's peculiar concept of "necessity." For Nietzsche, the necessity of an event does rule out alternatives, but simply from the standpoint of the "self-evidence" of the immediate event as such, with nothing *other* or outside it, whether that be a causal chain or a self-originating "will" or "substance." This is why Nietzsche says that "occurrence (*Geschehen*) and necessary occurrence is a *tautology*" (*WP* 639; *KSA* 12, 535–36). Necessity is counterposed not only to free alternatives but to any sense of mechanism, causality, or law: "Let us beware of saying that there are laws in nature. There are only necessities" (*GS* 109; *KSA* 3, 467–69). Necessity does not follow from the force of law but from the *absence* of law (*BGE* 22); it cannot mean some fixed relation between successive states (which violates the primacy of radical becoming) but simply that a state is what it is rather than something else (*WP* 552, 631; *KSA* 12, 383–86, 135–36). Necessity indicates that an occurrence "cannot be otherwise" *simply* by force of its immediate emergence, independent of any sense of causality—whether the self-causality of freedom, the final causality of teleology, or the efficient causality of determinism—since causality always looks *away* from an occurrence as such and in one way or another posits the idea of alternatives (if only to displace them). Nietzsche does not deny the possibility of causal thinking, only its primal posture as "explanation." Causality is an *interpretation* of experience that is useful for "designation and communication" (*BGE* 21–22). Necessity names the primal immediacy of events-in-becoming *as such*, for which in each case an "alternative" would not be "another event" but *no event* (see *WP* 567; *KSA* 13, 370–71).

9 For significant studies that emphasize Nietzsche's strategies of appealing to readers' lives rather than propositional knowledge, see Christopher Janaway, *Beyond Selflessness: Reading Nietzsche's Genealogy* (Oxford: Oxford University Press, 2007), David B. Allison, *Reading the New Nietzsche* (Lanham, MD: Rowman & Littlefield, 2001), and Alexander Nehamas, *Nietzsche: Life as Literature* (Cambridge, MA: Harvard University Press, 1985).

10 See the 1871 fragment "On Music and Words," found translated (by Walter Kaufmann) in Carl Dahlhaus, *Between Romanticism and Modernism*, trans. Mary Whittall (Berkeley: University of California Press, 1980). In "The Dionysiac World View," gesture and tone are originally instinctive, without consciousness, but not without purpose. See *The Birth of Tragedy and Other Writings*, eds. Raymond Geuss and Ronald Spiers (Cambridge: Cambridge University Press, 1999), p. 134.

11 See Kathleen Higgens, "Nietzsche on Music," *Journal of the History of Ideas* 47/4 (Winter 1986): 663–72. Nietzsche thought that the Greeks had a capacity largely lost in modern experience, namely a "third ear" that could hear the musical background of language (*BGE* 8). He even talks of an element of dance in writing (*TI* Germans, 7).

12 See *Friedrich Nietzsche on Rhetoric and Language*, edited and translated by Sander L. Gilman, Carole Blair, and David J. Parent (New York: Oxford University Press, 1989).

13 See my article "Writing Knowledge in the Soul: Orality, Literacy, and Plato's Critique of Poetry," *Epoche: A Journal for the History of Philosophy* 11/2 (Spring 2007): 319–32.

14 See my *A Nietzschean Defense of Democracy: An Experiment in Postmodern Politics* (Chicago: Open Court, 1995).

Editions used

The Antichrist, in *The Portable Nietzsche*, ed. and trans. Walter Kaufmann (New York: Viking Press, 1954).

Beyond Good and Evil, in *Basic Writings of Nietzsche*, ed. and trans. Walter Kaufmann, (New York: Random House, 1966).

The Birth of Tragedy, in *Basic Writings*.

Daybreak, trans. R. J. Hollingdale (Cambridge: Cambridge University Press, 1982).

Ecce Homo, in *Basic Writings*.

The Gay Science, trans. Walter Kaufmann (New York: Random House, 1974).

On the Genealogy of Morality, ed. Keith Ansell-Pearson, trans. Carol Diethe (Cambridge: Cambridge University Press, 2007).

Human, All Too Human, trans. R. J. Hollingdale (New York: Cambridge University Press, 1986).

Twilight of the Idols, in *The Portable Nietzsche*.

Untimely Meditations, trans. R. J. Hollingdale (Cambridge: Cambridge University Press, 1983).

The Will to Power, trans. Walter Kaufmann and R. J. Hollingdale (New York: Random House, 1967).

The Wanderer and His Shadow, Part 2 of *Human, All Too Human*.

Thus Spoke Zarathustra, in *The Portable Nietzsche*.

15

Nietzsche's Experimental Ontology: Political Physiology in the Age of Nihilism

Nandita Biswas Mellamphy

Nietzsche is and was a thinker of imminent nihilism, and in this regard, he is particularly interesting and important to those who, following Foucault's famous challenge, aim to engage in a diagnosis of the present. Nietzsche saw his culture, his environment, and their future in terms of the devaluation, self-destruction, and annihilation of humanity—its projects, people, and values. Instead of shying away from this destruction, he turned toward it. Nietzsche affirmed the symptoms of his time and engaged them by using them as tools for the development of a social machine that would produce the "Übermensch": the transformation of the "Human-All-Too-Human" into the "Overhuman." Why did he think this was important? For him, the "Overhuman" was both the *culmination* and the *overcoming* of nihilism. He saw nihilism not as an end but as a "transitional pathological phase" which, however destructive, could nonetheless trigger a "phase shift"[1] leading to the emergence of a new ontology beyond that of the human. Nietzsche wanted a politics conducive to this coming ontology, I argue, and I will suggest that his invention of the concept of "will to power" as a "physiological process" can be articulated within the framework of such a politics of emergent ontology.

One fundamental assumption of a Nietzschean political physiology is that the engine of transformation that drives the formation of individual personality, identity, and values in the human realm can also be found in other living forms or vital processes. Humans, in this regard, are like other organism and animals; but in having striven to forget and overcome their animality, humans have become sick organisms. Going back to the historical source of occidental thought, Nietzsche would find the illness of European culture at the speculative root of western civilization: "indeed, one may ask as a physician: 'how could such a malady attack this loveliest product of antiquity, Plato'?"[2] What were considered by most to be the signs of human flourishing—Platonic philosophy, Christianity, and parliamentary democracy—Nietzsche saw as signs of degeneration of a collective organism. Nietzsche would thus approach the fundamental political question of human beings—who rules and over whom?—as a malady to be diagnosed and treated. As pathological as Nietzsche's writings became over the course of his fertile but fragile thinking life, they are nonetheless exemplary in their attention to the particularly pathological nature of modern human existence.

The three stigmata of Friedrich Nietzsche

This chapter comes directly out of an extended argument I develop in my book, *The Three Stigmata of Friedrich Nietzsche: Political Physiology in the Age of Nihilism*. It is a speculative study that seeks to offer a possible and plausible theory of "political physiology" in Nietzsche's thought and so I beg your indulgence as I refer to it throughout.

This speculative study presents Nietzsche's political physiology by interrelating three concepts not usually taken and treated together by the secondary scholarship: first, in the domain of his political thought, the concept of "great politics"; second, in the phenomenological domain, his concept of "eternal return"; and finally, set against the backdrop of his materialist theory of the self-overcoming subject, the concept of "the philosopher of the future." These three key concepts are ill-defined in Nietzsche's work: none are given an explicit or systematic explanation, all of them are *stigmata* emblematic of other operations, and each of them is unequivocally a crucial strand of his thought. In drawing together these three concepts and attempting to examine them explicitly in light of one another, this study presents Nietzsche's speculative materialism as a politics of the transformation of the Human into the Overhuman directly within the context of the immanent intensification of nihilism.

Why do I call these three central but ephemeral Nietzschean notions "stigmata"? I invoke them as physiological symptoms, as bodily marks that resemble or mimic an*other* condition and as that which enables the dia*gnosis* of that condition. From this perspective, the three concepts under scrutiny are signs or symptoms of a larger vital process conceived as an entire living "theater" of contesting individuations. But stigmata are also "wounds," understood not in the sense of mere aftereffects but as virulent loci of active and actual suffering (*pathos*). The task of political physiology and of the philosopher-physician is thus to contend with a thought that "wounds" its thinker. As Alain Jugnon has recently claimed, Nietzsche's philosophy of life is a theater of material genesis that goes beyond a mere metaphorical description of movements and of the passions of the "soul." As a theater of material genesis, the operation of "pathos" is itself identified as the fundamental gesture and movement of living matter. Methodologically, according to Jugnon, this theatrical movement announces its own technique:

> In such a staging of life in which matter and movement are interposed, the central question of each and every aim and framework, of every open window on the real becomes: "What is underway? (*Que se passe-t-il?*) Like all spectators, philosophy gazes across a scene and manages to construct, by this movement, the mobility of the dramatic matter itself: like all actors, philosophy surveys the scene, mimes the sentiments, is penetrated by pathos, and attempts to establish by these displacements the very direction (*sens*) of drama."[3]

Nietzsche's political physiology: Nihilism and the pathology of health and illness

Political physiology begins with this virulence *in* and *of* Nietzsche's thought. As Nietzsche himself acknowledged, in the historical condition of nihilism (a condition in which Nietzsche found himself and in which we find ourselves today), health and illness are not so easy to distinguish and may lead to many misunderstandings:

> Health and sickness are not essentially different . . . In fact, there are only differences in degree between these two kinds of existence: the exaggeration, the disproportion, the nonharmony of the normal phenomena constitute the pathological state (Claude Bernard). Just as *"evil"* can be considered as exaggeration, disharmony, disproportion, *"the good"* may be a *protective diet* against the danger of exaggeration, disharmony, and disproportion.[4]

The politico-physiological perspective is attentive to the problem of "health" and "illness," psychophysiological states that are problematic for Nietzsche because "health and sickness are not essentially different." Although the concepts of "great politics," 'eternal recurrence," and "the philosopher of the future" are ill-defined in Nietzsche's thought and therefore can be said to be complicit with the very illnesses that Nietzsche sought to name, they are also "signs of health"[5] that are meant to be part of the curatives characteristic of "great health."[6] Because the difference between "health" and "illness" is *intensive* not *substantial*—that is to say, "health" is not a different substance forming a qualitatively different state than "illness," "health," and "illness" are only "differences in degree."[7] The symptoms of health and illness can only be distinguished by their toxicological effects on the organism in question (and in this passage, Nietzsche juxtaposes two symptomatic states that Deleuze would later strongly develop: "strong/active" and "weak/reactive").

The three stigmata of Nietzsche's thought—"great politics," "eternal recurrence," and "the philosopher of the future"—thus form a pathology, the politico-physiological force of which can be interpreted within the terms of "symptomotology," as Nietzsche himself notes in the preface to *The Gay Science* and as Deleuze reiterates in the introduction to *Nietzsche and Philosophy*. Following Nietzsche's declaration of the task of the philosopher-physician as interpretation of the "hints and symptoms of the body,"[8] Deleuze develops the critical force of Nietzsche's political physiology by emphasizing that this bodily symptomotology proceeds by way of a conceptualization of the relation between "active" and "reactive" forces that cannot avoid encountering a fundamental difficulty or confusion: if active forces "by nature . . . escape consciousness" and "consciousness is essentially reactive," then "it is inevitable that consciousness sees the organism from its own point of view . . . that is to say, reactively." "The real problem is the discovery of active forces without which the reactions themselves would not be forces."[9]

As Deleuze rightly shows, when the "whole of philosophy" is interpreted symptomologically, the political physiologist is forced to confront the untenability of maintaining the strict metaphysical opposition between "appearance" and "essence," as well as the scientific opposition between "cause" and "effect."

> A phenomenon is not an appearance or even an apparition but a sign, a symptom which finds its meaning in an existing force. The whole of philosophy is a symptomatology, and a semeiology. The sciences are a symptomatological and semeiological system. Nietzsche substitutes the correlation between sense and phenomenon for the metaphysical duality of appearance and essence and for the scientific relation of cause and effect.[10]

The mutual implication of "health" and "illness," the "active" and the "reactive," the "conscious" and the "unconscious" is the pathology of effects most pertinent to the politico-physiological perspective because it directly confronts and exposes these two central misunderstandings or "prejudices" of metaphysical and scientific knowledge (e.g., "appearance" and "essence," "cause" and "effect"—what Nietzsche calls in *Beyond Good and Evil* 2 the "belief in antitheses of values"). When viewed toxicologically, the relation between health and illness is not an issue regarding the qualitative and substantial properties of antithetical states, but rather it is a vital relation connecting a dynamic organizational network. The challenge of such a toxicological perspective would be to understand health not chiefly as the synthetic interplay of negativity or negation, but negativity itself as a poison that is necessarily part of the vital engine of an ongoing metastable process of becoming (in this sense, negativity becomes part of an experimental art/science in administering dosages of poisons).

From a politico-physiological perspective, "great politics" and "great health" are not substantive oppositions of "petty politics" and "illness"; rather they must be viewed as thresholds that form around vital sites of becoming (here we understand will to power as the ongoing formation of metastabilities). This is why for a Nietzschean political physiology, when understood as a vital theater of contesting tensions *qua* transformations, negativity and pessimism can be forces that strengthen as well as weaken: "Pessimism as strength – in what? In the energy of its logic, an anarchism and nihilism, as analytic. Pessimism as decline – in what? As growing effeteness, as a sort of cosmopolitan fingering, as 'tout comprendre' and historicism. The critical tension: the extremes appear and become predominant."[11] The cultivation of critical tensions is the affirmative work of opposing forces, of overcoming.

According to Nietzsche's own description in the unpublished works (viz., part one of Kaufmann's redaction entitled *Will to Power*), nihilism is a historical, epistemological, and psychophysiological condition in which the introduction of an externality into a system first functions to *fortify* it, but then triggers a cannibalistic response *against* it. The pathology proceeds as follows: what is first introduced into a system as an antidote preserving the unity of a system turns against itself and results in the dissolution of that system. (This is how modern immunology has characterized diseases of "autoimmunity"). The effect and the affect of this process? Nietzsche says quite succinctly: "The highest values devaluate themselves."[12]

> . . . In sum: morality was the great *antidote* against practical and theoretical nihilism.[13] . . . But among the forces cultivated by morality was *truthfulness:* this

> eventually turned against morality . . . – and now the recognition of this inveterate mendaciousness that one despairs of shedding becomes a stimulant . . . This antagonism . . . results in a process of dissolution.[14]

In the absence of *stasis* (the mechanisms of which impose *limitations*), the affirmation of nihilism becomes the curative force of the poison of nihilism. This is the operative difference between "passive" and "active" nihilism:

> Nihilism. It is *ambiguous:*
>
> A. Nihilism as a sign of increased power of the spirit: as *active* nihilism. B. Nihilism as decline and recession of the power of the spirit: as *passive* nihilism.[15]

For Nietzsche, nihilism "represents a pathological transitional stage"[16] in the evolution of a subject that is in the throes of dissolution. In this strong sense, Nietzsche's bodily thought is both a *product of nihilism* and a theater of production that seeks to *overcome nihilism* by *actively* thinking through nihilism. Active nihilism is the force of destruction/creation *qua* transformation. If we recall that for Nietzsche, reactive nihilism is a situation in which a system begins to eat itself by turning itself against itself (following the pathology of autoimmunity) hanging onto itself in order preserve even a minuteness of its discharge, then active nihilism becomes the *transformative* activity of force that no longer turns back onto itself. It is the force of *morphosis,* the "plasticity"[17] characteristic of active force in which nothing is carried over. It affirms by dominating, by commanding a weaker force to obey (in this sense force is always hierarchical), but its domination proceeds by expenditure not by recuperation (this is why the overcoming of nihilism for Nietzsche cannot ultimately proceed by Dialectics or by Fascism). Nietzsche even has a name for this active process: the active and most extreme form of nihilism—the process in which existence is lived and expended without limitation or recuperation : "Let us think this thought in its most terrible form: existence as it is, without meaning or aim, yet recurring inevitably without any finale of nothingness: the *eternal recurrence*."[18] It is, therefore, in Nietzsche's analysis of nihilism that we can start to chart the pathology of this dissolving subject.

The mnemotechnics of nihilism and the genesis of the "human"

Nietzsche had conceived of *Beyond Good and Evil* as a "prelude" to and anticipation of an impending civilizational and cultural "spectacle" whose enactment was still being put into place, but whose destiny had already inevitably been cast. This spectacle "of a hundred acts that will occupy Europe for the next two centuries"[19] is that of *nihilism.* Although the kind of nihilism he presaged had yet to reach its dramatic historical crescendo in his own age, Nietzsche identified its faint tonalities in his account of the genesis and pathologization of "bad conscience" in *The Genealogy of Morals.* My main aim here is to highlight that for Nietzsche, the "human" has from its very first emergence been constituted by mnemotechnics (the evolutionary development of a "memory of the will") which is simultaneously also a process of detachment and abstraction, or what Nietzsche describes as a process of intensive "spiritualization." The "human" first emerges as the relation between a religious subjective mode that operates by way of intensifications of "spiritualization" and the mnemotechnical ensemble of artifices without which the "human" could not be instrumentalized. This process of spiritualization results in the birth of the "priestly type" and according to Nietzsche, heralds the first dangerous movement toward the "domestication" of the human animal.

According to Nietzsche's account in *The Genealogy*, all aristocratic systems of value are ones in which the spectrum of value judgments are directly reflective of the power of the highest in social rank. In section 6 of *GM*, Nietzsche contrasts the political "aristocratic" and the priestly aristocratic: the political aristocratic expresses his power by exercising his material animal instincts; his rule is legitimized by his political superiority. The "priestly" type, on the other hand, does not exercise but controls his material nature through dietary restrictions, control of bodily processes, and forbidding of intermixing with the "impure." The priestly type was forbidden from externalizing and discharging his instincts and regulated them through strict adherence to a whole panoply of bodily prohibitions. Nietzsche says that this spiritual type embodies a kind of walking psychological contradiction: on the one hand, he feels his superior spiritual power over others, but compared to the warrior type, he also feels his material/physical impotence. Although the priestly types tried to overcompensate for this impotence by highlighting their *spiritual* superiority, this intensified spirituality was in fact a direct effect of a feeling of impotence, and therefore slowly festered into feelings of "arrogance, revenge . . . love, lust to rule, virtue – but it is only fair to add that it was on the solid of this essentially dangerous form of human existence, the priestly form, that man first became an *interesting* animal."[20]

This psychological separation between mental and physical power internalized by the priestly type actually had the effect of complexifying the consciousness of the human animal; this new human was less animal because he was able to repress his animality through intellectual controls; but this human was also less healthy, increasingly becoming "alienated" from the physical material basis of its animal state. According to Nietzsche then, the effects and influence of this priestification are both the first great *spiritualization* of the human animal and the first great moment of "domestication" of human animality.

Nietzsche's account of the emergence of "bad conscience" is a psychophysiological account of the political animal. In this argument, Nietzsche claims that that the founding of the first political societies required a constitutive moment of alienation at the level of the psychophysiological evolution of human beings, a kind of "archi-nihilism."[21] Historically then, nihilism was the catastrophic consequence generated by an "archi-nihilism" that itself first gave birth to and transformed the not-yet-human animal into a potential social and political agent:

> I regard the bad conscience as the serious illness that man was bound to contract under the stress of the most fundamental change he ever experienced—that change which occurred when he found himself finally enclosed within the

> walls of society and of peace. The situation that faced sea animals when they were compelled to become land animals or perish was the same as that which faced these semi-animals, well adapted to the wilderness, to war, to prowling, to adventure: suddenly all their instincts were disvalued and "suspended".[22]

The constitution of the political life, Nietzsche here argues, develops via psychic and physiological modifications in the human animal. According to Nietzsche, the constitutive moment of the *human* as "political" rather than merely "animal" occurs precisely at the moment in which the animal instincts cease to become discharged and instead become "internalized," sublimated and deployed *subliminally*. Nietzsche describes this process as the early psychophysiological transformation of the "hominid" into the "human" configured and given signification through an economy in which the renunciation of desire is made productive and meaningful:

> All instincts that do not discharge themselves outwardly turn inward—this is what I call the internalization [*Verinnerlichung*] of man: thus it was that man first developed what was later called his "soul." The entire inner world, originally as thin as if it were stretched between two membranes, expanded and extended itself, acquired depth, breadth, and height, in the same measure as outward discharge was inhibited. Those fearful bulwarks with which the political organization protected itself against the old instincts of freedom—punishments belong among these bulwarks—brought about that all those instincts of wild, free, prowling man turned backward against man himself. Hostility, cruelty, joy in persecuting, in attacking, in change, in destruction—all this turned against the possessors of such instincts: that is the origin of the "bad conscience".[23]

This transformation is a process of bifurcation in which a process of intensifying alienation resulting from the growing disconnection between the instinctive and sublimative registers results in the *complexification* of the animal into a human technical (tool-making), principally *mnemotechnical* (memory-making)—and hence a moralizing *political* subject. In the second essay of *GM*, Nietzsche characterizes the "human" with the ability to make promises, which itself requires the ability to ritualize pain by inscribing it into cultural memory:[24]

> How can one create a memory for the human animal? How can one impress something upon this partly obtuse, partly flighty mind, attuned only to the passing oment, in such a way that it will stay there?" One can well believe that the answers and methods for solving this primeval problem were not precisely gentle; perhaps indeed there was nothing more fearful and uncanny in the whole prehistory of man than his *mnemotechnics*. "If something is to stay in the memory it must be burned in: only that which never ceases to *hurt* stays in the memory" – . . . Man could never do without blood, torture, and sacrifices when he felt the need to create a memory for himself; the most dreadful sacrifices and pledges (sacrifices of the first-born among them), the most repulsive mutilations (castration, for example), the cruelest rites of all the religious cults (and all religions are at the deepest level systems of cruelties)—all this has its origin in the instinct that realized that pain is the most powerful aid to mnemonics.[25]

Just as in Kafka's stark tale of corporeal inscription in *The Penal Colony*, the "human" for Nietzsche is a mnemotechnical political animal. If the human animal can become political, it is because the arts of remembering, identifying, ritualizing, and symbolizing become the technical motor for the further psychophysiological evolution. For Nietzsche, the "human" is, constitutionally and constitutively speaking, mnemotechnical: its subjective and objective development is fundamentally linked to memory. The human develops subjectively into the priestly bad conscience by concretizing memory in the form of mnemotechnical objects. When read alongside Nietzsche's speculation regarding the "subject" as "fiction," the political animal is revealed to be a *prosthetic* engendered in tandem with the technical arts of remembering and forgetting.

The political and historical problem of nihilism, as such, is also a problem of the psychophysiological transmutation of the animal human. Specifically for Nietzsche, the archi-nihilism that founds the human and later develops into the monotheistic self-consciousness (the "bad conscience") becomes intensified and reified in modernity as the problem of willing:

> We can no longer conceal from ourselves what is expressed by all that willing which has taken its direction from the ascetic ideal: this hatred of the human, and even more of the animal, and more still of the material, this horror of the senses, of reason itself, this fear of happiness and beauty, this longing to get away from all appearance, change, becoming, death, wishing, from longing itself—all this means—let us dare to grasp it—a will to nothingness, an aversion to life, a rebellion against the most fundamental presuppositions of life, but it is and remains a will! . . . And, to repeat in conclusion what I said at the beginning: man would rather will nothingness than not will.[26]

"Willing" becomes the hallmark of the mnemotechnical human, in due course becoming a symptom of its decadence as well as the active battleground for its overcoming (i.e., the Overman or *Übermensch*). In the psychophysiological development of the human then as told by Nietzsche in *GM*, the process of sublimation eventually makes possible the production of knowledge and becomes the historical motor for the large-scale cultural decadence and degeneration characteristic of modernity (the "ascetic ideal").

Nietzsche's solution to the problem of nihilism is not, however, a declaration simply rejecting willing in favor of returning to the animal instinctual state (i.e., through the willing of an economy of drives); because willing is itself a product of sublimation, Nietzsche knows very well that a nostalgic yearning for a bygone psychophysiological state is both undesirable and (what is more) impossible. Rather he will suggest that the overcoming of nihilism must involve the violent playing-out of nihilism to its end, that is, an intensification of nihilism—one which will necessitate a politics of nihilism as a necessary corollary of a "philosophy of the future." Against this backdrop of nihilism, the "subject" becomes the political and mnemotechnical battlefield upon which the war of life is waged and played out. In order for Nietzschean political physiology to undertake the task of overcoming both the historical problem of nihilism and its constitutive foundations ("archi-nihilism"), the intensification of nihilism (a process of decadence and degeneration) will be forced to play out on the subjective plane. The overcoming of nihilism requires the affirmation of the most extreme form of nihilism itself, the overcoming of willing through the affirmation of nonwilling.

It is Pierre Klossowski's interpretation of eternal recurrence that forms the foundation for the theory of political physiology offered here. Klossowski understands the body to be an inchoate and primal battleground of affective drives that are translated and communicated into thought within the cultural code of everyday signs.

> The body is a production of chance; it is nothing other than the site of conjunction and conflict between a concrescence of individuated impulses which come together for that brief time span we call 'a human life', impulses which aspire only to de-individuate themselves.[27]

From this perspective, the eternal recurrence is twofold: on the one hand, it is an experience of the singular body; an ecstatic unveiling or revelation, a "forgetting" (of all identities, laws, and boundaries) into which all identity is absorbed and revealed in its inchoate multiplicity; and on the other hand, the eternal recurrence must be made intelligible and infinitely repeatable: it must be a necessity that is willed and re-willed.[28] Klossowski theorizes eternal recurrence in terms of wave phenomena that interrupt the normal inscription of memory necessary to sustain self-consciousness: all directed exertions of the will commingle and disappear in the multiple swells and surges of the impulses which entail and require a profound subjective amnesis. In the interruption of self-consciousness (the dissolution of "self" that is undergone in the experience of eternity), the subject as a stable entity becomes a fiction, the affirmation of which becomes the means for reconnecting with the joyful but terrible and potentially perilous forces of life. As an experience of the "suspension" of self-consciousness (and the emergence of the unconscious drives and impulses), the eternal recurrence is not primarily a conscious reasoning, a thought-experiment nor a doctrine, but instead, a mechanism of mutation that reorganizes forces within a system (the "in-formational" operationality of any system).

The eternal recurrence becomes a teaching only when it itself becomes a sign—a cultural imperative of a collectivity. In other words, the feeling produced by the experience of eternal recurrence must be translated into thought so that it can be re-willed anew and transmitted by those abundant enough to endure it. The eternal recurrence thus becomes not a return to some authentic or original state, but a dynamic and violent process of individuation in which the human animal literally undergoes a psychophysiological mutation, a playing-out that leads to the death of one form of existence (the decadent form of human as described for example in *The Genealogy of Morality*) into what Nietzsche hopes is the genesis of a new psychophysiological configuration of self-organization. When interpreted from the perspective of political physiology, the eternal recurrence becomes comprehensible as a process of *morphosis* in which both the physical and metaphysical mechanisms of subjectivity are forced to organize and individuate anew. It is in this operative sense that the eternal recurrence is the transformative mechanism driving Nietzsche's political physiology.

The pharmacological approach of political physiology

What kind of politics would be adequate to this? "What is to be done" politically when nihilism has become a "normal condition?" The political physiological perspective is ever vigilant in remembering that what is a cure can also be a poison, and what is a poison can be a cure. The boundary separating values—high/low, noble/base, good/evil, healthy/ill—can no longer be securely differentiated and Nietzsche himself points to this fact:

> "It is the value of all morbid states that they show us under a magnifying glass certain states that are normal -- but not easily visible when normal. Health and sickness are not essentially different, as the ancient physicians and some practitioners even today suppose. One must not make of them distinct principles or entities that fight over the living organism and turn it into their arena . . . "[29]

As the French philosopher Bernard Stiegler has recently said, the philosopher today must be a *toxicologist*[30]; and this echoes something that I have recently also said in relation to Nietzsche's call for a philosopher that is also a physician: in the politics conditioned by nihilism but which seeks to overcome nihilism by activating the potency of nihilism, the philosopher-physician must be a *homeopathic* toxicologist governed and guided by the principle of "*like cures like*" (*simili similibus curentor*), the administering of the poison as the curative force itself.[31] This kind of politics—is there, truly, any alternative to this?—is fraught with so many *moral* dilemmas precisely because its operative principle works without seeking to—without *having* to—ontologize the distinction between "true" and "false," "good" and "evil." This is also why for Nietzsche, the question of power is *not merely nor even primarily* a question of property or territory and the negotiating of its representations; but rather, power is a question of production, of *morphosis* and its transformations, the process of formation that emerges as the result of a tension of forces, the process that imposes "upon becoming the character of being."[32] Following Bernard Stiegler, the question of the "political" must necessarily proceed via a pharmacological perspective: we must look for the signs of health in the very illnesses of the human condition, as well as be able to recognize signs of illness in what may be considered by the majority as signs of "health."

Notes

1 A term used in wave mechanics to describe the differential effect of phase relations.
2 Friedrich Nietzsche, *Beyond Good and Evil*, trans. Walter Kaufmann(New York: Random House, 1966), preface.
3 [translation mine]. Alain Jugnon, *Nietzsche et Simondon: Le théâtre du vivant* (Editions Dittmar: 2010), p. 18.
4 Friedrich Nietzsche, *The Will to Power*, trans. Walter Kaufmann (New York: Random House, 1967), § 47.
5 *BGE* §154.

6 Friedrich Nietzsche, *The Gay Science* , trans. Walter Kaufmann (New York: Random House, 1974), §382.
7 *WP* §47.
8 *GS* Preface, §2.
9 Gilles Deleuze, *Nietzsche and Philosophy*, trans. Hugh Tomlinson (Chicago: Athlone Press, 1983), p. 41.
10 Deleuze, p. 3.
11 *WP*, §10.
12 Ibid., § 2.
13 Ibid., §4.
14 Ibid., §5.
15 Ibid.,§22.
16 Ibid., §13.
17 Deleuze, p. 42.
18 *WP*, §55.
19 Friedrich Nietzsche, *On the Genealogy of Morals,* trans. Walter Kaufmann (New York: Random House, 1967) III, §27.
20 *GM* I, §6.
21 I am grateful to Bernard Stiegler for this term. Roundtable Discussion with Bernard Stiegler, "Trans-individuation, Technology, Politics", *New French Thought* conference, Department of Philosophy, Villanova University, 3-4 April 2009.
22 *GM* II, §16.
23 Ibid.
24 *GM* II, *i.e.,* §3, 6; GM II: *i.e.*, §16, 17.
25 *GM* II, §3.
26 *GM* III, §28.
27 Pierre Klossowski, *Nietzsche et le cercle vicieux* (Paris: Mercure de France, 1975), pp. 52–3.
28 Pierre Klossowski, "Nietzsche's Experience of the Eternal recurrence," in David B. Allison (ed.), *The New Nietzsche* (Cambridge: MIT Press, 1985), p. 115.
29 *WP*, §47.
30 Questions About a General Pharmacology" Keynote address, *New French Thought,* conference in the Department of Philosophy, Villonova University, 3 April 2009.
31 Biswas Mellamphy, "Corporealizing Thought: Retranslating the Eternal recurrence Back into Politics," in Herman Siemens and Vasti Roodt (eds), *Nietzsche, Power, and Politics* (Berlin: De Gruyter: 2008), p. 760.
32 *WP*, §617.

16

"Let that be my love": Fate, Mediopassivity, and Redemption in Nietzsche's Thought

Béatrice Han-Pile

There is no doubt that Nietzsche considered the theme of amor fati (love of fate) of essential importance: he referred to it in his later work as his "formula for greatness in a human being" (EH: 258), "the highest state a philosopher can attain" (WP 1041), or again his "inmost nature" (EH: 325). Amor fati is often mentioned by commentators in connection with the eternal return and implicitly taken as an illustration of the sort of existential attitude characteristic of someone who would respond positively to the challenge of the daimon and affirm his or her life as worth living over and over again (Magnus 1978: 145; Hatab 2005: 49; Reginster 2006: 229–30). It is occasionally touched upon in relation with various themes, such as self-creation (Leiter 2001: 284) or the call for a reevaluation of all values. Yet (surprisingly given its importance for Nietzsche), there is very little secondary literature specifically devoted to it. Perhaps this initial surprise will lessen if one considers that for all its importance, there is very little material on amor fati in Nietzsche's work. All in all, I was able to identify only seven passages, four in the published work, one in the *Will to Power,* one in the *Nachlass*, and one in Nietzsche's correspondence. And if one tries to help oneself out by looking for separate elucidations of love, one does not fare much better. While critical passages about neighborly love or the love of women are not rare, Nietzsche says little about more positive forms of love. In one of his latest fragments, he cryptically declares that "I have never desecrated the holy name of love" (1888, LN1 286) and Zarathustra praises the "bestowing love" of the "predator of all values" (Z: 100) and of the "friend," but without expanding on the nature of such love.

As for fate, discussions in the secondary literature often focus on the issue of whether the doctrine of the eternal return commits Nietzsche to fatalism, with widely diverging conclusions (Hatab 2005: 127–33; Leiter 2001: 283–90; Reginster 2006: 209). In what follows, I shall restrict myself to examining Nietzsche's thoughts on fate exclusively in connection with amor fati: I shall thus adopt the minimal construal of fate directly entailed by *all* the references to the latter in the published work, namely, "what is necessary" (GS: 223; EH: 258; EH: 325) or "everything that is necessary" (NCW: 680). Interestingly, this understanding of fate as all-encompassing necessity is very close to the one put forward by the Stoa, whom Nietzsche clearly had in mind when he claimed that amor fati involves more than "merely bearing what is necessary" (EH: 258)—thus Aetius reported that "the Stoa describe fate as a sequence of causes, that is an inescapable ordering and connection" (Long and Sedley 1987: 336). For the purposes of this paper, I shall leave aside such issues as the relation between this conception of fate as necessity and its more archaic and pathos-laden understanding in the *Birth of Tragedy* or the status of necessity in general as a category in Nietzsche's work, to focus on the paradoxes and difficulties attached to having fate thus construed as the object of any love, let alone the highest possible form of love. In doing so, my aim will be fourfold: (a) to grasp both the structure of amor fati and the sort of love it involves, (b) to understand better the part played by the concept in Nietzsche's later work, (c) to identify some of the ways in which amor fati might be attained by us and (d) to question the sustainability and limits of such an ideal.

Unless it is construed counterintuitively, as a blind force devoid of any intentionality which moves us in a purely causal way (a possibility which Nietzsche would certainly reject), love involves a valuation of its object. Loving something or someone entails understanding this object or person as valuable. The usual assumption is that such valuation must be positive, which enables us to distinguish between love and negative emotions such a dislike or hate, in which the object repels us. So to love something entails understanding it positively, as worth loving. Yet this observation poses two structural problems for amor fati. First, it points toward a potential contradiction between the nature of the attachment and the putative value of its object. As Nietzsche puts it, "one will see that the problem is that of the meaning of suffering" (WP §1052). Even on the minimal construal evoked above (as necessity), fate is bound to entail at least some suffering and unhappiness for each of us. We shall lose loved ones, or see them hurt. We shall be harmed ourselves. And even if our life was as devoid of suffering as possible, fate will inevitably lead us to aging and death, possibly in painful or degrading circumstances. In order to love fate, then, one would have to accept the paradoxical possibility of loving a repellent object (either a fully negative one or one which on the best construal involves some very significant negativity).

Secondly, there are two main ways in which we can value a loved object: in relation to our own needs, for example, because we deem its possession or enjoyment highly desirable or even indispensable to our well-being or happiness; or in relation to the object itself, because it appears to us as endowed with intrinsic value. In the first case, we perceive the object of our love as something that we should seek to acquire or, should we be fortunate enough to have it in our possession already, prevent the loss of. In the second, we try to preserve or protect the beloved object for its own sake, regardless of our own happiness. Yet both these options raise further doubts about the suitability of fate as an object of love. Regarding the first, on either construal (Greek *moira* or necessity), fate is seen as indifferent to our needs and desires and would only fulfill them (or not) accidentally. We are aware that we cannot possess it and have no control over it. Furthermore, it is not even the sort of object we can actively *seek*: we are already under its sway and if anything cannot be rid of it. So how could we conceive of it as an indispensable component of our happiness? And if we were to value fate per se rather than in relation to ourselves (the second option), then a different problem arises, which was originally identified by the Stoa as *argos logos* (idle reason). Perhaps its best-known version is given by Cicero: "if it is your fate to recover from this illness, you will recover whether you call for the physician or not. Likewise, if it is your fate not to recover, whether you call for the physician or not, you will not recover. One of the two is your fate, therefore it is pointless to call for the physician" (Cicero: 28–9). Along similar lines, by definition, fate or necessity will unfold whether we love it or not, and it is not clear what difference our love could make. If this is the case, then amor fati would seem a rather futile form of love. Plainly put, why bother?

Thus prospective lovers of fate are faced with two paradoxes: (a) amor fati involves an apparent contradiction between the nature of love and the partly negative value of its proposed object and in particular, requires us to love something which is difficult, if not impossible, to value in relations to our needs or desires; (b) should we value fate for itself, there would seem to be no point in our loving it: whether we do or not will make no difference either to fate or to what happens to us. Given these structural difficulties, how can we make sense of amor fati, let alone regard it as a desirable ideal? To seek a solution to this puzzle, it may help to turn to the traditional distinction between four forms of love: eros, agape, caritas, and philia. Of these, only the first three are relevant to amor fati as philia (in its Aristotelian version) entails an element of disinterestedness from the part of the lover and reciprocity on the part of the loved object, two conditions which love of fate cannot satisfy. And since caritas, at least according to Nygren, is an Augustinian synthesis of eros and agape designed to solve a specific doctrinal problem (viz., whether human love can by its own strength ascend to God), I shall focus on the last two. Very interestingly, the main difference between eros and agape, Greek and Christian forms of love, concerns the relation between loving and valuing. Both traditions agree that love is not blind and involves a valuation of its object, but they disagree on the source and nature of such valuation. In a nutshell, erotic love is motivated by the perceived value of its object: we love someone or something *because we value them.* By contrast, agapic love bestows value on its object, and this regardless of the value previously attributed to it: we value someone or something *because we love them.* Agapic love is Christian in origin and finds its first formulations in the New Testament and John's and Paul's letters. According to Nygren, it has four main features: (a) it is a divine form of love; (b) it is spontaneous in the sense of not being externally motivated—God's undeserved (and undeservable, at least in the Lutherian tradition Nietzsche was familiar with) gift to man; (c) it is not motivated by the value of the object (Christ came for sinners and the righteous alike); and finally, (d) it creates value by transfiguring its object (the sinner becomes worthy by virtue of being loved by God).

It is difficult to know which (if any) of these two forms of love Nietzsche had in mind when he first coined the expression "amor fati": 'amor" is a fairly neutral choice of words, although interestingly, it is Luther's own in his redescription of agapic love against Augustinian *caritas.* Furthermore, eros and agape are idealized types and it is unlikely that Nietzsche's understanding of amor fati would fall squarely under either description. I have developed elsewhere an erotic reading of amor fati and offered reasons why I think that it cannot work.[1] In this chapter, I wish to focus on the possibilities afforded by an agapic reading. In the *Gay Science*, Nietzsche introduces the notion as follows:

> I want to learn more and more to see as beautiful what is necessary in things; *then I shall be one of those who make things beautiful. Amor fati: let that be* my love henceforth! (GS §276: 223, my italics)

This passage can be seen as laying out a quasi-Platonic strategy for overcoming the perceived negativity of fate and thus making amor fati possible. However, two elements plead in favor of a different interpretation: first, on an erotic construal, the second part of the statement is rather mysterious: it is presented as a consequence ("then") of amor fati. The only interpretation that an erotic reading allows for is rather literal: having learned to see things as beautiful, I would be in a position to create beautiful things. But the expression "making things beautiful" (*die Dinge schön machen*) clearly refers to *existing* things, which rules out the idea of a physical poiesis whereby nice things would be produced. The alternative is to understand this making beautiful of things as an agapic transfiguration of their value brought about by our love for them. This central feature of agapic love, namely, its ability to transform the former value of its objects, is explicitly identified by Nietzsche as one of the characteristic of the Overman: "verily, a predator of all values must such a bestowing love become; . . . . May your bestowing love and your knowledge serve towards the meaning of the earth! . . . . *And may the value of all things be fixed anew by you*!" (Z: 101–2, Nietzsche's italics). I shall try later to specify how this bestowal works in the case of amor fati; for the moment, let me point out the second aspect of GS 276 which favors an agapic reading of love.

It concerns the peculiar modality of the expression "let that be my love." First, although it is, grammatically speaking, an imperative, it can also be read in a nonprescriptive way, as an expression of hope for the coming of agapic love rather than as an erotic call for action. Secondly, the sort of act it refers to (letting be) is neither fully active nor passive: it suggests that the love may come to and through the agent (who has to "let it" happen—perhaps, in this case, precisely by hoping for it), but that it cannot be fully *caused* by the agent. Although most Indo-European languages only allow for passive and active modes, ancient Greek had a third mode to refer to such cases where agency is ambiguous. The middle voice was meant to capture the modality of situations in which the agent is both active and passive, in such a way that s/he participates in the action but without being in control of it.[2] Gonda (1960: 53 sq) underlines this peculiar active/passive mode of the middle voice in relation to a particular example in ancient Greek, that of marrying someone. The active form (*gameô*) was standardly used by men and denotes an action in which the agent is fully in control, namely, the taking of a wife. This is grammatically reflected by the fact that the complement is in the accusative. The middle voice form (*gameomai*) was normally used by women: it denotes activity (the woman takes a husband) but also passivity (she gives herself over to him, a fact which is grammatically expressed by the complement being indirect and in the dative). Furthermore, the middle voice has an eventive dimension: it indicates that "the process of marriage befalls the subject" (59), in such a way that she participates in it without controlling it.

In my view, this mediopassive modality is typical of Nietzsche's reinterpretation of agape as a human form of love. The letting be of agapic love displays precisely the two features pointed out by Gonda: first, it is both active and passive, requiring, perhaps, the development or cultivation of a particular receptivity to such love, but without any guarantee that the presence of such sensitivity will generate our love. Secondly, it has a marked eventive dimension (love happens to us, as expressed by the locution "to fall in love"). This mediopassive mode is often found in passages devoted both to amor fati and to the eternal return. For example, Nietzsche's autobiographical observations in *Ecce Homo* recount how the revelation of the eternal return came to him on the background of the "yes-saying pathos *par excellence*" then "alive in me to the highest degree" (EH: 296; note that GS276 also refers to loving fate as being able to say yes to it, a point I shall comment upon later). The modality of this "being alive in me" of the "yes-saying pathos" is very similar to that of the "letting be" of amor fati: it suggests that Nietzsche's attitude was instrumental to the yes-saying "pathos" being alive, perhaps in the sense that he was self-aware enough to perceive its existence in him and offered it propitious conditions without which it would have died; yet the expression makes it clear that both the pathos and its life were neither generated nor controlled by Nietzsche himself.

This agapic interpretation is further suggested by the two following passages:

> Ten years—and nobody in Germany has felt bound in conscience to defend my name against the absurd silence under which it lies buried . . . . I myself have never suffered from all this; what is *necessary* does not hurt me; *amor fati* is my inmost nature. (EH: 325, Nietzsche's italics)
>
> What is most intimate in me teaches me that everything that is necessary, viewed from above and interpreted in the direction of a *superior* economy, is also useful per se—one needs not only bear it, but also *love* it. . . *Amor fati*: this is the bottom of my nature. (NCW: 680, Nietzsche's italics).

Amor fati is now presented in the first person, and not as an ideal but as a *realized* state ("my inmost nature," "the bottom of my nature"). Nietzsche does not offer any reasons to try to convince us of the desirability of loving fate, but a reflective description of how things appear to someone who is in such a state. This reflects his conviction that philosophy is a way of life rather than a theory about life: it has to be lived through to be genuinely understood. Significantly, the passage which explicitly links amor fati to the eternal return is introduced as follows: "philosophy, *as I have hitherto understood and lived it*. . . . Such a *philosophy as I live* . . . wants to cross over to a Dionysian affirmation of the world (etc.)" (WP §1041, my italics). It follows from this that the meaning of amor fati is not reducible to a pure conceptual content: it is inseparable from the first-person experiences that are both expressive of and governed by it.

This, however, makes the issue of genesis more acute. If amor fati cannot be rationally motivated or willed into existence, how will it come into being? Note that by virtue both of its irreducibility to a conceptual content and of the lack of rational justification for it, there cannot be any *de jure* answer to these questions, only empirical accounts such as the autobiographical observations made by Nietzsche about his own experience of amor fati. I shall now explore two possible ways that emerge from his writings. The first one is the eternal return, construed this time not as a thought experiment but as an imaginative and emotionally charged scenario meant to generate amor fati in a performative manner. The second, paradoxically, consists in the experience of suffering itself, understood under certain conditions. On this agapic reading, the eternal return should not be understood as a thought experiment meant to give us a standpoint from which we can rationally assess the value of our life and come to a decision, but as a poetic scenario that we are meant to enact imaginatively, in a way that reveals to us how we feel about our life in a single, potentially life-changing moment. This performative dimension of the eternal return is explicitly referred to by Nietzsche: "if this thought gained possession of you, it would *change you as you are* and perhaps crush you" (my italics). On such an interpretation, the eternal return has "disclosive force" (Hatab 2005: 99): the internalization of the scenario is *per se* an operator of existential change. In this respect, note that the possibility of a positive answer is introduced by a reference to the "*experience* of a tremendous moment" (my italics). In *Ecce Homo*, Nietzsche describes the revelatory power of such moments as follows: "with indescribable certainty and subtlety, something becomes visible, audible, something that shakes one to the last depths and throws one down." (EH: 300) Notice also that the demon does not start by asking a bare-faced question such as "would you want to live your life all over again?" (such as Clark's question: "would you want to marry me all over again?"). On the contrary, he presents us with a metaphorical and powerful description of what it might feel like for us to have this particular moment, "even this spider and this moonlight between the trees," recur. And significantly, the possible "answers" outlined are neither "yes" nor "no" but specific attitudes ("gnashing our teeth," being "crushed" or on the contrary becoming "well disposed to oneself and one's life"). While these may be seen as expressive of a propositional content, they do not state it and it would be difficult to construe them as conclusions reached through hypothetico-deductive reasoning. Correlatively, the yes-saying mentioned by GS341 should not be construed as a constative speech act (in this case an assertion), but in a performative way: just as the "yes" of the marriage vow both expresses our love and actualizes our commitment, in the same way, saying "yes" to the eternal return is not judging our life worth living again and again and assenting to what is entailed by that judgment, but committing ourselves to living in the light of that experience. Yet there is an important asymmetry between the "yes" of the marriage vow and the "yes" to the eternal return. While the first is fully up to us, the second comes to us (or not) at the peak of our imaginative internalization of the eternal return. Nietzsche makes this clear in his description of his own experience: "one hears, one does not seek; one accepts, one does not ask who gives; like lightning, a thought flashes up, with necessity" (EH: 300). Once more, the mediopassive modality typical of agapic love is in force: we can decide to "play the game" and take the scenario seriously (rather than inquire about its validity conditions), and how intensely we internalize it does matter, but we do not control the process and its outcome is not up to us.

Yet even if the commitment to amor fati did arise in us, there would seem to be an inherent fragility to it. It may be entirely sincere at the time it is made, and yet fade away once the rather dramatic conditions of its genesis have disappeared. The thought may "gain possession of us" in the paradoxical instant of our performative commitment, but can it retain its hold on us durably? Perhaps, but perhaps not. However there is another, possibly more durable way: suffering itself. Nietzsche offers a very rich, first-person phenomenology of suffering, and his narratives are both the expression and the illustration of the transfiguration of the negative which is characteristic of agapic love. Consider the following passage:

> Here it happened in a manner that I cannot admire sufficiently that, precisely at the right time, my father's *wicked* heritage came to my aid—at bottom, predestination to an early death. Sickness *detached me slowly*: . . . It bestowed on me the necessity of lying still, of leisure, of waiting and being patient—but that meant, of thinking. (EH: 287, Nietzsche's italics)

From an erotic standpoint, "predestination to an early death" would probably be one of the strongest possible objections to loving fate, and so would having the sort of sickness that may cause our death. Yet in Nietzsche's narrative, both are perceived as blessings ("in a manner that I cannot *admire* sufficiently . . . it *bestowed* on me . . ."). How is this agapic reversal possible? Three things are worth noting from the outset: first, not any suffering will do. Only protracted and intense suffering, an "icing up in the middle of youth," (GS: 32), that "long slow pain in which we are burned like green wood" (NCW: 680) may have a transfiguring effect. The reason is presumably that unless it is intense or long-lasting enough, the suffering will be discounted as an annoying but insignificant hindrance. And if it can be lessened, we are much more likely to seek any possible course of action (traditional or alternative medicines, surgery, etc.) that might bring about its decrease than to undergo an existential change. Our focus will be outward, not inward. By contrast, the need to "patiently resist a terrible, long pressure (. . . patiently, without submitting, but also without hope" (GS: 33) may open the possibility of loving fate for the sufferer. Secondly, should amor fati come to us, this would *not* mean the end of our pain: the sort of overcoming of suffering and of the self that Nietzsche describes does not involve moving to a painless state, an important point to which I shall come back. Finally, and importantly, note that just like that of agapic love, the modality of our relation to suffering is mediopassive: that we suffer is beyond our control, and there are limits to what we can do about it; yet crucially, we can to some extent influence the manner in which we exist our pain.

It is this ability to exist our pain in particular ways which opens up the possibility of fostering amor fati. This may sound paradoxical as it is by definition impossible to know in advance its shape or effects, and its advent is not within our control: so how can we prepare for it? Nietzsche's autobiographical reflections suggest that in response to suffering we can develop three features which are propitious to amor fati because they thwart the alternative existential possibilities which constantly threaten the sufferer, namely, self-pity, resignation, and self-deception. The first two of these features are courage and moral strength. Amor fati is not the outcome of a quietist attitude to suffering: on the contrary, Nietzsche remarks on the "long war such as I then waged with myself against the pessimism of weariness with life" (HH II: 212–3). Another passage refers the "ultimate, most joyous . . . yes to life' of amor fati to 'courage, and as a condition of that, an excess of strength" (EH: 272). Along the same lines, an unpublished passage about amor fati mentions "courage, severity towards oneself, cleanliness towards oneself" (WP §1041). These qualities are needed to counteract the rise of self-pity or nihilistic resignation. To my knowledge, Nietzsche does not say much about the first (although he has a lot to say about pity for others, none of it positive), perhaps because he does not seem to have experienced its temptation himself. Yet self-pity would make amor fati impossible for three reasons: first, it implies that one feels "hard done by" or treated in an unjust and undeserved manner. This, in turn, entails assumptions about providence (in particular, the idea that one should be treated in proportion to one's perceived merits) which Nietzsche finds both unwarranted and undesirable. Secondly, self-pity tends to divert our attention to favored alternative scenarios and thus to foster resentment toward the existing situation. Finally, it reveals deep existential limitations on the part of the sufferer, in particular the desire to protect oneself from pain at any cost without realizing that the most valuable things in human life can only come to us if we open ourselves up to the possibility of being hurt: "if you refuse to let your own suffering lie upon you even for an hour and if you constantly try to prevent and forestall any possible distress way ahead of time; if you experience suffering and displeasure as evil, hateful, worthy of annihilation, and as a defect of existence, then it is clear that besides your religion of pity you harbour . . . the religion of comfortableness. How little you know of human *happiness*" (GS: 269). Like the Last Men in *Zarathustra*, the self-pitier seeks to "move south" rather than risk hardship cultivating harsher lands. Yet it is only from such risks that higher human possibilities, including the "new kind of happiness" brought by amor fati, can arise.

Nietzsche is more explicit about resignation, which is presented as the antithesis of amor fati: "such an experimental philosophy as I live anticipates even the possibilities of the most fundamental nihilism: but this does not mean that it must halt at a negation, a No, a will to negation. It wants to cross over to the opposite of this . . .—my formula for this is amor fati" (WP §1041). For lack of space, I will not develop Nietzsche's arguments against Christianity or Schopenhauer; of more interest here is the thought that one must not "*halt*" at a negation. This can be understood as an allusion to his interpretation of Schopenhauer's position in the history of Western philosophy (he is supposed to have improved on the Christian world view by replacing the idea of a benevolent God with the will as doomed by its very structure to suffer endlessly). But it may also refer to a specific feature of Nietzsche's own experience of suffering, namely, the "Russian fatalism" described in *Ecce Homo.* Russian fatalism is a response to certain situations where the courage and strength of the sufferer find themselves overwhelmed by pain and sickness: "one cannot get rid of anything, one cannot get over anything . . . , everything hurts. Men and things obtrude too closely; experiences strike one too deeply; memory becomes a festering wound" (EH: 230). Such situations are bound to arise in the course of a long illness: suffering and powerlessness foster a greater sensitivity and vulnerability both to events and to people; one is hurt by details that the healthy do not even notice. One's memories of happier times, far from being comforting, become obsessive reminders of what was lost. The time comes when even the greatest courage and strength of mind must fail. In such times, the appropriate response is that of the "Russian soldier who, finding a campaign too strenuous, finally lies down in the snow. . . . . No longer to take anything, no longer to absorb anything—to cease reacting altogether" (ibid). Yet while this may look like a Schopenhauerian form of resignation (similar to the death by attrition sought by the ascetic), the function of such fatalism is the very opposite: "to preserve life under the most perilous conditions by reducing the metabolism" (ibid). Rather than being invaded and used up by negative reactions ("ressentiment, anger, pathological vulnerability, impotent lust for revenge"), it is best "not to react at all anymore" until one finds the courage and strength to measure oneself against one's pain in a way that transfigures both the suffering and the sufferer. Although it is meant to be discarded (perhaps to be adopted yet again later) as soon as our vitality is "rich and proud" again, Russian fatalism is thus a moving (and perhaps unexpected) acknowledgment of human finitude from Nietzsche's part. While, by definition, it prevents the sort of positive commitment of amor fati, it nevertheless fosters the right sort of attitude and can perhaps been seen as its precursor: "I displayed the 'Russian fatalism' I mentioned by tenaciously clinging for years to all but intolerable situations . . . . It was better than changing them, than *feeling* that they could be changed—than rebelling against them" (ibid).

The third feature that may encourage the birth of amor fati is the clarity of vision sometimes fostered in us by the need not to give up when faced with protracted suffering. This is rather paradoxical as pain is often said to cloud judgment. Yet should we display the courage and strength mentioned above, then suffering may prove itself to be the "ultimate liberator of the spirit (. . .) [that] forces us (. . .) to descend in our ultimate depths" (NCW: 680). In another passage, Nietzsche mentions the "supreme sobering up through pain" that is the means of "extricating [us] from the perilous world of fantasy" in which the healthy live (D: 69–70). As noted by moralists, suffering often strips human relations and events of their social trappings and reveals to us what matters most to us. "He who suffers intensely looks *out* at things with a terrible coldness: all those lying little charms which things are usually surrounded when the eye of the healthy regards them do not exist for him; indeed, he himself lies there before himself stripped of all colour and plumage" (ibid). Such clarity of mind is a defense against the mendaciousness of idealism or self-pity and thus may reinforce our courage in the face of suffering (by removing the temptation to dwell on alternatives). It is also per se a way to endure pain. For those who are strong enough, pain has a "spiritualising" effect: such individuals are able to overcome their native aversiveness to it by focusing on the increased lucidity that it may bring. Thus "the tremendous tension imparted to the intellect by its desire to oppose and counter pain makes him see everything he now beholds in a new light; and the unspeakable stimulus . . . is often sufficiently powerful to defy all temptation to self destruction" (ibid). Nietzsche lucidly points out that such awareness carries with it the danger of Faustian arrogance: "our pride towers as never before: it discovers an incomparable stimulus in opposing such a tyrant as pain is, and in answer to all the insinuations it makes to us that we should bear witness against life, in becoming precisely the *advocate of life* in the face of this tyrant" (D: 70). Yet for him such pride is preferable to resignation or self-pity in that it fosters a positive attitude toward this life: in this, it too can be seen as a precursor of amor fati, not because it conveys the right sort of understanding of fate, like Russian fatalism, but because of the commitment to life it denotes.

So how does one experience one's life if one has come to love fate, be it through an instantaneous, performative commitment to the eternal return or the long, difficult experience of suffering? To try to describe the experience of amor fati, one needs to focus on its main feature, the agapic bestowal of value. For Nietzsche, such bestowal is the correlate of a transfiguration of the self: "man becomes the transfigurer of existence when he learns to transfigure himself" (WP §821). As we have seen, suffering is instrumental to such "learning" because (in the best of cases) it helps us to develop the qualities (courage, strength, lucidity) which will allow us to overcome its adverse effects. The extent of the agapic transfiguration of existence is in direct proportion to the transformation of the self: "the tragic man affirms even the harshest suffering: he is sufficiently strong, rich and capable of deifying to do so. The Christian denies even the happiest lot on earth: he is sufficiently weak, poor, disinherited to suffer from life in whatever form he meets it" (WP §1052). Very importantly, such affirmation is not the assertion of a propositional content—it is perhaps best described as a commitment to living our lives in the light of our "deifying" love. Nor does it operate by holding in front of us the prospect of a life without any disorder, irrationality, or pain: this would only replicate the dichotomous structure of ascetic ideals by contrasting implicitly our currently wretched condition with a happy ever-after under the sway of amor fati. Whatever it does, agapic transfiguration does not work by ignoring the darker, chaotic, and irrational sides of human existence (which is perhaps why courage is so important in the fostering of amor fati). It does not diminish our aversiveness to pain, nor dispel the painful character of our more difficult experiences; yet through an existential transformation that makes us stronger and "more profound," it somehow enables us to love these experiences as fated, and this in spite of the suffering they cause us. This is not tantamount to recapturing them within the sort of eroticizing, providential narrative criticized in GS277. No justification or reasons are involved at all: we feel the pain that attaches to such experiences but find ourselves able to love them *nevertheless,* without holding them as objections to life. As Zarathustra says, "we love life, not because we are used to living, but because we are used to loving" (Z: 68). Amor fati, like Angelus Silesius' rose, has no why.

Yet amor fati is not only characterized by the ability to transfigure one's own suffering; it is also a positive state. Nietzsche indicates that "a full and powerful soul not only copes with painful, even terrible losses, deprivations, . . .; it emerges from such hells with a greater fullness and powerfulness; and most essential of all, with a new increase in the blissfulness of love" (WP §352). How is such an "increase" experienced? Another passage indicates that from the "abysses" of suffering, one returns "newborn, more ticklish and malicious, with a more delicate taste for joy, . . . with merrier senses . . . more childlike and yet a *hundred times subtler than before*" (GS: 37, my italics). The increased strength, sensitivity, and lucidity brought upon us by suffering do not disappear with the pain itself. They remain with us and transform our perception, not just of suffering, but of our whole life. We experience the "happiness which could only be invented by a man who was suffering continually" (GS: 110). We become more attentive and do not take anything for granted: the "smallest, tenderest, most fleeting moments life gives us" (HH II: 213) now stand out, and we delight in the little nuances and details we would not have noticed before. To those who "love life, it seems that butterflies and soap bubbles, and whatever is like them among men, know most about happiness" (Z: 68). We experience a constant sense of gratitude. Our demands on existence are much more modest; we know the "happiness of eyes that have seen the sea of existence become calm, and now they can never weary of the surface and of the many hues of this tender, shuddering skin of the sea" (GS: 110).

In this paper, I have tried to shed some light on the oft-mentioned but rarely discussed notion of amor fati. I have identified two central paradoxes (love of fate requires us to love a negative object, and we are supposed to achieve it knowing that our love will not make any difference to its object) and outlined two possible ways of understanding such love (erotic and agapic). I have developed the second in the light of the mediopassive modality used by Nietzsche in relation to amor fati, which, like the middle voice in ancient Greek, signals that love of fate is an existential attitude which requires our participation but which does not fully depend on us. On such an agapic construal, the modality of Nietzsche's remarks on amor fati is descriptive; his comments about the value of suffering are not meant as arguments to convince us that fate is lovable and thus trigger a quasi-Platonic ascent of love, but as observations made from the perspective of someone who already experiences amor fati. Importantly, this agapic construal of amor fati solves *both* the above paradoxes: loving a negative object is not a problem since agapic love is not dependent on the previously apprehended value of its object: furthermore, such value is positively transformed by the love itself. Secondly, while our love may not make any difference to the unfolding of fate which was not already preincluded in the latter (our loving fate, if it happens, is part of that fate itself), it will make a substantial difference to *us*. Our perception of the events that befall us (and of ourselves) will be greatly transformed. As we saw, this existential transformation will in turn allow us a sort of happiness which neither resignation nor rebellion could ever bring us. We experience "an equilibrium and composure in the face of life and even a sense of gratitude towards it" (HH II: 212–3). Although this cannot count as a motivation for loving fate (since this would be subscribing to the erotic logic which, as we have seen, ultimately fails), it is enough to rebut the objection that such a love is pointless.

By way of conclusion, I now wish to discuss a number of objections. The first two concern, one way or another, the limitations of human agape, and the fourth its status as an ideal. To begin with, consider that in Luther's version the transfigurative powers of divine love are infinite; there is nothing, past, present, or future, that God's love cannot redeem. But is such a love humanly possible? I may think that I can genuinely transform my whole life: but how do I know that I am not self-deceived about the extent of my powers? Self-deception is a notoriously problematic topic in that it is equally hard to describe the phenomenon appropriately and to present a coherent account of the psychological factors that supposedly make it possible. In fact, the difficulty is such that some are inclined to deny its existence altogether (in which case, however, there would be no objection to answer here). Furthermore, the sort of description and explanation available varies considerably depending on how weak or strong the cases envisaged are: instances of weak self-deception are very close to wishful thinking in that they can be construed as requiring no self-deceptive intent and no violation of our normal epistemic standards. The subject, although he is motivated by a negative affect, has no intention to deceive himself and does not know that he is doing it.[3] By contrast, strong cases are sometimes said to exhibit both an intention to deceive oneself (although it does not take the self-defeating form of a conscious choice) and a failure of reflective self-knowledge. Without entering into these debates, it seems possible to describe amor fati as a case of self-deception operating along the following steps (artificially separated for the sake of clarity): (1) faced with the experience of pain or suffering, which I see as a consequence of my fate, (2) I experience a negative affective response to the latter (such as anger, resentment, or hatred). This negative affect is in itself painful because it expresses an unpleasant truth about myself or my situation—hinting perhaps at my powerlessness in the face of my fate, my inability to cope with it, or at weaknesses in my character such as self-pity or cowardice. (3) In order to prevent this painful secondary affect and what it expresses from coming to reflective awareness, I deceive myself into believing that I love my fate. This instrumentally adopted belief allows me to think that I envision my pain in a positive light and that I am genuinely endowed with the sort of virtues which I wish to have (e.g., being a strong, generous and powerful individual who is capable of overcoming pain). (4) The whole process is made possible by the fact that neither my negative secondary affect nor my motivation to deceive myself is reflectively available to me at the time.

It would seem hard to deny that although it is not without difficulties, this model has some intuitive plausibility. Cast in the light of self-deceptive intent, the eroticizing narrative presented by GS277 could be seen precisely as the sort of rationale we might unwittingly use to persuade ourselves of our love for fate, and conversely that our fate is loveable at the scale of our whole life.[4] However, it does not follow from the fact that self-deception is possible that it is necessary. To go back to the original objection, it is certainly the case that we would have to be mistaken or more likely self-deluded if amor fati required of us that we should literally transform our whole lives, including our past. As human finitude precludes us from doing this, loving our fate would turn out to be an impossible task and we could only convince ourselves to have achieved it through sustained illusion or self-deception. But as we saw, such a radical ability is *not* required by amor fati: what is at stake is an existential transformation of the self and of our relation to our present (rather than our past). So just as there is no principle ground to rule out self-deception, in the same way there is no a priori reason to deem such self-transfiguration impossible. In cases of genuine amor fati, there would be no need for self-deception because we would be transformed in such a way that step (2) would simply not present itself: the agapic transfiguration of our aversiveness to pain would prevent the secondary negative affect from forming, and without it there would be no motivation for the rest of the process to take place.

Given that self-deception is not a necessity, let us grant that amor fati is, at least in principle, possible. This, however, raises a second difficulty, which concerns its sustainability over the course of a human life. Even if one grants that it can be agapic (in the modified sense above) and that it needs not involve self-deception, the question remains of the extent to which it can hold sway on us. Nietzsche clearly thought that he did experience it, and this seems evidenced in some of his writings. Yet his moving remarks about Russian fatalism also make it clear that he did not think that he himself was able to sustain amor fati all his life. We saw that it requires us to develop certain qualities (such as courage, moral strength, and lucidity), which may appear in response to the various challenges that life throws at us, in particular suffering, and evolve in proportion to the intensity of our ordeals. Yet there is no guarantee that we shall find it in ourselves to be equal to *all* the sufferings that may come to us. We cannot rule out the prospect of being faced with an ordeal that we *cannot* love, not for want of trying, but simply because it is beyond our strength. Russian fatalism may aid us to a point but there may come a time when all that is left to us, all the strength we can muster, is the "courage to die" (EH: 230). The courage to die, yes, but perhaps not that of loving the approach of our own death. Ultimately, amor fati may, as in Luther's description of *agape* (although for different reasons) turn out to be a "lost love (*verlorene Liebe*) . . . and the kindness thrown away." Like all human loves, it may wither and die, no matter how hard we try to keep our commitment to it—a significant dysanalogy with divine agape. This, however, needs not be seen as an objection against amor fati. The key is to note that it could only count as such on the romantic assumption that the most appropriate kind of love for us is a love that would overcome all obstacles, vanquish death, and last forever after. Yet this is precisely the sort of mendacious idealism that Nietzsche repudiates. For all his talk of the Overman (or perhaps because of it . . .), and like all those who have suffered considerably in their lives (Pascal comes to mind), he is keenly aware of the limitations of the human condition. Seen in this light, the fact that amor fati may not last forever simply reflects the fact that it is the love of finite beings, and is not a reason to reject it because of unrealistic and undesirable requirements. It may or may not come to us; we may not be able to sustain it forever. But if and while we have it, it saves us from bitterness and resentment as well as from Schopenhauerian resignation. Its redemptive powers may not be infinite, but they are the best we can hope for.

The final objection concerns the status of amor fati as an ideal. The previous acknowledgment of its limits does not detract anything from its desirability; but is loving fate the right thing to do when it comes to morally challenging situations? In particular, what about the suffering of others? Especially that of the people who are dear to us? Is *that* something that we should love as fated? In this respect, two things are worth noting: first, just as the agapic loving of our own suffering is not an exercise in masochism (our aversiveness to pain does not disappear), in the same way the potential love of the suffering of others should not be interpreted as a sadistic relishing of their pain: in neither case would we derive any pleasure from the loving, and both present us with a very significant challenge. Secondly, there are reasons to think that Nietzsche envisaged amor fati in the first person, as a suitable response to what befalls *us*, not others.[5] He did not say that we could (or should) love the fate of others. Nor does loving one's fate logically entail loving the fate of other people: love is not necessarily transitive (although it can be so, at least up to a point, e.g., if our love for someone extends, in time, to individuals this person cherishes). Common experience shows that we can perfectly well love someone or something without loving all the circumstances that made them what they are, nor everything that will happen to them in the future. In fact, our very love is likely to make us deplore the events that harmed or may harm those we love, and no one would deem our attachment less true for that. So while loving my fate does entail my being strong enough to love even the pain that it brings me, it does not commit me to loving the suffering of others, even though there may sometimes be a direct causal link between the pain I feel and the suffering they endure (e.g., if I am deeply saddened because someone I love is seriously ill): I can try to love my fate, hard as that may be, without loving theirs, even though my fate is necessarily linked to theirs.

Yet the objection can be reformulated in a way that makes it relevant even to this first-person perspective. There may be occasions when our feelings of anger or powerlessness in the face of the suffering of those we love will oppress us to such a degree that it will simply seem impossible (and even indecent) to us to love a fate that put us in such a position. This connects to an objection which is often made in relation to the eternal return: to will the recurrence of all things entails willing the return of some of the most abhorrent events in human history, and this may be seen as morally unacceptable. What then? One possible reply is to emphasize once more the mediopassive mode specific to amor fati. Whereas willing the return of morally repellent events is fully within our power, whether we love fate is not. Because of this deep asymmetry between willing and loving, the issues of moral responsibility and choice do not arise in the same way: we are not accountable for our love in the way we are for a decision. Yet this mediopassive feature of amor fati cuts both ways: while we cannot start or stop loving at will, the previous analyses have shown that we still have a part to play in fostering amor fati. So the question can be rephrased: not should we love fate, since this is not up to us, but should we try to *foster* such love? I can think of two answers, one of which is Nietzschean in spirit and the other, not. The first consists in pointing out that should we prove strong or lucid enough to try to foster love for our anger or powerlessness, and should amor fati arise in us, then the agapic nature of such love would transfigure the formerly negative value of such feelings. The situation itself would be perceived in a totally new light. How it would be then experienced is impossible for us to determine so long as we have not undergone a similar existential transformation ourselves.[6] Yet the important point is that arguing against the desirability of agapic love in the name of our existing conception of morality presupposes precisely the standpoint that would be invalidated by the transfiguration of values resulting from such a love. Our current moral repugnance is the very thing that amor fati would overcome and is thus no decisive objection to it. The other, non-Nietzschean, answer would consist in resisting this agapic logic and holding that it is not desirable in principle that certain things, such as powerlessness in the face of the suffering of the people that are dear to us, should come to be loved. One would then need to clarify the source and type of normativity entailed by this claim (what would ground such a principle? A robust conception of human nature? A substantive commitment to objective, universal values?) and it is not difficult to think of Nietzschean arguments against this sort of reply and endeavor. I cannot enter into this debate here but should one wish to uphold the objection, then one thing to note is that the very defeasibility of amor fati, the fact that there are empirical situations that may be beyond our power to love, may then come to be seen not simply as the unavoidable consequence of our human finitude but as a moral advantage. It may be construed not simply as expressive of the limits of our strength, but as a safeguard against the dangers of the potential excesses of love.

Notes and references

1 These have largely to do with what I have called the "motivational gap" between loving and willing. See B. Han-Pile, "Nietzsche and Amor Fati," *European Journal of Philosophy*.

2 There is a large amount of secondary literature on the middle voice, and the one thing scholars seem to agree on is that it is a very elusive notion (cf. e.g., Andersen 2004: 10: "there are as many definitions of voice or diathesis as there are theoretical frameworks in the relevant literature," S. Kemmer 1993: 1: "there is no generally accepted definition of the middle voice"). One of the reasons for this is that the Greek themselves did not elaborate on the matter. Andersen notes that the first grammar to use the three categories is a work attributed to Dionysios of Thrax. He focused on the opposition between active performance (*energeia*) and passive experience (*pathos*) and introduced *mesothes* as an intermediate category that applies to verbs that have a grammatical form which does not fit in either of the two previous ones (e.g., active verbs with a passive ending, such as deponents). Roman grammarians, in particular the Stoa (Zeno of Citium, the founder of the Stoic school) reappropriated this active/passive distinction by referring it to agency. Current grammar manuals of ancient Greek emphasize that the middle voice refers to actions that the subject performs on or for himself. See, for example, Smyth's *Greek Crammar* (Cambridge: Harvard University Press, 1956, §1713): "the middle voice shows that the action is performed with special reference to the subject: *loumai* (I wash myself)." Such actions often involve an ambiguous form of agency, neither fully active nor fully passive, as one is both the agent and the recipient of the action. Benvéniste (1966: 172 sq) and Gonda (1960: 30–67) picked up on this particular feature of the middle voice. According to the first, the middle voice does not so much indicate that the subject has an interest in the action as it points toward the fact that s/he is the medium in which something takes place. It indicates that the subject is part of a process (expressed by the verb) to which s/he participates but which is not reducible to such participation. To emphasize this dimension, he introduced the notion of internal diathesis (as opposed to the external diathesis of the active mode, in which the subject accomplishes an action which is under his control and carried out outside of him. For a useful account of the various conceptions of the middle voice, see Eberhard (2004), in particular: 'The middle voice from a Linguistic Perspective' and 'Philosophical Perspectives on the Middle Voice' (pp. 7–31).

3 See for example Mele's self labeled 'deflationary' account (Mele 1997: 91 sq). A standard example is that of the anxious husband whose anxiety and desire to be reassured about his marriage cause him to disregard potential evidence of deceitful behavior from his wife and to over-interpret elements in her conduct that may assuage his worries. For a criticism of this interpretation of self-deception, see Poellner 2004: 54–7.

4 And so could, more polemically, Nietzsche's reconstruction of his own life previously quoted in EH: 287.

5 Thus *all* the seven excerpts which mention amor fati do so in the first person. While one of them seems to envisage fate from a general perspective (WP §1041), the last two published passages (in *The Case of Wagner* and *Nietzsche contra Wagner*) strongly suggest that Nietzsche is talking about the love of his own fate, and the remaining quotes can be understood either way. On balance I have made the interpretive choice to emphasise the first person and am well aware of its theoretical costs, in particular the exacerbated tension with Nietzsche's claim in WP §1041 that the whole world must be affirmed as it is; note, however, that the passage refers to an *affirmation* (not love) of the world which is connected to amor fati but not identified with it. It could also be suggested that this was an unpublished observation and that affirmation, contrary to love, is transitive in nature (e.g.: I cannot affirm a proposition as true and deny its implications). On the first person reading of amor fati, what "fate" picks out is *existential* (rather than metaphysical) necessity, for example the perceived ineluctability of what happens to me from a personal standpoint rather than the interconnectedness of all things, which by contrast is emphasised by the eternal return. Still, for those who wish to reject this first person focus, then note that the Nietzschean rebuttal of the ethical objection suggested on p. 230 would apply in either case.

6 One may find examples in the writings of Christian mystics: under the sway of agapic love, powerlessness is welcomed as a reminder of our dependency on God. Anger is transformed into gratitude. Examples of such agapic transfigurations are not rare: see Saint John of the Cross: "oh that it may be perfectly understood how the soul cannot attain to the thicket and wisdom of the richness of God, which are of many kinds, save by entering in to the thicket of many kinds of suffering, and by setting thereupon its consolation and desire." (in Katz 1983: 49); see also Meister Eckhart: "if my suffering is in God and God is suffering with me, how then can suffering be sorrow to me" (in Sells 1994: 176) and Teresa of Avila (1957: 113): "yet at the same time this pain is so sweet, and the soul is so conscious of its value, that it now desires this suffering more than all the gifts that it used to receive." While the resulting values may not be what Nietzsche has in mind, the sort of transfiguration performed is exactly what is entailed by the structure of amor fati. On the relation between Nietzsche and Christian mystics, see Roberts 1998, chapter 6.

References

List of abbreviations

a) For Nietzsche's works

BT *The Birth of Tragedy*, trans. W. Kaufmann. New York: Vintage, 1967.

PT *Philosophy and Truth: Selection from Nietzsche's Notebooks of the Early 1870's*, trans. D. Breazeale. London: Humanity Books, 1999.

UM *Untimely Meditations,* trans. R. J. Hollingdale. Cambridge: Cambridge University Press, 1997.

HH *Human, All Too Human,* trans. R. J. Hollingdale. Cambridge: Cambridge University Press, 1996.

D *Daybreak,* trans. R. J. Hollingdale. Cambridge: Cambridge University Press, 1997.

GS *Gay Science,* trans. W. Kaufmann. New York: Vintage, 1974.

BGE *Beyond Good and Evil,* trans W. Kaufmann. New York: Vintage, 1989.

Z *Thus Spake Zarathustra,* trans. R. J. Hollingdale. London: Penguin, 1969.

TI *Twilight of the Idols,* trans. R. J. Hollingdale. London: Penguin,1968.

EH *Ecce Homo,* trans. W. Kaufmann. New York: Vintage, 1990.

NW *Nietzsche Contra Wagner,* in *The Portable Nietzsche,* translated and edited by W. Kaufmann. London: Penguin, 1968.

WP *The Will to Power,* trans. W. Kaufmann. New York: Vintage, 1968.

K *Kröners Taschenausgabe.* Stuttgart: Alfred Kröner Verlag, 1956 (2 volumes) (the translations of KSA and K included in this paper are mine).

KSA *Nachgelassene Fragmente.* Berlin: Walter de Gruyter, 1978.

SL *Selected Letters of Friedrich Nietzsche,* transl. C. Middleton. Indianapolis: Hackett, 1996.

b) For Schopenhauer's works

WWR *The World as Will and Representation,* transl. E. F. J. Payne, New York: Dover, 1958. Volume I contains the original text, and volume II the Supplements.

Other works

Andersen, P. K. (2004), *Empirical Studies in Diathesis.* Münster: Nodus Publikationen.
Benvéniste, E. (1956), *Problèmes de Linguistique Générale I.* Paris: Gallimard.
Cicero, *De Fato,* http://www.thelatinlibrary.com/cicero/fato.shtml.
Eberhard, P. (1982), *Middle Voice in Gadamer's Hermeneutics.* Tübingen: Paul Mohr Verlag.
Frede, D. (2003), "Stoic Determinism," in B. Inwood (ed.), *The Cambridge Companion to Stoicism.* Cambridge: Cambridge University Press, pp. 179–206.
Gonda (1960), "Reflections on the Indo-European Medium." *Lingua* 9/4: 233–52.
Hatab, L (2005), *Nietzsche's Life Sentence: Coming to Terms with the Eternal Recurrence.* London: Routledge.
Katz, S. (1983), *Mysticism and Religious Traditions.* Oxford: Oxford University Press.
Leiter, B. (2001), "The Paradox of Fatalism and Self Creation in Nietzsche," in B. Leiter and J. Richardson (eds), *Nietzsche* (Oxford Readings in Philosophy). Oxford: Oxford University Press.

Long, A. and Sedley, D. (1987), *The Hellenistic Philosophers*, volume 1. Cambridge: Cambridge University Press.
Magnus, B. (1978), *Nietzsche's Existential Imperative*. Bloomington: Indiana University Press.
Mele, A. (1997), "Real Self-Deception." *Behavioral and Brain Sciences* 20: 91–102.
Nehamas, A. (1985), *Nietzsche: Life as Literature*. Cambridge: Harvard University Press.
Poellner, P. (2004), "Self-Deception, Consciousness and Value," in D. Zahavi (ed.), *Hidden Resources*, special issue of the *Journal for Consciousness Studies*, pp. 10–11, 44–65.
Reginster, B. (2006), *The Affirmation of Life: Nietzsche on Overcoming Nihilism*. Cambridge: Harvard University Press.
Roberts, T. (1998), *Contesting Spirit: Nietzsche, Affirmation, Religion*. Princeton, NJ: Princeton University Press.
Sells, M. (1994), *Mystical Languages of Unsaying*. Chicago: Chicago University Press.
Stambaugh, J. (1994), *The Other Nietzsche*. New York: SUNY Press.
Teresa of Avila, (2004), *The Life of Saint Teresa by Herself*. New York: Penguin.

17

"Not to Destroy, but to Fulfill"

Eli Friedland

It is tempting, with Nietzsche, to be drawn—dazzled, puzzled, or simply perplexed—toward his visions of future human possibilities and to lose sight of what is close at hand; that is, to the conditions of the present which must be worked with if future possibilities are to be achieved. Nietzsche himself, especially with his *Zarathustra*, understood this temptation only too well. Indeed, in *Ecce Homo*, he writes of "forcing" his eye to focus on the "nearest things, the present time," in *Beyond Good and Evil*,[1] which is why that book is the necessary counterpart to the visionary *Zarathustra*.

This is not to say that in *Zarathustra*, Nietzsche presents the achievement of a future spiritual transfiguration as *ex nihilo*, or from some *tabula rasa*. We might think here of Zarathustra's repeated metaphors of the human being as a continuity, as "a bridge," for example (*Z* Prologue 4; III.12.2), and as a "rope, fastened between beast and Overhuman—a rope over an abyss./A dangerous across, a dangerous-on-the-way, a dangerous looking back, a dangerous shuddering and standing still" (Prologue 4).[2] What happens when one *leaps over* the human on the rope (the rope that he also *is*) is illustrated to Zarathustra by the jester, on his first day in the Motley Cow (Prologue 6). And while Zarathustra's longing for the "Overhuman" may indeed, at this early point, have serious affinities with the impatient destruction of that jester—who sends the "human" falling to his death when he leaps over him on the tightrope—it is crucially important to the drama of *Zarathustra* that he only achieves his own highest hope by coming to deeply understand and experience the purely destructive foolishness of attempting to achieve the future by leaping over the present. Thus the wiser, almost-convalescent Zarathustra of the third book will still insist that "the human is something that must be overcome," but he immediately appends this consideration:

> There are many different paths and ways of overcoming – look *you* to them! But only a jester thinks: "The human can also be *overjumped*." (Z III. 12. 4)

What is implied in this transformation of Zarathustra's own understanding is that *therapy*, and not some "great leap forward," for example, is fundamental to his sense of overcoming the present human. Just because the human "is a bridge" and "a rope," the overcoming of the human, all-too human is a process that can only be achieved by its continued attachment to the possibilities and proclivities of the present human condition. And this means that the new health toward which Nietzsche the physician and therapist is pointing can only be understood in its necessary relation to the entire bridge over the abyss, including especially its foundation in the starting side. Our perceptions, whether of new or of old "tablets," are value-laden and always-evaluating accesses to the world—and are our *only* accesses to the world—one cannot abstract from the drives and necessities of one's being in the act of "perceiving." Paths of therapeutic transfiguration therefore depend fundamentally on the material that is at hand to be transfigured, regardless if the transfigurative genius himself would be able to work with almost any material he had at his disposal (cf. *Dawn* 8 with 540; and 38). As St Bernard tells the pilgrim Dante, a good tailor must "fit the dress he makes to cloth he has" (Dante, *Paradiso* 32.140–1).[3]

In what follows, I hope to gesture at some of the important continuities with the past that Nietzsche uses in his attempt to open on to his "philosophy of the future." In particular, I want to highlight those continuities with respect to the concepts and practices of Christianity, as they have unfolded over two millennia, in order to suggest that Nietzsche's "anti-Christianity" is very far from a naïve attempt to abandon the deep psychophysiological drives that have informed—and that continue to inform—the religious consciousness that requires the Christian moral and metaphysical dispensation. Indeed, Nietzsche does with respect to Christianity what Jesus said with respect to Judaism: "I come not to destroy the law, but to fulfill it" (Matt. 5:17). And it is through that fulfillment that his therapeutic transfiguration of those drives hopes to open the future to new possibilities.

What this means is that Nietzsche intended the interpretation of his published writings to have therapeutic consequences in and of itself (a lesson from Plato). To borrow the words of another scholar, from another context, Nietzsche's books, like Plato's, are not "book[s] of whose content one can merely take cognizance without undergoing a change."[4] Attending to Nietzsche's deliberate appeal to Christian consciousness opens new interpretive possibilities for his deliberately difficult (*BGE* 27, *WS* 71. *D* Preface 5) "written and painted thoughts" (*BGE* 296), possibilities whose consideration both require and at the same time assist in enacting a transformation in his careful reader (cf. *WS* 87). This is of course not to suggest that there is anything automatically therapeutic about reading Nietzsche: as with any therapy, one must work very hard and take it very seriously.

Obviously, I cannot provide here a full exploration of this therapeutic effort. Instead, I will limit myself to drawing out some oft-overlooked affinities between Nietzsche's most important symbols, and Christianity's, with the hope of laying some groundwork for a new and fruitful approach to Nietzsche's therapy. Implied in this approach is a profound affinity between Nietzsche and his greatest philosophical rival (and greatest friend), Plato, with respect to their understandings of the mimetic nature of the human animal. Within this understanding, one would not expect an "ideal" described to be achieved, but rather, through its engagement with existing "dispositions and capacities for representation/imitation (*mimêsesi*)" (Plato, *Laws* 655d3), to excite and partially direct new self-transfigurations whose results are necessarily open-ended, multiple, and not entirely predictable. One would not, for example, expect the figure of the

Übermensch or Zarathustra to "produce" replicas of Zarathustra, just as one would not expect the Christian figure of Jesus to produce Jesus's, nor the Homeric Achilles to produce Achilles's.

For this reason, we should note that this is not something that can be genuinely approached from a strictly analytic point of view. Even in terms of terminology, Nietzsche's use of words and grammar is always essentially transformative (open-endedly transforming the terminology he uses), so to reduce what he supposedly said to a static description—however precise—will always miss the most important aspects of his efforts. The dual nature of the Socratic question that opens the *Phaedrus* must be continually attended to in Nietzsche's therapeutics (and indeed, this is precisely why his work *is* therapeutic): "Where *to*, and where *from*?" (227a1: *poi dê kai pothen?*). There are a number of terms in Nietzsche's work that are extremely difficult to fully grasp without undergoing a profoundly transformative experience—transformative of both oneself *and* the meaning of the term. This sentence can, and should, be taken in both of its senses: on the one hand, if one *does* come to grasp these terms, that in itself will lead to such an experience; on the other hand, one needs to experience such a self-transformation *in order* to fully grasp what Nietzsche is doing with these terms. This suggests a paradox, but fortunately, being human, what we can only describe in paradoxical terms is very often something we can live—indeed often cannot help but live—in a seamless (which does not mean an easy) way.

What does it mean to fulfill in order to go beyond—to go beyond *by* fulfilling? In the first place, we must understand that no one is "free" to have or not have a belief. A belief is a sign, a symptom of what "the great reason of the body (*Leib*)," to use Zarathustra's term (*Z* 1.4), is *doing*—it is not an independent conceptual structure for which an "individual" is "responsible." A belief may in some sense organize and direct behavioral conditions for those whom the belief *has* (*sic*), but it neither organizes nor directs (except into limited conscious expression) the fundamental psychophysiological requirements and capacities that lie beneath and give rise to that belief in the first place (what Aristotle called the *hypokeimenon*). A belief, to say the very least, is merely the tip of an iceberg. And while that tip may be in plain sight, it is not for that reason in control.

This is why a merely rational refutation of a belief, for example (as heard all too frequently from modern zealous atheists), simply cannot suffice to transfigure how we experience life and why. And this is also why any genuine process of cultural transfiguration is a project of *centuries* (*HH* 1.450), involving and requiring a slow shift in the deep structure of language, thought, desiring, expectations, and goals[5]—a shift that must at one and the same time *fulfill* the psychophysiological requirements of nihilistic consciousness (one could also call this Paulist consciousness), *and* accomplish by so doing what we might call a persuasive redirection of its psychic momentum. "Great politics," as Nietzsche conceives it, is cultural therapy, not the immediate problem-solving that "politics" has largely been reduced to today (*HH* 1.438, 449).

The philosophers who take this task in hand—and for Nietzsche, taking this "difficult, unwanted, unrefusable task" in hand *just is* philosophy (*BGE* 212)[6]—will "employ the preparatory work of *all* philosophical laborers, *all* subduers of the past.

With creative hands they reach towards the future, and *everything that is or has existed* becomes their means, their tool, their hammer" (*BGE* 211, my emphases; and cf. *BGE* 61). And clearly, "everything that is or has existed" now includes, in a major way, Christianity.

The first point that we should note, then, is that the three "major" transfigurative moves in Nietzsche's writings are all signified with profoundly Christian terms (which most Christians, especially those who do not read German, may not immediately recognize). These are: the *Übermensch* (Overhuman—often mistranslated as "superman"), *ewige Wiederkunft/kehr* (eternal recurrence/return), and *Wille zur Macht* ("will to power"). The words Nietzsche uses to name these moves are all standard German translations of Greek and Latin words, the discourse and debate about which have defined what it is to be Christian. In the ecclesiastical literature, the Greek *hyperanthrôpos*—directly translated into German as *Übermensch*—very often refers to Jesus himself (especially in the Orthodox tradition); the expected "second coming" of Christ is, in German, *Wiederkunft/kehr Christi*—though the "translated" Greek word is *parousia* (presence); and "will"—*Wille*—is a crucial Christian conception that grounds "original sin," beginning with (but not ending with) Augustine, who uses the Latin terms *voluntas* and *arbitrium*.

In strictly Christian terms, then, these are words often used to discuss Christ,[7] his return as savior and redeemer, and the Roman Catholic doctrine of original sin (which fundamentally depends upon the notion of "will"). It is extremely difficult to believe that Nietzsche, especially with his theological and philological education, could have been unaware of this, and we must therefore consider why he used these terms to name what were, for him, transfigurative movements *beyond* Christianity.

Of course, linguistic affinities are not negligible in their consequences, but without deeper structural affinities, they cannot alone suffice. Nevertheless, before turning to the "deeper" level, we must take note of a particular strategy at the level (itself already deep) of language: Nietzsche is claiming a space for the redefinition of the words he uses by creating irresolvable debate about "doctrines" in his work that employ those words, doctrines *that are not there*. The point is not to defend the doctrines, but to let a debate *about* them redefine the words (cf. *BGE* 4 with 18; Horace, *Ars poetica* 69–72). This is a lesson he learned from Plato, whose supposed doctrines of the "Forms/Ideas," immortality of the "soul," etc., simply are not present *as doctrines* in the Platonic dialogues. Similarly, there is in fact no consistent *doctrine* of eternal recurrence, of will to power, or of an *Übermensch* to be found in Nietzsche's published work. But there are powerful impetuses to suggest that there are, and to provoke both advocacy *and* refutation, subtle interpretation *and* less thoughtful doctrinal adherence. The debate that is thereby stimulated, and not some decisive interpretation attained therein, is everything in this regard (cf. *BGE* 18, and its implications for *BGE* 19). In the *activity* of that debate, the terms that initially define and confine it can come to be redefined—revalued—themselves. For historical examples, one may think of the long debate opened by Augustine's notion of "will" (*arbitrium* or *voluntas*), and how it eventually eclipsed the previous meanings of the terms he used; as well as the debate opened by Plato's reimagining of the "soul" (*psuchê*), and how it eventually transformed the Homeric sense of the same word. For contemporaries of Augustine and of Plato, their new conceptualizations presented the difficulties of understanding. But for we moderns, it is the more ancient conceptualizations that are difficult—if not almost impossible—to grasp.

This is, of course, the point of such a strategy, a strategy that deliberately invites contemporary confusion in order to therapeutically shape a future human consciousness in its crucible. Perhaps better: in order to provoke and direct (in a limited way) a *self*-shaping of future consciousness. *Not* an "opposition" of one concept to another, both having the same name, but the intensification and spiritualization of the highest possibilities of the present concept in the future understanding.[8] And this strategy at the level of words and concepts is likewise deployed by Nietzsche in his broader "polemics," including those directed against Christianity in general.

It has been noted, by Foucault among others, that a polemic is defined by what it is a polemic *against*. And this is most certainly true. But we harbor a hope—and Nietzsche knows this—that what is implied in this realization is that one might somehow, some day, achieve a point at which one escapes the "against" completely. For lack of a better word, let us call this aspiration "freedom" (please note the quotation marks). This is not, however, what Nietzsche means. For Nietzsche, the polemic remains permanently, though its status in our consciousness can change. Whatever we are able to overcome through a polemic, in Nietzsche's sense of both words, becomes part of the bedrock of our consciousness, part of the "deep-down stupidity (*Dummheit*)" that structures—that alone *allows* a structure for—the flourishing of new life and life-possibilities (cf. Graham Parkes' chapter in this volume). Every such battle is permanently preserved and will not cease to inform who we are. Thus, for example, Homer's moral and religious dispensation remains a part of western Europeans, despite (and because of) Plato's victory over that dispensation. Likewise, Nietzsche's aspirations for victory over Plato's dispensation in no way include a fruitless annihilation thereof. This *a fortiori* applies as well to that most notorious of Nietzsche's "Platonic enemies," Christianity. Nietzsche has no hope or desire that Christianity might or should be "overcome" *in Christianity's sense of the word* (i.e., an ultimate purging from the universe, physical and metaphysical, of the polemicized principle—the final triumph of "good" over "evil," or "evil" over "good"), as such a desire would preserve in deed what it opposes in word—just as the Manichaean dualism that came to so characterize Western Christianity crept into it through Augustine's very efforts to refute and refuse it. By the very act of opposing Manichaeism itself as an evil doctrine (as, e.g., in *Confessions* 8.10.22) as compared to a "true" one, Augustine cemented the very dualism that he was attempting to deny—in Christian terms, one could say that the flesh of his argument is willing, but the spirit weak. In more Nietzschean terms, Augustine *said* No to Manichaeism, but *did* Yes.

What is the consciousness with which, and upon which, the philosopher must work? It is the ramifications of this question that almost break Zarathustra, for it requires accepting and *affirming* the very meagerness of human reality—the "All-too-small" and "All-too-human" reality of even the greatest human beings (*Z* 3.13). He must *love* this all-too-human smallness, must *love* what he despises, must *love* his enemy.[9] Only as such—only, that is, by fulfilling this Christian principle too—can he overcome *his own* nihilistic, Paulinian "loathing for all existence" (ibid), a loathing that makes *his* greatness too "all-too-small." To go beyond Christianity, Zarathustra must become the first Christian, and this is his tragic moment *par excellence*, the moment of realizing and celebrating himself as a *fate*—as a *Christian* fate. Without doing so, his own seeming opposition to modern Christian human-being would be the equivalent of Augustine's anti-Manichaeism: he would *say* No, but *do* Yes, and his great loathing would be the greatest self-loathing and earth-loathing imaginable.[10] "O my soul," Zarathustra, Odysseus-like, says to himself, "I taught you the despising that does not make things wormeaten, the great, the loving despising that loves most where it despises most" (*Z* 3.14).

The metaphysical residuum that had remained, until this point, in Zarathustra's loathing for the smallness of human beings was the implicit assumption that in this smallness, humans had failed in some way—which implies an ideal of the human *an sich*, of consciousness *an sich*, by which such a failure might be assessed in the first place. In other words, it implies that there is another world, a "world behind" (*Z* 1.3) this one whose total economy of life has a different, *better* structure, and by which *this* world can and must be judged wanting. And as Lampert rightly points out, until Zarathustra's truly redemptive "Yes-saying" to even the smallest humans, in the third book, he in fact harbors and embodies a secret need (secret from himself) for "sweet revenge on the small and vengeful"; and his own accusation against life's accusers is itself "an accusation . . . against life insofar as it seems to need what is low."[11]

So long as we consider Christianity as the conflictual multiplicity it is, and has been over the millennia, rather than as the supposedly conclusive judgments about what "true" Christianity is that has emerged from that conflict, in the forms of various churches' doctrines, then we can see that Nietzsche's philosophy mirrors Christianity in an uncanny way. The very debate concerning the ambiguity of Nietzsche's *Übermensch*—that is, whether the term refers only to one "Overhuman" who leads the other humans, or whether it implies a possibility of several or even every human being bringing him or herself up beyond their present "self"—tracks almost exactly the ambiguities exploited by Christian theologians over the centuries, who used the image of Jesus as *the* Übermensch to tempt believers toward an overcoming of themselves, and to thereby realize the Übermensch (i.e., what is "over" and "beyond" their specific "humanness") that they also could be. And as with the Christians, so with Nietzsche: there is no mutual exclusivity to these different possibilities; rather, they are symbiotic.

Consider as well, in this regard, the concept (perhaps better, the conception), of "eternal recurrence." It is critically important to remember that in the book in which Nietzsche devoted most attention to this concept, Zarathustra *rejects* the Spirit of Heaviness' suggestion that time is a circle (*Z* 3.2.2), and the implication is strong that when his animals interpret this thought of "eternal recurrence" to him in a similar manner, Zarathustra sees them as foolishly misunderstanding it and, like Socrates in the *Timaeus*, simply does not respond to the "cosmology" that has been related to him (*Z* 3.13). When Nietzsche later, in *Ecce Homo*, "defines" eternal recurrence as the "*unbedingten und unendlich wiederholten Kreislauf aller Dinge*" ("Books," *BT* 3)—the "unconditional and infinite repeated circulation of all things"—he appends an important comment that must send us back to carefully consider what is meant: the Stoics, he says, had only *traces* (*Spuren*—the Latin etymology of which is noteworthy) of this teaching. But the Stoic teaching is precisely of infinite repetitions of the same (see, e.g., the fragment from Zeno in *Stoicorum veterum fragmenta* 1.109 [Leipzig 1903–24, von Arnim, ed.]). If only "traces" of Zarathustra's teaching are to be found in Stoic teaching, Nietzsche does not consider them identical, as infinitely repeating cycles of the same.

It is of course true that the original, meditative, questioning aphorism in which the thought first occurs (*GS* 341) mentions "*unzählige Male*"—"innumerable times"—of repetition and appears to have much more affinity with (and is perhaps identical with) Stoic exercise. But this would not be the only time that Nietzsche preserves the "traces" and "tracks" of the path of becoming of his thought, and we should note that when he discusses this aphorism as the "fundamental thought"—"*Grundgedenken*"—of *Zarathustra* already there in the *Gay Science* (*EH* "Books" *Z* 1), he is quite specifically discussing it as embryonic; that is, as a not yet fully developed part of the not yet fully developed (infant) *Zarathustra*. The gestational process took him 18 months (after August 1881), he tells us, and therefore *GS* 341 was written and published *antepartum*, as it were, while still in the process of maturing. Nietzsche goes out of his way to stress the metaphor of pregnancy in this section, which indicates we should treat it very seriously. One example of this is the word he first uses to describe what the thought of eternal recurrence was in relation to the book *Zarathustra*. He calls it the *Grundconception*—the "fundamental conception"—of the work. But "*Conception*" in Nietzsche's German evokes the Latin *conceptio* (and English "conception"), which has an immediate ambiguity that "*Konzeption*" does not in modern German—it suggests both the mental activity we associate with "conceiving" of a notion or idea, *and* the act of conceiving a child, and this is why Nietzsche chose to use it. So we should not necessarily chain ourselves to resolving, in the sense of finding compatible definitions, *GS* 341 entirely with Nietzsche's later work.

It is fruitful, at this point, to consider this *from a Christian perspective*, and offer an interpretation from that perspective. Is one of the thoughts that Nietzsche is trying to provoke a *single* recirculation of all things that lasts unconditionally and eternally? *Ewige Wiederkunft* not as an eternally repeating process of recurrence, but as a return *forever*—just as the anticipated *Wiederkunft Christi* ("return of Christ") forecasts the return forever of Jesus Christ? The Greek word translated in Luther's Bible as *Wiederkehr* or *Wiederkunft* (and it seems to me that this is precisely why Nietzsche will use both terms to describe the "eternal return"[12]) is *parousia*,[13] which means not "return," but "presence" (e.g., 1 Thes 3:13). A presence in which the angel of the Apocalyse promises that "*chronos ouketi estai*"—"time shall be no more" (Apoc. 10:6). Is the "eternal *presence* of the same" suggested, and suggested precisely to Christians, by Nietzsche's ultimate affirmation of life?

Nietzsche's interpretation of Jesus as the "son of man" in *The Antichrist/ian* (aph. 34) is revealing. This concept, he writes, is of "an 'eternal' actuality, a psychological symbol *redeemed from the concept of time*."[14] In fact, this direct experience Jesus had of himself as eternal—as literally having no concept of time (*Zeitbegriff*)—is crucial to

Nietzsche's picture of him (*A* 33, 34, 41). There is something essential here. The very belief in a transcendental God—who always was, is, and will be—contains within it an intimation that time as human beings experience it is somehow false, a "moving image of eternity," as Plato's Timaeus puts it (*Timaeus* 37d; cf. Job 10:5, Psalms 90:4, 2 Peter 3:8). In *The Antichrist/ian*, the *Übermensch*, the "sense of the earth" (*Z* 1.4, p.12), just *is* Jesus, but Jesus understood as a *hyperanthrôpos*, an Overhuman, and not the personified son of the one true God. This is Jesus the rabbi, the teacher, whose example[15] offers the possibility of a new and fruitful tragic being-in-the-world, in the duplicitous antagonism and cooperation with Dionysus that was once, in the tragic age of the Greeks, engaged by Apollo (it is important to remember that, for Nietzsche, it was the Apollonian aspect that perished at the hands of Socratism, not the Dionysian). And it is the *life*, not the death, of this Jesus that matters for Nietzsche (see *A* 33–35 especially). This is what Nietzsche gestures at in the last line of *Ecce Homo* (and perhaps the difficulty of understanding this is why he so obsessively keeps asking if anyone has understood him throughout that work, including in this last line): "– Hat man mich verstanden? – *Dionysos gegen den Gekreuzigten* . . ." – "– Has anyone understood me? – *Dionysus versus the crucified one* . . ." This final phrase is what in the first sentence of *Ecce Homo* Nietzsche has referred to as "*die schwerste Forderung*"—"the most difficult challenge"—that he will soon confront humanity with. And perhaps the greatest part of that challenge (and I am making this sentence intentionally ambiguous) is not to destroy the religion that has so enervated European humans, but to fulfill it. The *Christian*/Dionysian tragedy that *Zarathustra* is, takes this as its task, and by so doing inaugurates the possibility of a new—very different—tragic age.[16]

***

It is worth noting that even if one interprets Nietzsche's "anti-Christianity" as a complete polemic against a truly hated enemy, one cannot (or anyway should not) ignore Nietzsche's own awareness of the possible irony involved therein, an irony he highlights in the last two sections of *The Antichrist/ian*. In the penultimate §61, Nietzsche excoriates Luther for restoring the Christian church *by attacking it*. Only after this excoriation does Nietzsche offer, in the last section (§62), his own tremendous condemnation and attack on Christianity and the Christian church (cf. also *EH* "Books" Wagner §2)—a juxtaposition so striking that it simply *begs* the reader to bring the criticism of Luther to bear on Nietzsche's own effort.[17]

The famous statement by Nietzsche in *Ecce Homo* in which he says, "I am the Antichrist"? Well, he doesn't actually say this, and the qualifications he introduces are noteworthy. What he writes there is: "Ich bin, *auf griechisch*, und nicht nur auf griechisch, der Antichrist" ("Books," 2; KSA 6, 302, my emphasis)—"I am, *in Greek*, and not only in Greek, the Antichrist/ian." Now the word "anti," in Greek, does not mean what it does in German (or English, for that matter). There is no sense of being an opposite, for example, in the Greek, nor does the Greek imply any lethal enmity—indeed, all it really means, *in Greek*, is to be standing directly before another, facing him or her. And this comes in a section in which Nietzsche disavows being able to think or feel German!

It is, of course, not easy to read Nietzsche as a Christian. This is largely because, particularly in his most powerful and direct attacks on Christianity, like *The Antichrist/ian*, his comments are felt so keenly precisely because they cannot be dismissed—they are at the least trenchant, and what is more, seem to spring forth from a profound compassion (among other things, of course). It is not easy to read that, in the opinion of this obviously extremely intelligent and insightful former-theologian, during the entire time of Christianity, "there have been no Christians" (*A* 39). It is more difficult still if one wonders whether this might in fact be true. For Christians provoked to such a thought, Nietzsche's therapy may in fact be as rewarding as it is difficult.

Notes

1 *EH* "Books" BGE §2.
2 All translations from *Thus Spoke Zarathustra* are from Graham Parkes' superb translation (Oxford, 2005), though I have on rare occasions modified these to draw out the nuances that I want to highlight. All translations from Nietzsche's other works are listed at the end of my chapters, though I have frequently modified them.
3 Alighieri, Dante. 1970. *Paradiso*. ed. G. C. Sansoni. Firenze: G. Civelli, 842. My translation.
4 Strauss, Leo., *What is Political Philosophy? and Other Studies* (Chicago: Chicago University Press, 1988), p. 144.
5 We could also think of this in terms of what Rancière calls the "redistribution of the sensible" (*The Politics of Aesthetics*, pp. 13–17).
6 Cf. the description of the task of Hyllos—to burn his father Heracles alive—given him by Heracles in Sophocles' *Trachiniae* (lines 1262–3): *hôs epicharton/teleous' aekousion ergon*—"a joyfully accomplished, unwanted task."
7 The concept of Jesus *qua* extraordinary or overhuman being, and particularly as a model of striving for other human beings, is found in many earlier works of Christian philosophy and theology, including those of the second century "heretic" Montanus (who is said by Epiphanius to have called Jesus simply "*hyperanthrôpos*"—see *Panarion* 48: 10, 3; note that the only English translation of this misconstrues this entirely), but also William of Ockham and Nicolas of Cusa. The principle behind such a model can be summed up by the Scholastic dictum (and readers of *Zarathustra* may well hear echoes of this in the idea of man as "a bridge," and "an overcoming") "*homo non proprie* [or: *naturaliter*] *humanus sed superhumanus est*"—"man is not, strictly speaking, human, but overhuman" (attributed to Thomas Aquinas, *Quaestiones disputatae in virtutibus*, since at least Saint Alfonso Maria de Liguori in the eighteenth century—see the latter's *Homo apostolicus* 5.1.101; however, I do not find this phrase in Thomas' work). The Latin *superhumanus*, like the Greek *hyperanthrôpos*, is directly translated by the German *Übermensch*.

The necessity of faith for Christians is also, in a curious analogy to the power of the Sirens' song, described as an "overhuman power" (*dunamis hyperanthrôpon*) by Clement of Alexandria in his *Stromata* (II.ii.9.7.1).
8 Cf. the different evaluations of the "uses and abuses" of "blood" in *Z* 1. "On Reading and Writing" and 2. "On Priests."

9 In *Ecce Homo* ("Books" *Z* 8), Nietzsche will write that "man" can*not* be "an object of love" for Zarathustra, which should give us pause here. And when earlier in the same work (*EH* "Wise" 8) he had given the words that Zarathustra uses to describe his "*redemption* from disgust," what he quotes is not "The Convalescent" from book 3 of *Zarathustra*, but "On the Rabble," from book 2. But the latter specifically describes the redemption that Zarathustra only *thinks* he has achieved, but which is in fact a way of being that he actually *needs* to redeem—as illustrated by *Z* 3.13 and 14 (see also *BGE* 258, in which the "healthy aristocracy" is said to act in much the same way as Zarathustra's "redemptive" vision in "On the Rabble." That aphorism too *seems* to be a wholesale advocacy of such an aristocracy, but then Nietzsche goes out of his way to draw an analogy between it and the "Java"—actually Amazonian—vine, the *sipo matador*. As its name implies, this vine uses a host tree to attain its height, but in the process it kills that tree, and in so doing kills itself as well). It is significant that the latter two chapters (and those following) are *never* mentioned by Nietzsche in *Ecce Homo*—he will write only of chapters up to the immediately preceding one, "On Old and New Tablets" (save one very brief mention of the fourth book as a whole - *EH* "Wise" 4). Nietzsche leaves it to his reader to consider why this seemingly glaring contradiction is there, and my suggestion is that the answer lies in the explicitly stated purpose of *Ecce Homo*, which is for Nietzsche to say who *he* is (*EH* "Foreword" 1), and by telling *himself* his life ("Foreword" Conclusion) with "extreme honesty" ("Wise" 8). And as he makes clear in the first sentence of the "Books" section, "I am one thing, my writings are another." Nietzsche is, with "extreme honesty," acknowledging that he is not Zarathustra, nor capable of what Zarathustra *is* (a lesson from Plato and his Socrates?). The character of Zarathustra, or rather, the *type* Zarathustra (*EH* "Books" 1, 6), is imaginable by him, yearned for by him, but also *beyond* him, and therefore when he honestly appraises himself in relation to his creation, he speaks only of what *he*—Nietzsche—is capable of when he speaks of Zarathustra. And he is capable of *writing* Zarathustra, and to a certain extent writing himself *into* Zarathustra, but he is not capable of *being* Zarathustra. The last four chapters of book 3 of *Zarathustra* are not mentioned in *Ecce Homo* because these are the chapters in which Nietzsche writes *beyond* and *over* himself. There is a lesson here *about philosophers*: they too write beyond themselves, live beyond themselves, "live posthumously" (*EH* "Books" 1, *A* Foreword).

10 Lampert too draws attention to this fundamental struggle of Zarathustra, though without noting (I do not necessarily say without *noticing*) its Christian implications. See Lampert, Laurence, *Nietzsche's Teaching* (Yale: Yale University Press, 1986), pp. 216–18 and 94–5.

11 Lampert, p. 217.

12 For a particularly deliberate example of Nietzsche taking up both terms, though not interchangeably, see *TI* "Ancients" 4 and 5. The first aphorism (with *Wiederkehr*) takes up (Christian) sexuality, the second (with *Wiederkunft*) takes up (Christian) longing for eternal life *per se*.

13 *Parousia* is translated as *adventus* by St. Jerome in the Vulgate Bible, which does indeed mean something more like "coming" or "arrival." But Nietzsche was a philologist *par excellence* and would certainly have noticed the difference.

14 "*Eine 'ewige' Thatsächlichkeit, ein von dem Zeitbegriff erlöstes psychologisches Symbol.*" (KSA 6, 206).

15 By this I do not mean the example as illustrated in *BGE* 269, where Nietzsche on the surface seems to suggest that Jesus needed so badly to be loved by everyone that

he invented hell as a place to send those who did not do so. Nietzsche is not writing about Jesus himself there, but about the "holy disguise and fable" of Jesus—which is to say he is talking about *Paul*.

16 The first introduction of *Zarathustra*, at *GS* 342, is titled "*Incipit tragoedia*," usually translated as "the tragedy begins." While this translation is not wrong, and is certainly also intended to be applied to the specific tragedy of *Zarathustra*, it does not attend to the ambiguity that Nietzsche clearly intended (Nietzsche never writes in Latin only to look smart!). *Incipit tragoedia* also means more generally, "tragedy begins"—that is, tragedy in general as a new form of art and way of life—the "Birth of Tragedy from the Spirit of Nihilism."

17 This technique of undermining the force of his own argument by juxtaposition is one that Nietzsche uses with some frequency. Cf., for one striking example, *BGE* 18 with 19.

Editions used

All translations of Nietzsche's work have been used inasmuch as they are in accordance with and frequently modified according to: Nietzsche, Friedrich. *Kritische Studienausgabe* (KSA). Giorgio Colli and Massimo Montinari, eds. Berlin: de Gruyter (1980).

A *The Antichrist*. Trans. J. Norman. Cambridge: Cambridge University Press (2005).

BGE *Beyond good and evil: prelude to a philosophy of the future*. Trans. R. Hollingdale. England: Penguin Books (2003).

EH *Ecce homo: how to become what you are*. Trans. D. Large. New York: Oxford University Press (2007).

GS *The gay science*. Trans J. Nauckhoff. Cambridge: Cambridge University Press (2007).

HH *Human, all too human: a book for free spirits*. Trans. R. Hollingdale. Cambridge: Cambridge University Press (2007).

GM *On the genealogy of morals: a polemic*. Trans. D. Smith. New York: Oxford University Press (1996).

TSZ *Thus spoke Zarathustra: a book for everyone and nobody*. Trans. G. Parkes. New York: Oxford University Press (2005).

TI *Twilight of the idols: how to philosophize with a hammer*. Trans. D. Large. New York: Oxford University Press (1998).

Index